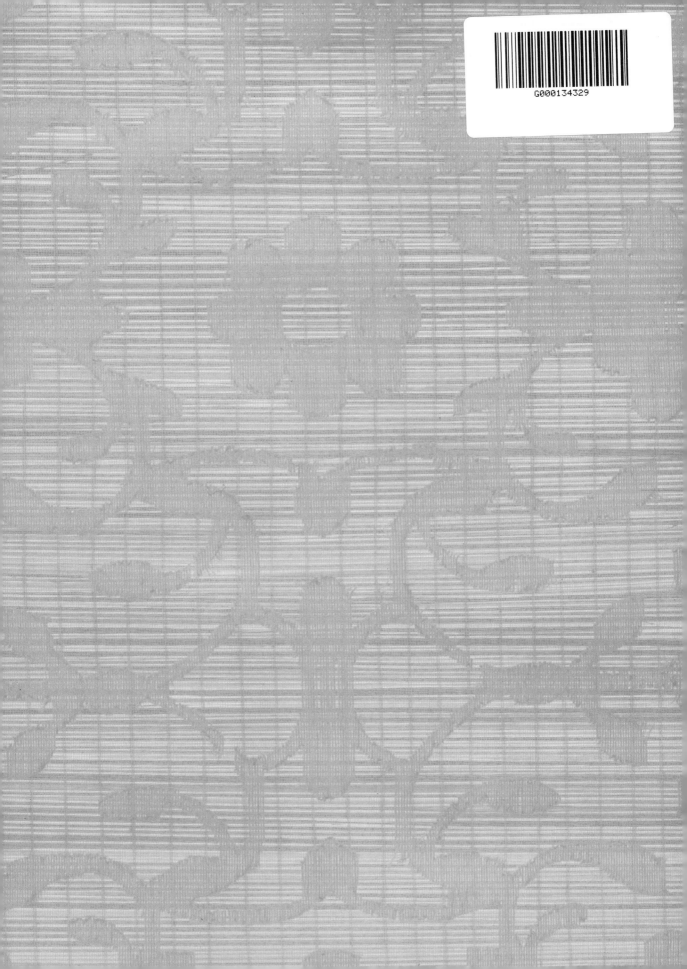

The Indian Spa

ayurveda | yoga | wellness | beauty

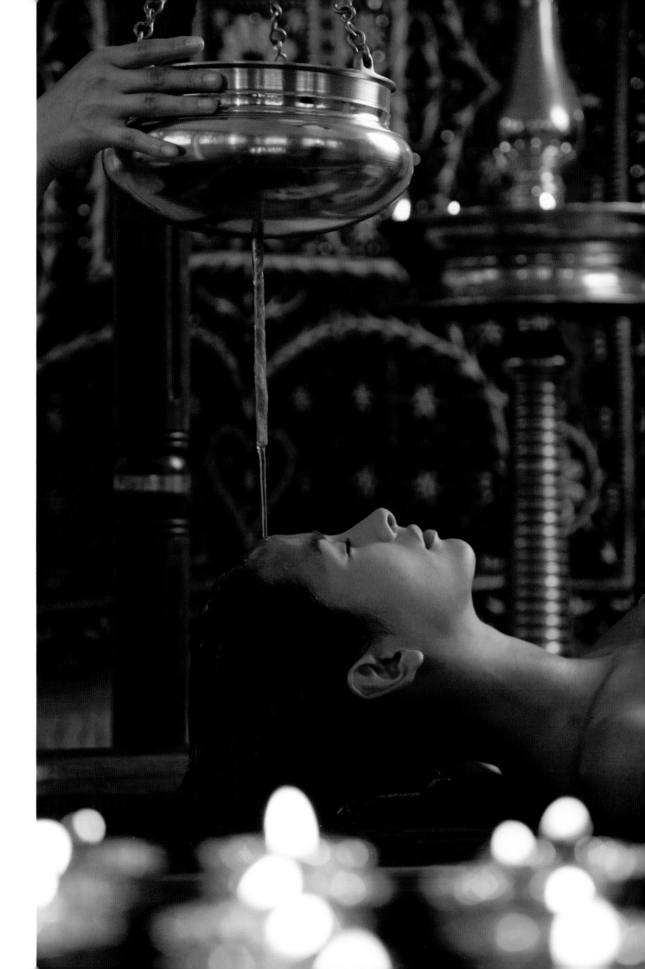

The Indian Spa

ayurveda | yoga | wellness | beauty

Kim Inglis

photography by Luca Invernizzi Tettoni

Talisman

Published in 2008 by
Talisman Publishing Pte Ltd
52 Genting Lane, Ruby Land Complex 1
#06-05 Singapore 349560
Tel: +65 6749 3551
Fax: +65 6749 3552
Email: customersvc@adpsing.com
www-apdsing.com

Texts © 2008 Kim Inglis www.kiminglis.com
Photos © 2008 Luca Invernizzi Tettoni www.tettoni.com

ISBN 978-981-05-9353-7
Printed in Singapore

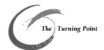

Created by The Turning Point. Designer: Don Siegel

The techniques outlined in this book are meant for
information only, and are not intended to replace
diagnosis and treatment by a qualified medical
practitioner. The author, photographer and publisher
accept no liability with regard to the use of techniques
contained herein.

Page 2: A candlelit *sirodhara* session in the luxurious
Ayurvedic Penthouse at the Oriental Spa has the hushed
atmsophere of a devotional ceremony.

Right: Udaivilas is a spa resort on the shores of beguiling
Lake Pichola: A private sun deck with cascading
bougainvillea and glittering pool is inviting and cooling.

Overleaf: A morning yoga session amongst the ruins of
a temple at the deserted Rajput outpost of Bhangarh
sets up Amanbagh guests for a day of calm and quiet.

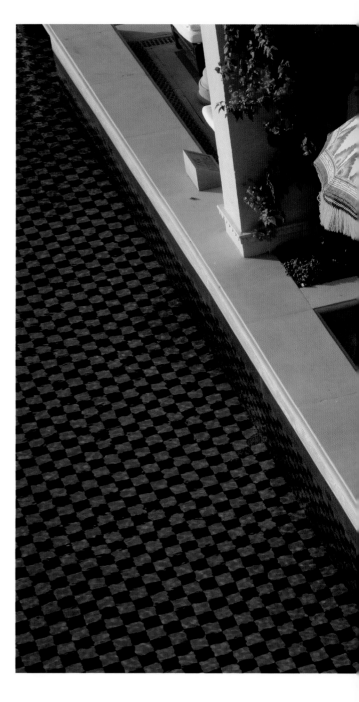

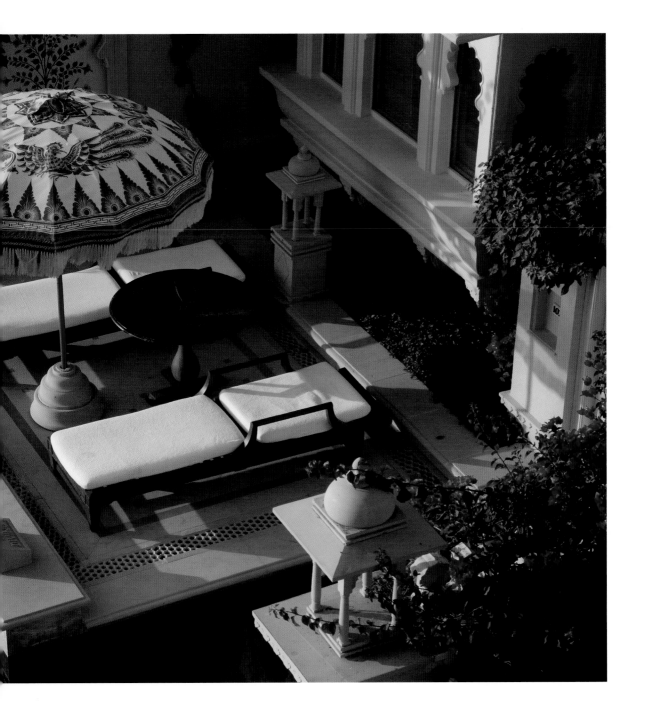

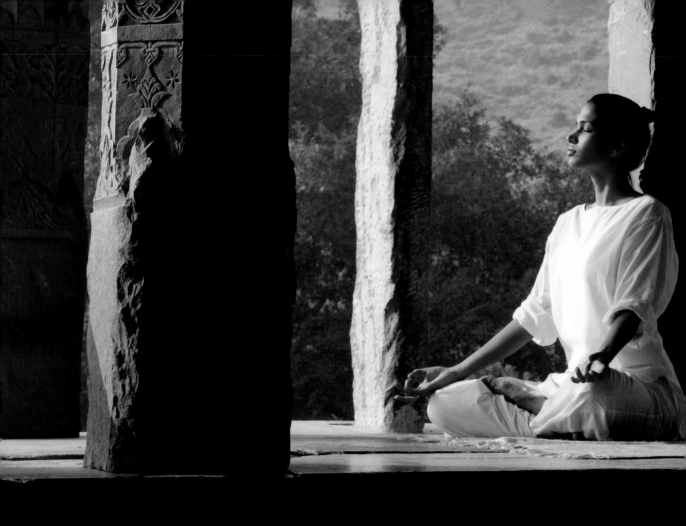

Contents

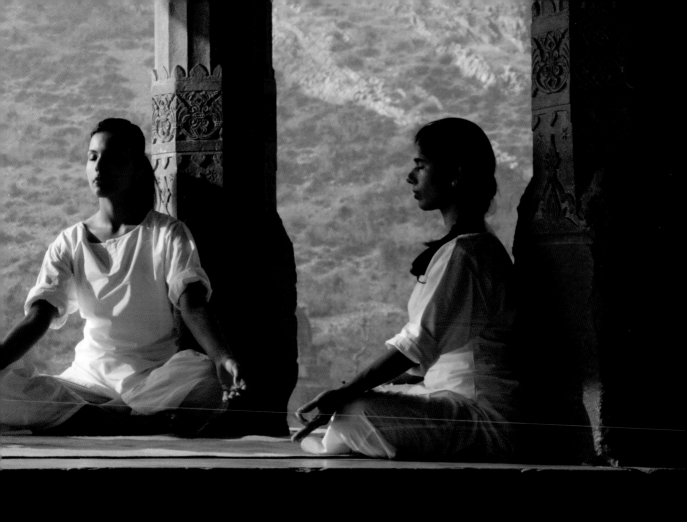

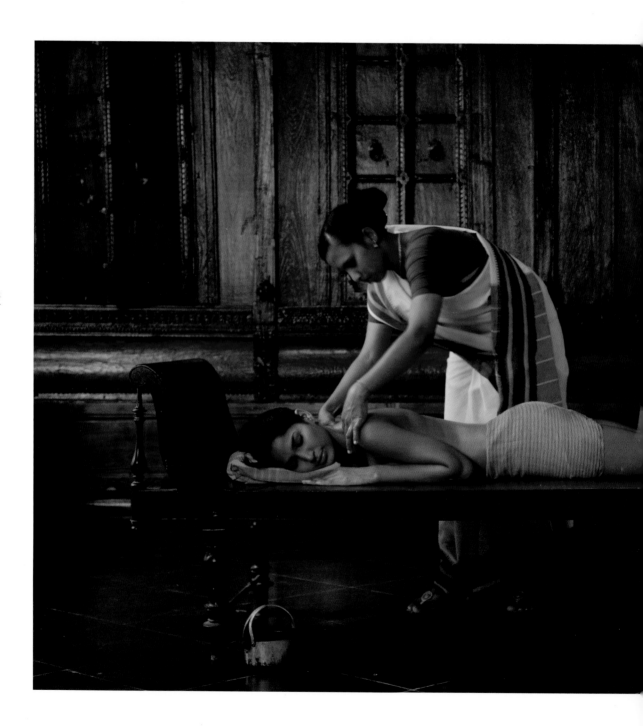

Introduction

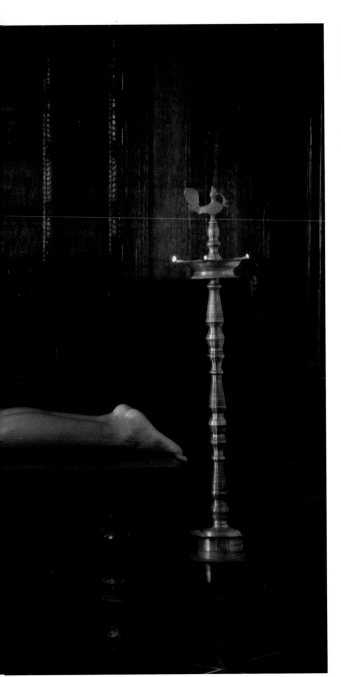

At no time in the history of the planet have India's stress-busting, all-encompassing therapies had more relevance. While we strive to improve material gains, we often neglect the spiritual, the physical, the mental and the emotional. Taking time out to concentrate on ourselves is no longer just a treat – it's a necessity. This is where India's age-old traditional practices come in.

Whether you travel to India to visit a spa, to try to "find yourself", to receive some medical care, or to spend time relaxing with friends or family, you are almost certain to come across these ancient wisdoms. They permeate through all levels of society and are found in every walk of life. Even though the country is modernising at a rapid rate, everyone – on some level or another – is tied to its deep-rooted traditions.

Ancient Healing

Many of these age-old traditions are explored in this book. We get to the core of the country's medical systems – Ayurveda, Unani and Siddha – and explore its history of herbal healing and ancient beauty procedures. The mind, body, spirit practices of yoga, meditation and *pranayama* are showcased in depth. Related cultural phenomena like astrology, palmistry, temple and household habits, martial arts and gemology are also covered.

Left: A beautiful Gujerati wooden screen that comprises a panel from an old house serves as a fitting backdrop for an oil massage session in the spa at Neemrana Fort Palace. This property is one of India's most atmospheric, where authentic architecture and service is combined with wonderful hospitality.

Some of these terms will be familiar to readers, while others will be totally new. We'll take you through the myriad of wonders that has emerged from this extraordinary subcontinent, simultaneously explaining how past wisdom has relevance in today's world.

Ayurveda and yoga are probably the most well known of the ancient disciplines outside India – and both seek to encompass much more than physical wellbeing. They are covered in depth in the ancient texts or *Vedas* and there are countless written instructions for both. Even though they weren't traditionally practiced together, today they are finding synergy. "What's interesting about India's systems," explains one Ayurvedic physician, "is that they often incorporate more than one regime. Methods of healing like Ayurveda include a lifestyle regimen, aroma, meditation, gems, amulets, herbs, diet, *jyotish* (astrology), colour and more." It is this holistic approach that is so inspiring.

Natural Therapies

Rejuvenating the body, soothing the mind, nurturing the spirit – India's therapies open up possibilities we never realised we had. Many aim to help a person reach their maximum potential, while others utilise the country's pharmacopoeia for relaxation, beauty care and rejuvenation. "Over centuries of usage, it has been seen that herbs and other natural

Right: India is home to a vast pharmacopeia of healing plants, some of which are showcased here at the spa at Mandarin Oriental Dhara Devi. "Plant ingredients contain vitamins, minerals and enzymes, which are imperative for good health," says Shahnaz Husain. "Old Ayurvedic recipes are now supported by scientific research and information – and are increasingly popular."

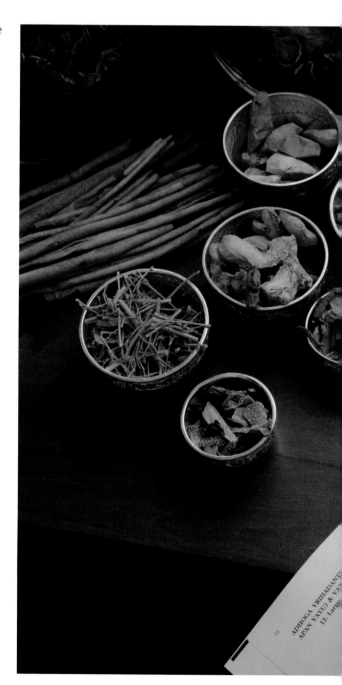

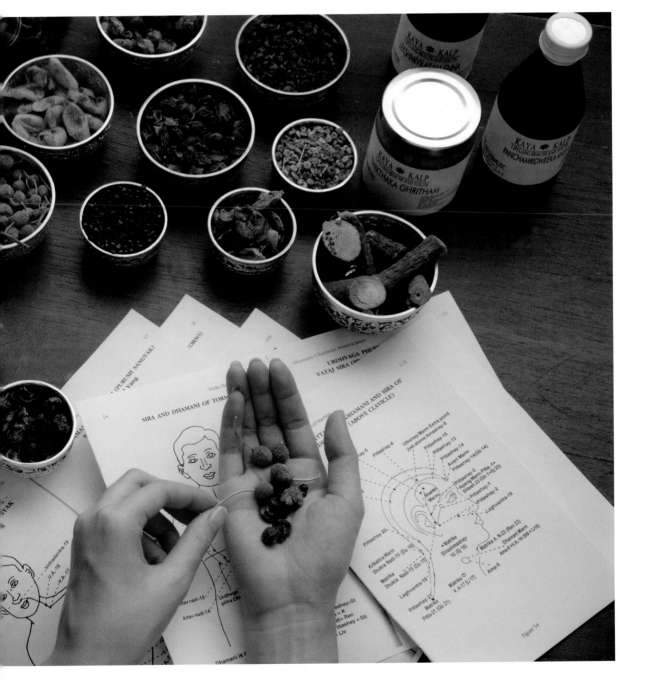

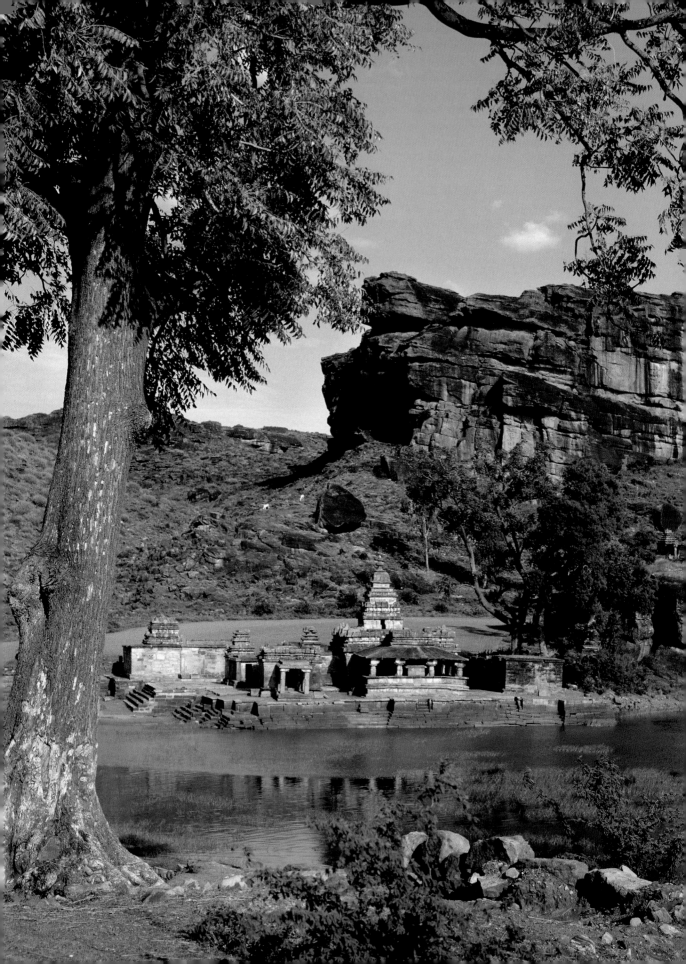

substances not only have curative powers, but many beneficial properties for both health and beauty," explains Shahnaz Husain, one of India's top herbal manufacturers. "Apart from their powerful and specific healing properties, these ingredients have a long history of safe human usage. The body responds extremely well to natural substances and has an in-built resistance to synthetic, chemical ones."

In *The Indian Spa* you'll find therapies and treatments that for the most part utilise natural ingredients – from the obvious plants, flowers and essential oils to such unusual products as mercury, diamonds, gold and more. Husain's 24 Carat Gold range, Diamond Collection and Astro-Gem Therapy range are a case in point. Even more obscure are some of the Ayurvedic *vasthi* therapies, whereby warm oil is poured into garam flour "reservoirs" placed on specific points of the body. Or try the sublime *pizichil*, a treatment apparently formulated for royalty: here medicated oil is poured on the body and massaged in by two or more therapists to activate the nervous system. Detoxifying, cleansing, beautifying, regenerating, balancing – they're all designed with total wellness in mind.

Spas, Retreats, Resorts and More

Along with explanations of plants and products comes a chapter dedicated to India's cornucopia of gorgeous spas, retreats, resorts, hotels and even clinics. Previously, Vedic knowledge was the preserve of Brahmin scholars based in the country's ancient, enduring temples. All that is changing now, as the new India emerges. Alongside its age-old culture and history is a rapidly expanding economy, with huge advances in technology, manufacturing and the service industries. Investment in tourism is one of these growth areas: improved airports, better infrastructure, new facilities and more hotel rooms are desperately needed. The country's movers and shakers are making inroads in these areas – and a plethora of new or revamped properties is beginning to emerge.

Opposite: Temples, such as this extraordinary example at Badami, hold the secrets to India's ancient culture.

Below: A type of massage whereby the masseur uses his feet to activate pressure points is one of India's more exotic offerings.

13

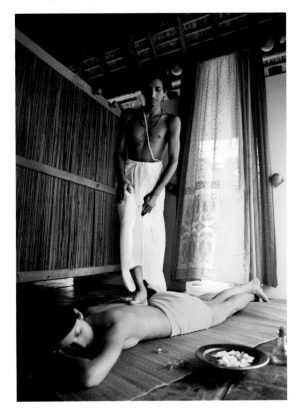

We bring you the best of the best. Secluded retreats, renovated forts, *havelis* (mansions) and palaces imbued with atmosphere and élan, Himalayan hideaways, metropolitan day spas and stylish beach resorts are all showcased. Most have first-class service and facilities now; the days of indifferent food, erratic plumbing and poor service have been banished along with the Raj.

The somewhat lackluster hotels of the past have been replaced by a host of world-class properties that compete more than adequately on the global stage. Oberoi Hotels' top-tier Vilas properties in Rajasthan are fairy-tale fortresses, palaces and tented encampments. Combining modern facilities and service, they nonetheless retain a respectful sense of place. The Neemrana group has gone the restoration route "taking the ruins of history and turning them into jewels", while Taj are still wowing visitors with their combo of grand city hotels, beach resorts and historic palaces. In addition to these, you'll find many owner-operated properties, where an individual's vision ensures a stay of exceptional quality. In conjunction with the growing global trend for wellness, all the hotels have attached spas or can be viewed as complete spas in themselves.

Extraordinary India

Domestic travel in India has also improved beyond recognition, so the possibility of substituting the tried-and-tested Delhi-Agra-Jaipur triangle with locations further afield is no longer just a pipe dream. Kerala is now a hot destination for the Ayurvedic aficionado offering both modish rustic estates and sybaritic sea, sand and sun resorts. Rich in culture and natural history, it is proving more than popular. Similarly, Karnataka is marketing itself as a yoga destination with some extremely well-run yoga *salas* (schools) and retreats. Rajasthan is now home to some truly stunning properties that offer peace, privacy and top-rate facilities in drop-dead gorgeous surrounds.

Spas and retreats are not only on the rise in India. Globally they are experiencing enormous growth as increasingly sophisticated consumers seek soul-soothing places to escape to. The need for meditative surrender and total chill-out is a real phenomenon – and India is well placed to cater to the demand. This is partly because many of the experiences that people desire – yoga, meditation, beauty and body treatments – originated in this vast country, and partly because it has the diversity of landscape and quality of personnel to deliver them. After all, where else can you find a yoga master, an Ayurvedic doctor, a highly-trained beauty therapist and a masseuse from a family of traditional healers in one location?

Above: A trip on a Keralan houseboat makes for a relaxing and rejuvenating sojourn in south India.
Right: Goa's beaches are home to some fabulous hotels and spas.
Overleaf: View from soul-soothing Udaivilas across Lake Pichola at dusk. Can you think of a better place to spa?

14

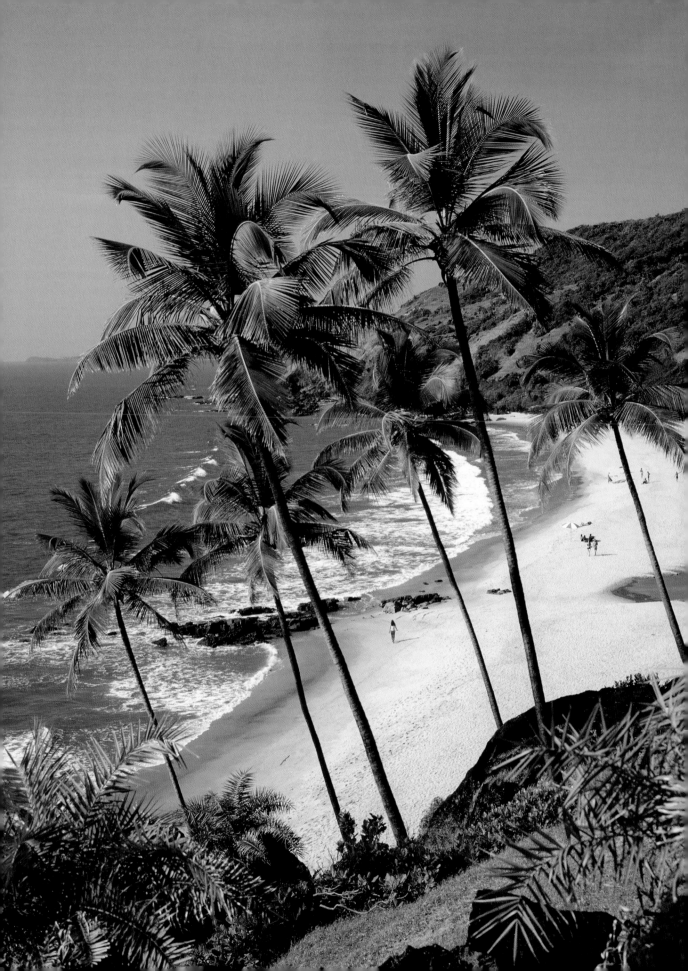

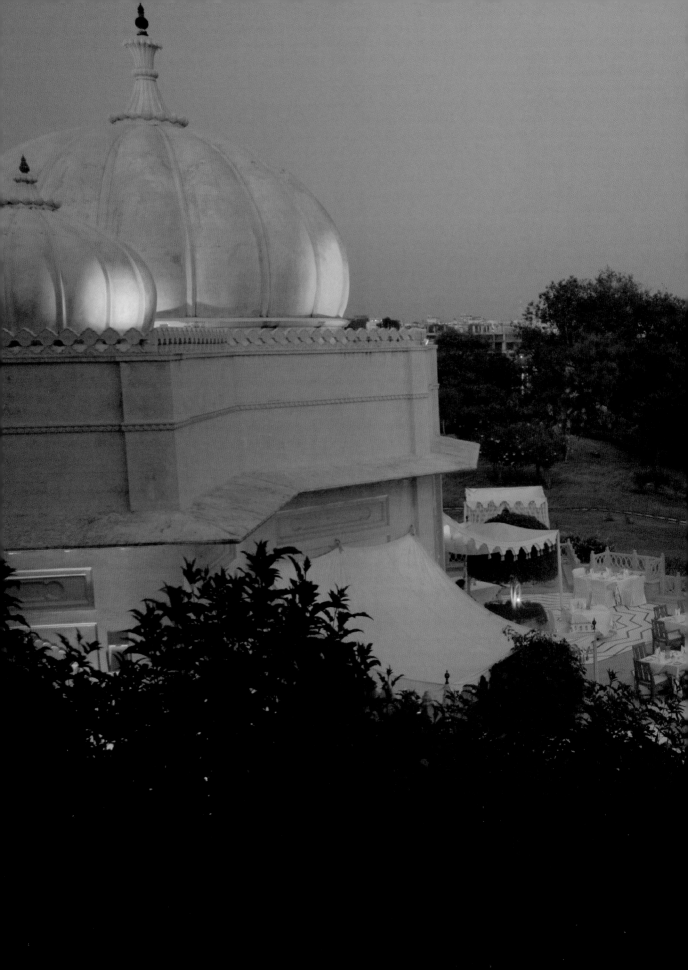

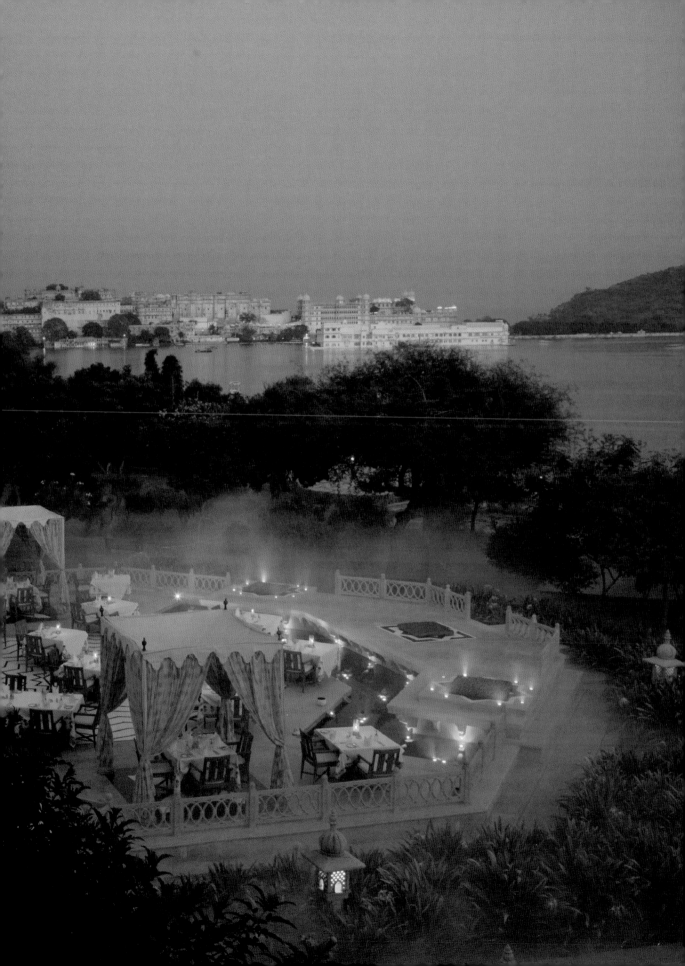

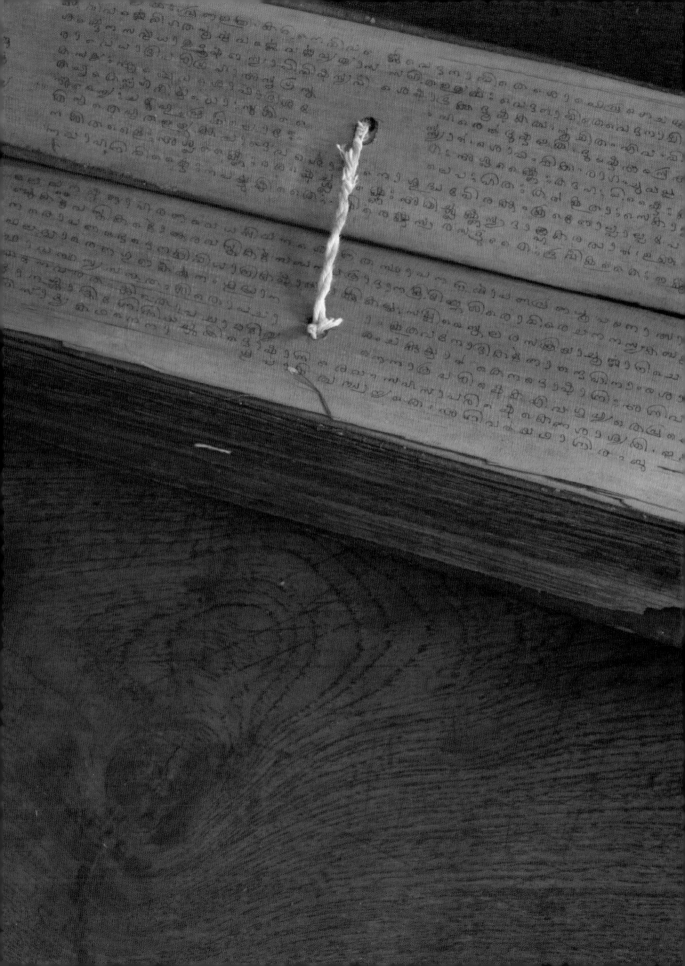

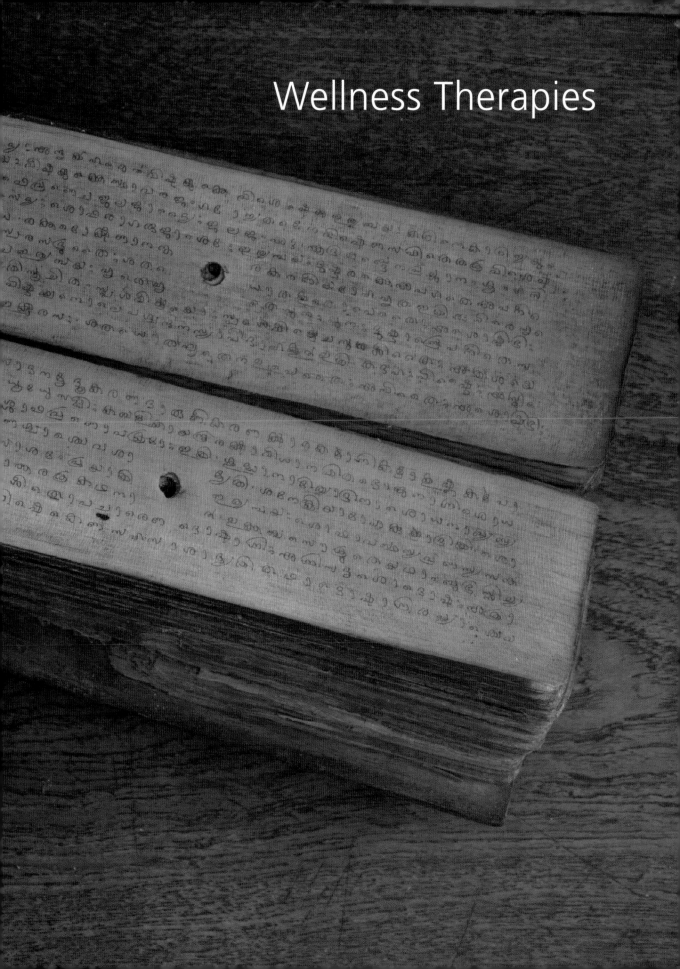

Wellness Therapies

Ayurveda

"The three – body, mind and soul – are like a tripod, the world stands by their combination; in them everything abides. It is the subject matter of Ayurveda for which the teachings of Ayurveda have been revealed."

— *the* Sutrasthana *of* Charaka Samhita *(1.46–47)*

To non-Indians, knowledge of Ayurveda is scanty at best, downright wrong at worst. Even though it originated in India thousands of years ago, Ayurveda only recently became popular in the West when certain treatments began to be included on spa menus. Perhaps the best known is *sirodhara*, the therapy whereby warm oil is poured continuously on to the third eye or middle of the forehead (see pages 56–59). Because it was new, different and exotic, Ayurveda became lauded as the latest spa phenomenon – although it is, in fact, an ancient form of natural medicine.

Hijacked by the *hoi-polloi* and popularised by the Press, Ayurveda became the new buzzword for beauty, rejuvenation, reinvention – with wellness and weight-loss thrown in for good measure. It was touted as a wonder cure from the East, a panacea for all Western ills. As with all such "discoveries", there was some truth in the tittle-tattle – and a lot of hype. In the ensuing kilometres of copy dedicated to the subject, Ayurveda was diagnosed, dissected and discussed. So-called Ayurvedic spas sprang up on every continent. Conventions were held and "experts" consulted. In the process, this exported Ayurveda became so distorted and diluted, that it came barely to resemble the real thing.

Sirodhara became *de rigeur* for the stressed executive. The fact that it was traditionally used as part of an overall wellness strategy in conjunction with other treatments, spiritual discipline, a special diet and more, was conveniently forgotten. After all, what could be more liberating than lying on a soft massage bed with lashings of soothing, comforting liquid pouring over the top of your head? Similarly, some Ayurvedic massages, originally therapeutic in context, became one-off, hour-long energisers, or relaxants, or whatever else the client decided he or she wanted.

So, what exactly is Ayurveda? Where and how did it originate? What is its history? And most importantly, is it relevant today?

The Roots of Ayurveda

Translated from Sanskrit as the "Science of Life", Ayurveda was first mentioned in the verses of the *Rig Veda*, the first of the Vedas or Hindu sacred texts. Here there is reference to *panchamahabhut* (the five basic elements of creation, see page 80), and the three *doshas* or primary forces of *prana* or *vata* (air), *agni* or *pitta* (fire) and *soma* or *kapha* (water and earth) as comprising the basic principles of Ayurveda. However, there is much more detail in one *upaveda* (subsection) of the *Atharva*, the fourth *Veda*, written some time during 3,000 to 2,000 BC. Here, Ayurveda is documented more specifically: it is described as knowledge of self-healing or holistic healing, with the idea that everything is interrelated, yet still unique. The texts stated that if Ayurveda was applied on an individual

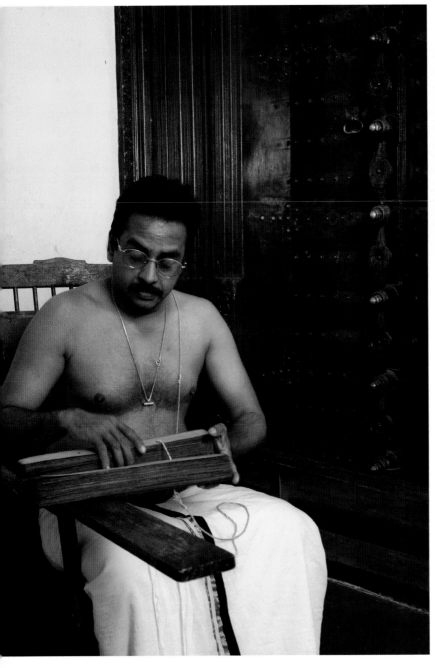

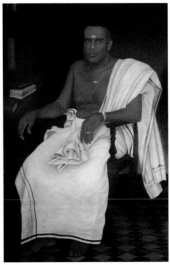

Legend has it that Ayurveda was first revealed to the seven *rishis* or saints who congregated in the Himalayas to receive the secrets of the "Science of Life" for the benefit of mankind. Today, Kerala is considered the centre of Ayurveda in India, because it is believed that 18 families of Keralan Brahmin scholars were entrusted with the secrets of Ayurveda to preserve its wisdoms for posterity. Each of these families contained physicians that had mastered all eight branches (*ashtanga*) of Ayurveda. They became known as *ashtavaidyas* (*vaidya* translates as "physician"). Today only five of these families remain.

On *left*, sitting on the porch of the family home, is Ashtavaidya Shankaran Mooss, the head of one of these remaining families; *above* is an oil portrait of his grandfather painted in the 1930s. The previous page shows a close up of the palm leaf manuscript the *ashtavaidya* is studying: written in Malayalam from Sanskrit, it covers selected formulations.

basis in people's everyday lives using diet, massage, oils and herbs, exercise and yoga, practitioners could be healthy and disease-free.

Around the turn of the first millennium BC the treatise known as the *Charaka Samhita*, the most well-known Ayurvedic text on internal medicine, appeared. Believed to have been written by the great sage-physician Charaka, it explained the logic and philosophy of Ayurvedic medicine. Composed in the form of a symposium wherein groups of Ayurvedic scholars take up a series of topics for discussion, it is written in verse in keeping with the Vedic oral tradition of conserving knowledge. It therefore seems likely that Ayurveda had been in existence for many hundreds, if not thousands, of years before.

Around the same time, the *Sushruta Samhita* appeared. It comprised knowledge about prosthetic surgery, caesarian operations, cosmetic surgery and even brain surgery. Sushruta is famous for his innovation of rhinoplasty, cosmetic surgery for the nose, an interesting fact as he was alive two centuries before the Greek Hippocrates who is regarded as the father of medicine. Around 500 AD, the physician Vagbhata compiled the third major Ayurvedic treatise, the *Ashtanga Hridaya*. It contains knowledge from both previous books, but also new information on diseases and cures. It is the text of choice for many practicing Ayurvedic physicians today because it is a precise condensation of the two earlier texts.

Naturally, many other useful reference texts were written, and it is documented that Ayurveda became entrenched in Indian life between 1,000 BC and 800 AD. Both Hindus and Buddhists maintained the academic study of Ayurveda, and also ensured that the science was made as publicly available as possible. Medicinal herbs were planted, hospitals were founded, the art of nursing (as described by Charaka) was widely systematised. But it wasn't until the Buddhist period (323 BC to 642 AD) that Ayurveda began to be exported outside India's shores. During this time, Buddhist missionaries and monks took knowledge of Ayurveda, along with other aspects of Indian culture, to Europe (Rome and Greece), the Middle East (Baghdad) and China. Closer to home, the neighbouring countries of Sri Lanka, Tibet, Burma, Thailand and Indonesia all accepted its teachings. In fact, its influence can still be seen in many Asian healing systems: Acupressure, for example, is a direct descendant of *marma* massage (see pages 38–39).

Above: A typical *thaliyola* or palm leaf Ayurvedic text in the Dravidian script. The words would have been inscribed on to the leaves with a *narayam* (sharp needle) by scholars.

Opposite, clockwise from top: A revered Ayurvedic doctor in Trivandrum waits for his patients. A copy of the *Ashtanga Hridaya* in Sanskrit: the page is open at Chapter 16. Chapters 1 to 15 contain knowledge of the basics of Ayurveda; chapters 16 to 30 are on treatments. Ancient Ayurvedic equipment including a medicine box or *marunnu petty*, a mortar and pestle, and oil and powder containers.

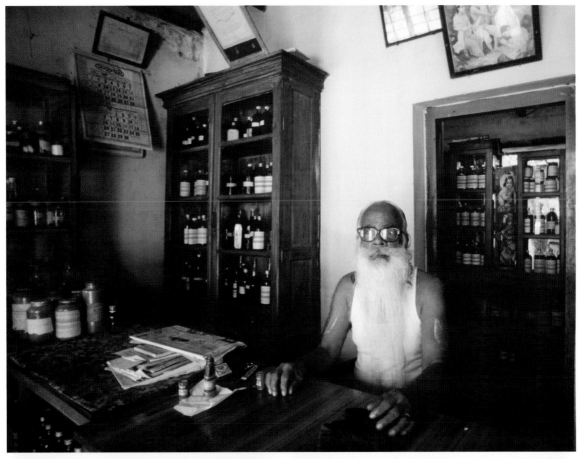

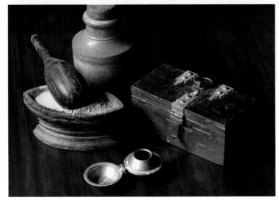

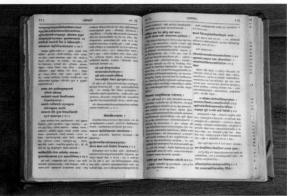

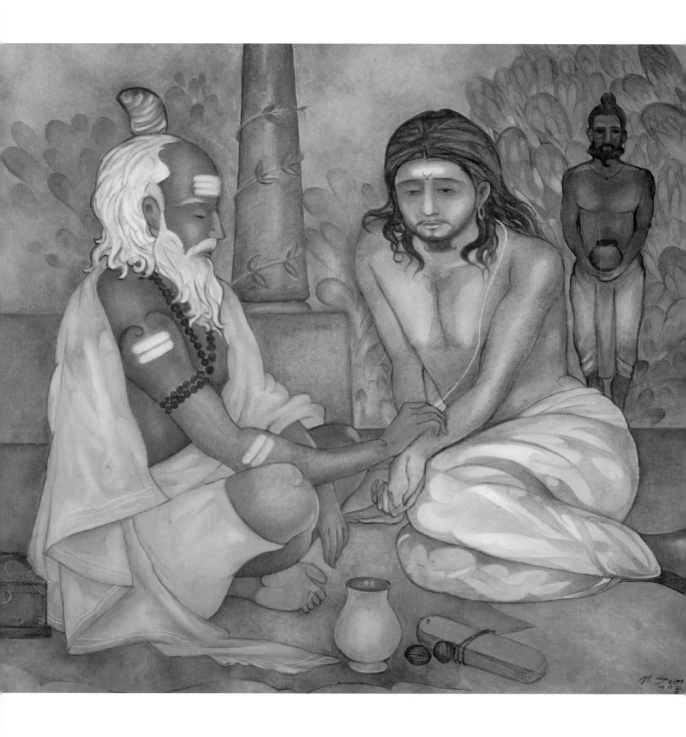

In India, Ayurveda's heyday was probably from the 6th century to the 10th century AD. During this time, universities and teaching hospitals catered to students from all over the world, and there are numerous references to the efficacy of the Indian system of medicine. But by the end of the 12th century, Ayurveda's influence had begun to wane. In north India, from the 10th to the 12th centuries, waves of Muslim invaders, bringing their own physisians and philosophers, burned books, destroyed hospitals and libraries, and slaughtered Hindu sages and Buddhist monks as infidels. They replaced them with their own Unani doctors, a form of medicine formulated by Arabian physicians combining Greek and Ayurvedic practices, (see pages 68–71) and so the system fell into decline.

This decline was further exacerbated by the arrival of the British. The East India Company denied state patronage to Ayurveda, closed down schools and medical colleges, and substituted it with Western medicine. Of course, at a local level, Ayurveda continued to be practiced, but it wasn't until Indian Independence in 1947 that official initiatives were taken to revitalise indigenous medical forms – and Ayurveda once again became popular.

Left: A painting from Ayurmana in Kerala depicting a supplicant seeking medical and spiritual aid from an ascetic doctor.

Above: A patient consultation at Kalari Kovilakom, a Keralan palace that has been converted into an Ayurvedic retreat.

Overleaf: A therapist administers *sirodhara* to a guest beneath soaring arches at the dramatic Neemrana Fort Palace.

What is Ayurveda?

Ayurveda advocates that each person is born with a basic constitution or genetic make-up called *prakruti* in Sanskrit. If there is a changing nature or situation in the body during one's life (*vikruti*), imbalance occurs. This may pass over time or may become a disease. The aims of Ayurveda are *ayus* ("long life") and *arogya* ("diseaselessness") with ultimate spiritual goals. Health is achieved by balancing what are known as the bodily humours or *doshas* at all levels, according to an individual's constitution, lifestyle and nature. There are many similar holistic medical systems in other communities, including the Chinese, North and South American Indians, and Africans.

Diagnosis

Before any form of Ayurvedic treatment may be prescribed, patients first of all undertake a consultation with an Ayurvedic physician to ascertain their body type and present health status. "In Ayurveda, body type is the variation in percentage of *vata*, *pitta* and *kapha* (air, fire and water) in our body," explains Dr Yogesh at Udaivilas Spa. "Based on the present *dosha* state or *vikruti*, suitable oils, medications, therapies, advice or more may be prescribed."

Ayurvedic physicians point out that Ayurvedic treatments vary from place to place, doctor to doctor and according to the nature of the client/doctor relationship which makes it confusing.

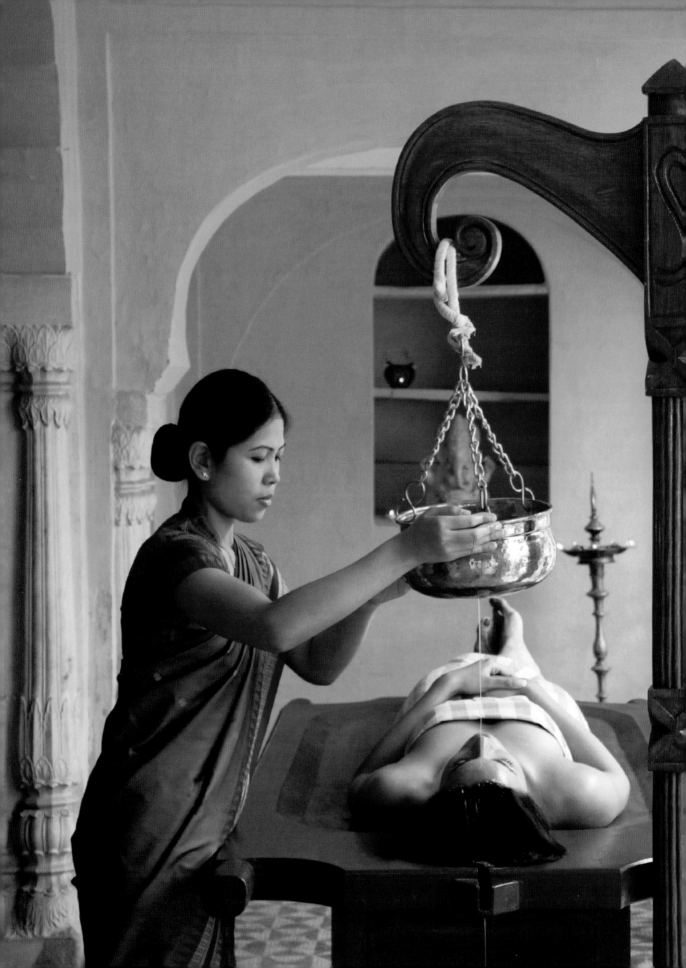

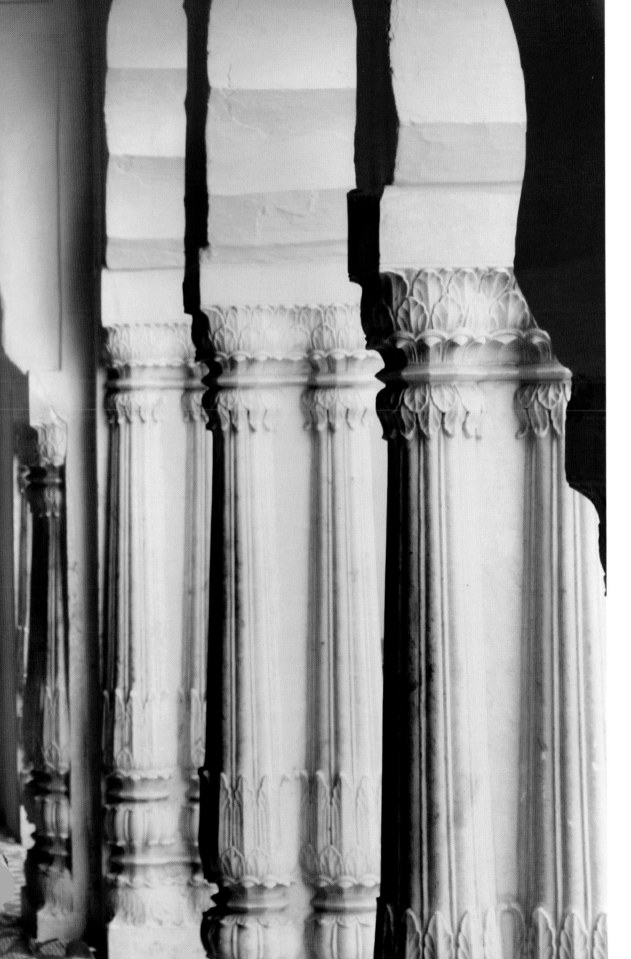

It also makes it difficult to analyse, research and compare to other medical systems. "However, the purpose is always the same," explains Dr Raphel from Rajvilas: "Each body has its own defined constitution from birth to death. It is affected by diet, climate, activities, bath, food, how we think and more. With different treatments, we doctors try to bring the body back to equilibrium: we find out what is lacking and modify it, we add things and we request changes in diet, stress levels, life-style habits and more." He goes on to add that the body has the power to cure itself; Ayurveda simply helps it with the healing process.

Diagnosis is an extremely important part of Ayurveda. In a clinic or hospital, it is undertaken first thing in the morning before the patient has consumed anything. The doctor inspects the tissues and the skin; examines the "nine doors" (two eyes, two ears, two nostrils, mouth and throat, anus, and penis or vulva) and their secretions; takes faeces and urine samples to assess the *analam* or digestive fire; takes the patient's pulse and body temperature; questions the patient on their sleep patterns, health, life-style, climate preferences and more; and generally takes a great deal of time to consider the patient as a whole. Nothing can be prescribed without this extremely thorough consultation.

For those who simply want to try an Ayurvedic treatment at a spa, the consultation will be shorter, but is still an important part of the whole process.

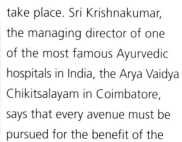

"At a spa, we look at *darshana* or appearance, *sparshana* or touch (ie pulse and body temperature), and undertake *prasnai* or discussion," explains Dr Yogesh, "this gives us enough information to decide on a patient's basic imbalances and which medicated oils we should use in a treatment."

Prognosis and Treatment

After diagnosis, the doctor decides which of four categories the disease or complaint falls into: Curable with ease, curable with difficulty, ameliorable, or incurable. At this point an astrologer may be consulted to find the best time and place for treatments to take place. Sri Krishnakumar, the managing director of one of the most famous Ayurvedic hospitals in India, the Arya Vaidya Chikitsalayam in Coimbatore, says that every avenue must be pursued for the benefit of the patient. "Everything is inter-related," he explains, "mind and body, person and universe, disease and lifestyle. A consultation with an astrologer may bring up something that the doctor has not noticed."

This is one example of how Ayurveda may be difficult for non-Indians to grasp. Skepticism of such practices like astrology runs high in the West, even though looking holistically at patients and their problems is increasingly gaining credence. Some treatments are equally problematic.

Treatments are multi-faceted and depend on a huge number of factors including disease, client personality and habits, *dosha* imbalance,

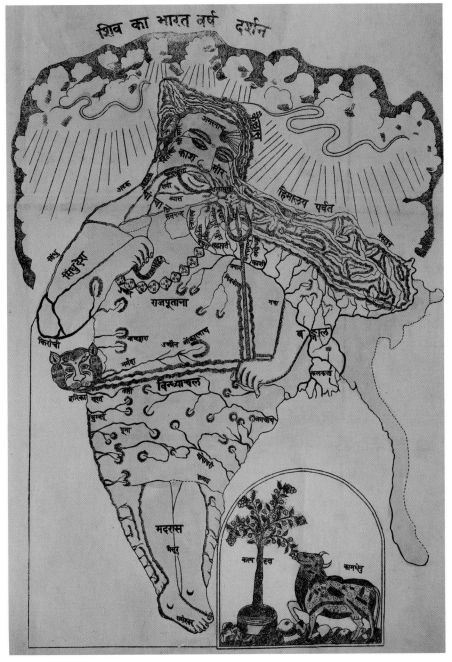

Opposite: The eye therapy known as *netra tarpanam* (see pages 54–55) is useful for eye strain, myopia and general tiredness in the eye area. Medicated ghee is poured into a secure area round both eyes to nourish and soothe.

Left: An old map of India is transposed with an illustration of the body of Shiva, the Indian god of yoga. The various geographical areas of the subcontinent are aligned to different parts of Shiva's body. For example, his head which symbolises intellect, imagination, consciousness, is depicted in the Himalayas, his spiritual home, while his feet, indicating grounding, comprise the southern tip of the subcontinent.

Overleaf, left: A student of the Vedas in Sanskrit at Ananda – in the Himalayas.

Overleaf, right: One of 318 plates of Rama's story, taken from the *Citraramayana* ("Picture Ramayana"), the only known illustrated manuscript of the *Ramayana* in Malayalam. Called *Aushadha Saila* or "Medicine Mountain", it depicts the story of the monkey god Hanuman retrieving a mountain of herbs that help his fellow monkeys regain consciousness after a battle. Even in the epics, much is made of India's healing herbal heritage.

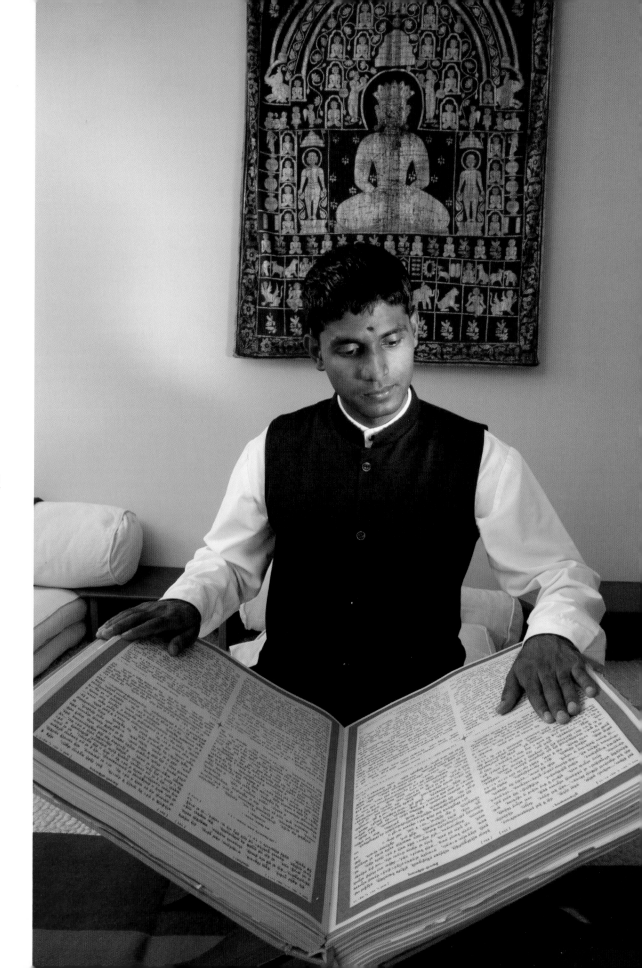

climate, and many more. The basic premise is to cleanse and detoxify the body and balance the *doshas*, restoring them to their original state of equilibrium. But how this is achieved varies wildly. There are hundreds of levels of practice, from folk to official, and thousands of prescriptions. One thing remains constant: a course of treatments is rarely shorter than three weeks, and after the course is completed, follow-up is very important.

In the following pages we cover many common therapies, but if you visit an Ayurvedic doctor, expect to be prescribed any, or even many, of the following: purification therapies, special diet, herbs and minerals, medication, massage and other body work, exercise, yoga, meditation, aromatherapy, flower and gem essences, advice on lifestyle and climate, and acupressure. All the medicines, oils and powders used in treatments are 100 percent natural and rely on India's huge pharmacopoeia. "Ayurvedic texts contain details of a staggering number of plants, minerals, metals and other natural substances, along with their properties, methods of collection and extraction, as well as specific combinations of complementary herbs," says Shahnaz Husain, Indian herbal ambassador and manufacturer. "The specific processing methods and well-known combinations enhance the efficacy of the treatments. Many of the formulations are still used with success today."

Ayurveda in Spas

Even though some treatments are less common now, many are still to be found both at grassroots level and in the country's 2,100 Ayurvedic hospitals.

They are also increasingly finding their way into spas and retreats. Husain notes: "Ayurvedic treatments are ideal for spas, because they counteract degenerative processes, environmental pollution, toxic build-up and mental stress, all of which have become

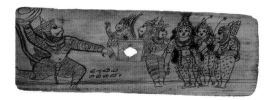

undesirable features of modern life." She notes that many people visit a spa particularly to address such afflictions, and with Ayurveda taking total wellbeing into consideration, its treatments are in line with the aims of most spas.

Some diehard Ayurvedic doctors, with their emphasis on authenticity, frown on this relatively new spa phenomenon. They believe that Ayurveda should remain wholly in the realm of medicine. Others, however, feel it is a trend to be encouraged as it advertises the benefits of this ancient system. "As long as doctors is such spas differentiate between the clinic and the spa, it is fine," one doctor told me.

There is a problem with standardisation, however, and many doctors admit that the Ayurvedic experience ricochets from clinical, by-the-book treatments to unhygienic practices and others driven only by monetary gain. But the government and the medical community are working to rectify this – and standards are improving. In *The Indian Spa*, we only recommend reputable establishments and differentiate clearly between the medical and the recreational.

Ayurvedic Massage

"Give yourself a full body oil massage on a daily basis. It is nourishing, pacifies the *doshas*, relieves fatigue, provides stamina, pleasure and perfect sleep, enhances the complexion and the lustre of the skin, promotes longevity and nourishes all parts of the body."

— *from the* Charaka Samhita

As with other forms of massage in Asia, Ayurvedic massage is a therapeutic massage, not a relaxation tool. Its primary aim is to encourage the movement of toxins (including vitiated *doshas*) from the deeper tissues into the gastrointestinal tract where they can be efficiently eliminated later. It is also given to stimulate circulation of the blood and lymphatic fluid. It is rarely considered a complete therapeutic cure in itself, but is used in conjunction with other therapies.

Massage is first mentioned in the 5,000-year-old *upaveda* of the *Atharva*, although was almost certainly practiced before this. Later, in the two major Ayurvedic treatises, the *Charaka Samhita* and the *Sushruta Samhita*, both believed to have been written at the turn of the first millennium BC in Sanskrit verse, it is discussed in depth with exhaustive listings of positions of the body and measurements of oils, pastes and powders. These two encyclopaedic works are considered the most authoritative writings on Ayurveda, covering the theoretical knowledge behind the healing of the mind, body and soul of the patient.

In the *Charaka Samhita*, discussion of massage as a real purification method to alter the chemical processes in cells is detailed and comprehensive. In the essay on *panchakarma* (see pages 62–63), various methods for the evacuation of toxins and the restoration of *prana* or cosmic energy to the body via lymphatic drainage are outlined. The *Sushruta Samhita*, on the other hand, is a treatise on surgery; it is here that methods of acupressure on the meridian points, magnetism of the *chakras* and the positive spiritual and mental effects of massage are covered.

Both works go a long way towards explaining why an Ayurvedic massage can have such amazing all-round benefits: accumulated stress and toxins in the mind as well as the body are expelled, thereby recharging and rejuvenating the entire person both physically and mentally.

Abhyangam

Taken from the root word *ang* meaning "movement" and the prefix *abhi* meaning "toward" or "into", *abhyangam* refers to both the movement of toxins into the alimentary canal for elimination, and the moving of energy within the body. It is the standard Ayurvedic massage. Traditionally performed with lashings of medicated herbal oil chosen according to one's *dosha* and state of health, it is designed to be performed by one, two, four, or more therapists simultaneously.

Right: At the Ayurvedic Penthouse in the Oriental Spa, Keralan *abhyangam* is performed by two therapists. This style of synchronised massage uses harmonious strokes, rhythm, speed and pressure from head to heel. "The experience of being cocooned in caring warmth with the therapeutic effect of the oil balances all the three levels of physical, mental and spiritual wellbeing, creating deep relaxation," says a spokesperson.

32

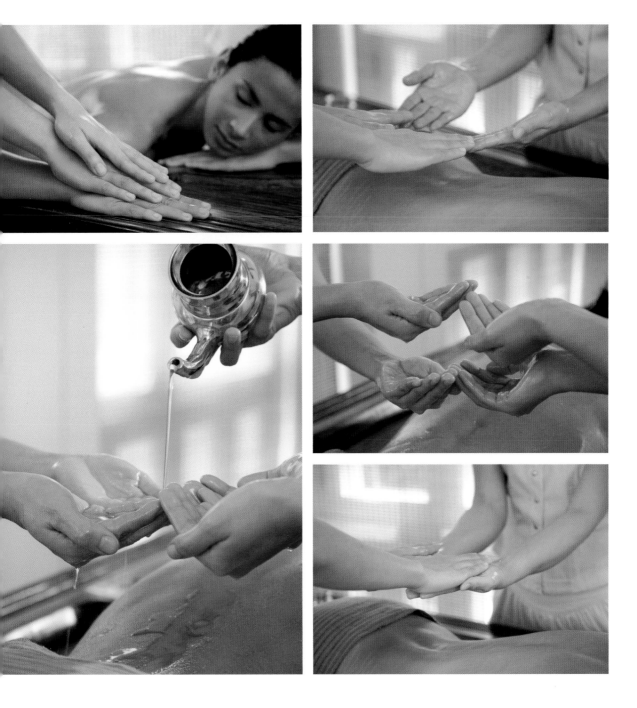

"*Abhyanga* massage uses long strokes mainly with full palm involved," explains Dr Yogesh from Udaivilas. "All the pressure movements will be in the direction of blood circulation, what we call *dosha anuloma*, from the trunk to the extremities and up to down. The reverse hand movements are passive (without pressure). This is to pacify imbalanced *doshas*." He goes on to add that the massage is not meant to be particularly relaxing, but "feelings of relaxation will come after."

The classic texts outline five different positions that the client should adopt during *abhyangam*, with postures 1 and 2 being repeated at the end, thus making a total of seven. These are:

1. Seated with both legs extended
2. Lying on the back
3. Lying on the left side
4. Lying on the stomach
5. Lying on the right side
6. Seated with both legs extended
7. Lying on the back.

Therapists generally spend an equal amount of time on each posture, but if there are particular areas that need special attention, these will definitely take precedence.

It is recommended that everyone have an *abhyanga* massage as part of their daily Ayurvedic ritual; it should be done in the morning, so that toxins accumulated during sleep may be expelled, and should be followed by an *ubtan* scrub made from pulses or grains (see page 175) and steam bath or shower. Typically, the massage starts with a head massage to render the mind relaxed and open and is followed by a body massage.

If you have *abhyangam* at one of the Oberoi Spas, the therapist soon gets a feel for your body, and concentrates on repeated strain-injured areas (RSIs) to increase benefits. Dr Yogesh says that this physical therapy has a direct connection to the mental and the spiritual: by the end, you should be physically and mentally relaxed – yet alert and rejuvenated also. Outside India, the Oriental Spa in Bangkok has an extremely authentic Ayurvedic floor where Keralan-trained masseuses perform *abhyangam* as a duo (see opposite). Their timing and synchronicity are quite astonishing – giving both muscles and mind a marvelous boost.

As with other Asian massages (Balinese very much comes to mind on this point) Ayurvedic massage involves a positive energy transfer from the therapist to guest's body. "For this," explains Dr Yogesh, "the therapists need to have a total mental involvement in the process. We suggest that therapists self meditate for a minute or two just before starting the treatment, in order to be fully present and involved."

Benefits of good *abhyanga* massage include increased circulation, improvement in muscle tone, calming of the nerves, increased mental alertness, soft, smooth skin and, of course, the elimination of impurities from the body.

Right: Staff at the Ayurvedic Penthouse at the Oriental Spa believe that authentic Ayurvedic equipment, such as the copper tub and teak massage bed seen here, as well as skilled therapists and correct oils, promote deep healing inside and out.

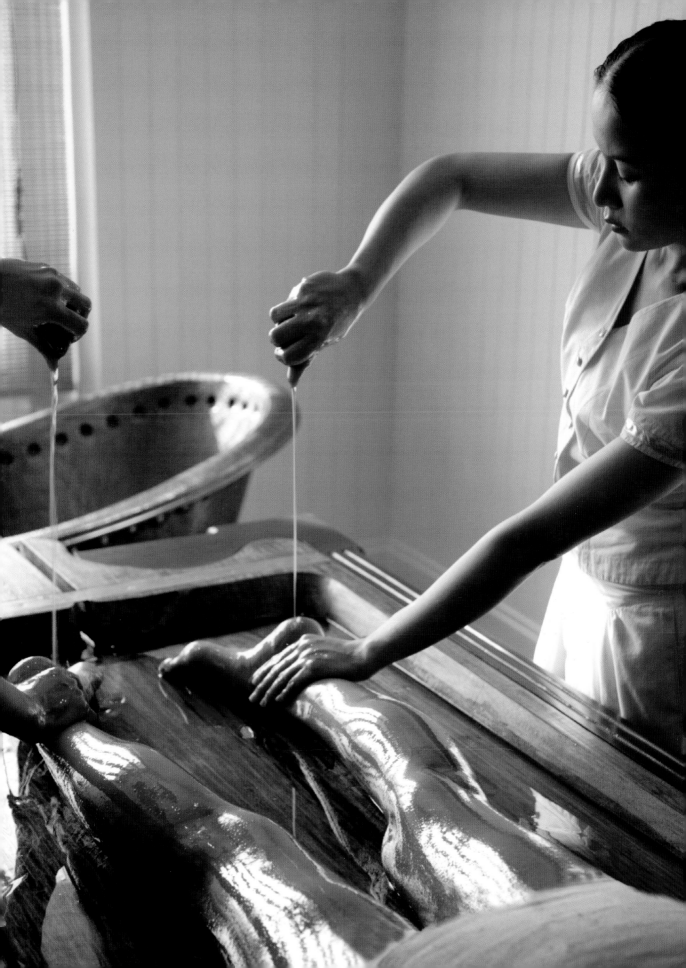

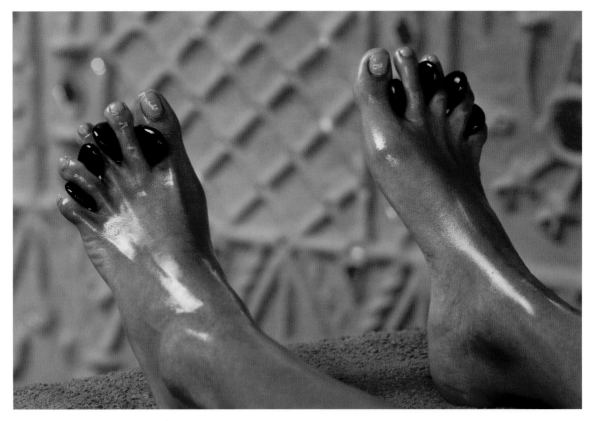

The stones used in hot stone massage are often basalt, a black volcanic rock with a high iron content, that absorbs and retains heat well. The heated stones placed on specific points of the body improve the flow of energy in the body. Small stones between the toes are delightfully indulgent, while larger ones placed on the plams and body impart feelings of warmth and security.

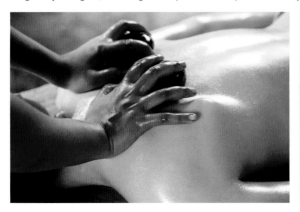

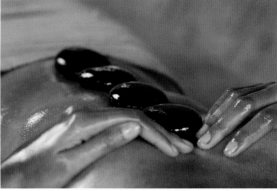

Hot Stone Abhyangam

Some spas and clinics in India are known for their experimentation with Ayurvedic practice. "The old ways aren't always the best for modern times," confided one doctor, who then immediately requested anonymity as if afraid of appearing disloyal to his profession. Dr Mathai at Soukya, the holistic medical centre near Bangalore, has no such qualms advocating such an idea. His aim to create integrated therapies that combine wisdoms from different fields in order to fully service clients is both forward-looking and logical. "We want to take the best that holistic medicine has to offer," he declares, "and give it to the world with quality, honesty and heartfelt Indian humility."

One example of such an integrated treatment is the deeply penetrating, all-over body blast he terms hot stone *abhyangam*. Employing the healing medicated herbal oils and massage movements of Ayurveda with the warmth and nurturing qualities of hot stones developed by both Native American Indians and Tibetans (separately of course!), it is one and a half hours of pure bliss.

There is simultaneously a therapeutic element and a feel-good factor to this treatment, so you can relax cocooned in the warmth emanating from the hot stones knowing that what is taking place is good for you. The long, firm strokes the masseuse employs encourages the elimination of toxins from the deeper tissues and also stimulates peripheral circulation of both blood and lymph. This, along with the heat from the stones, enables the medicated oils to be absorbed to do their work.

Naturally, as with all Ayurvedic treatments, oils are chosen according to the client's constitution, imbalance and/or ailment.

One therapist is in charge of heating and re-heating the stones, while the other alternates between oil massage, stone massage with oil, and placing stones at key points on the body. As the treatment progresses, a rhythm is established. One part of the body is being massaged, while a strategically placed stone sends heat deep into another part of the body; as the stone cools, it is replaced or taken away and another stone is placed elsewhere. After the back, legs and arms have been treated, the client turns over, and is then invited to lie down on eight stones that run up either side of the spine. The heat is then twofold: coming up from below through the back, and down from stones on the front.

With soothing music, the quiet efficiency of the therapists, firm massage strokes and the wonderfully nurturing warmth from the smooth stones, this is an experience to savour. The mind wanders and returns, the body sighs in acceptance, the spirit is soothed. Tension is released, muscles relax, the circulatory system speeds up and the system's vital energy channels are unblocked. This enables the body's vital energy or *prana* to start to flow freely again.

Unfortunately, it seems all too soon when the treatment comes to an end. Nonetheless, the benefits linger: and if this therapy is prescribed as a daily treat during a long-term stay, they are magnified considerably.

Marma massage

In India pressure points are known as *marmas* and are similar to Chinese acupressure points. Translating from the Sanskrit as "secret" or "hidden", they are found at junctures of the body where two or more tissues, muscles, veins, ligaments, bones or joints meet.

In Traditional Chinese Medicine (TCM), there are thousands of pressure points, but only 107 exist in the Ayurvedic system. Consisting of major *marmas* that correspond to the seven *chakras* and minor points that radiate out along the torso and limbs, they are measured by finger units (*anguli*) to detect their correct locations. There are 22 points on the legs, 22 on the arms, 12 on the chest and stomach, 14 on the back and 37 on the head and neck. The mind is sometimes considered the 108th point. In the *Sushruta Samhita* each point has a Sanskrit name.

Ayurveda states that each and every *marma* point is placed at a junction of different channels of *prana* movements in the body. *Prana* is considered the subtle vital energy that pervades every part of the system, nurturing cellular structure. If *marma* points become blocked or ruptured, *prana* flow is interrupted and organs may become diseased. If they are clear, *prana* is free to travel the meridians unchecked – and the body is healthy.

The idea of massaging the *marmas* began in Kerala at around 1,500 BC when masters of *kalari payattu*, the ancient martial art, first discovered the power of *marma* points (see pages 130–133). They identified the *marma* points as vital targets to attack. It was only a matter of time before physicians realised that these points could also be used for healing –

and began to experiment with massaging the points to trigger a restorative flow of energy. Today, *marma* massage is practiced at clinics and spas for varying reasons, be it therapeutic, relaxing or revitalising.

Marma massage generally combines flowing, soft movements (*abhyangam*) with pressure point therapy. For the latter, the therapist uses one or more fingers depending on the size of the *marma* point, and either presses directly or in circular motions on that particular point. It is believed that clockwise movements stimulate and energise a *marma* point while counterclockwise motions

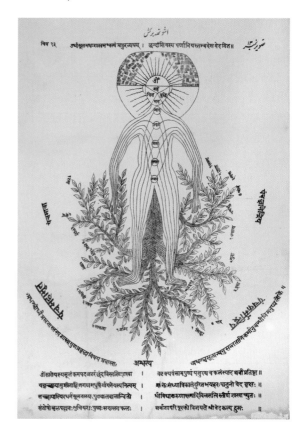

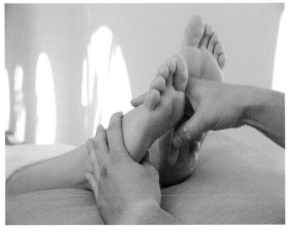
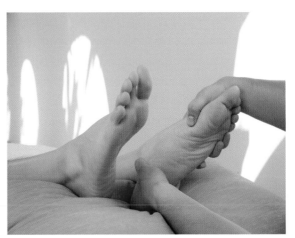

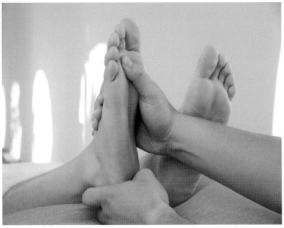
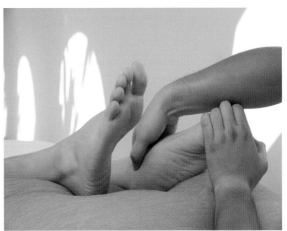

break up blocked energy and toxins. The practice is incredibly similar to Japanese *shiatsu* and Chinese acupressure, and it is believed by many that the origins of both lie in Ayurveda.

Benefits of regular *marma* massage are both physical and mental. The body is strengthened, toned and firmed; the mind is invigorated and energised. The result is a clear, confident outlook and a general sense of wellbeing and clarity.

Opposite: An educational drawing that shows the location of the seven *chakras*, rising from the base of the spine to the crown, and the key meridian lines in the body. It is believed that *prana*, the body's vital "air" or energy that is similar to *chi* in Traditional Chinese Medicine, flows along these lines, nourishing the cellular system, as well as the mind and spirit. A key component in *marma* massage is the invigoration of free pranic flow: in early Hindu philosophy, *prana* was held to be the principle of vitality that could survive a person's last breath for eternity or until a future life – so the effects of *marma* massage are long term.

Above: As with TCM, it is believed that the *marma* points on the feet are linked to an internal area or organ, so *marma* massage has benefits both internally and in the immediate localised area.

Indian Head Massage

In spite of its name, Indian head massage involves work not only on the head but on the upper back, shoulders, neck, scalp and face too. In the same way that both TCM and *marma* massage dictate that certain points on the feet are directly aligned to internal organs, Ayurvedic texts coordinate certain parts of the head to other body parts and/or symptoms or diseases. Therefore, a *champi* or head massage does not only affect the immediate areas massaged: it can be a healing, rejuvenating and thoroughly stimulating experience as well.

The moment a baby is born, the fontanel on the top of its head is covered immediately with cloth soaked in oil with a *bala* root decoction to

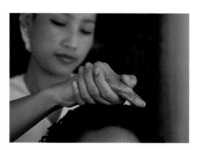

strengthen the head, sight and intelligence. Mothers massage their babies' heads to facilitate strong skull and brain development, and later, give their daughters head massages to stimulate the scalp. Men are used to receiving a scalp rubdown at the barber's shop and another place you are likely to receive an Indian head massage is in a salon or spa.

The massage normally takes from 30 to 60 minutes and is given seated in a chair. It may be dry, or nourishing oils may be used, to both condition

hair and calm the nervous system, as hair roots are connected to nerve fibres. Techniques vary, but the therapist usually starts by gently kneading upper back, shoulder and neck muscles, then works up to the head. Here, the scalp is squeezed, rubbed and tapped and hair may be combed or pulled. The therapist then locates the *marma* points along the head and spends time tugging and pressing earlobes, before moving on to the face. Facial massage is usually a mixture of acupressure and gentle manipulation, ending with soft stroking.

When the East India Company began its trade in spices and cotton in the 16th and 17th centuries, it wasn't just commodities that were in high demand. There was a fascination with Indian practices too, especially amongst the upper classes, and some enterprising Indians exported their wares and skills to Europe. An 18th-century history of British seaside resorts talks of a certain massage therapist called Sake Deen Mohammed who became the talk of Brighton with his "Indian Vapor Bath and Art of Shampooing"! Interestingly, the Hindi word for "head massage" (*champi*) was manipulated into the English word "shampoo".

Today, Indian head massage continues to be popular in Britain, and indeed around the globe, as it is easy to receive and has many benefits. People who suffer from headaches, migraines, insomnia,

Above and right: The 60-minute *urdwangam* or Indian head massage offered on the menu at the Ayurvedic Penthouse at Mandarin Oriental is a deeply relaxing and rejuvenating experience. Pressure point massage stimulates the vital energy points in the skull to increase the flow of subtle energies in the body; the client is left feeling extremely comforted and nurtured.

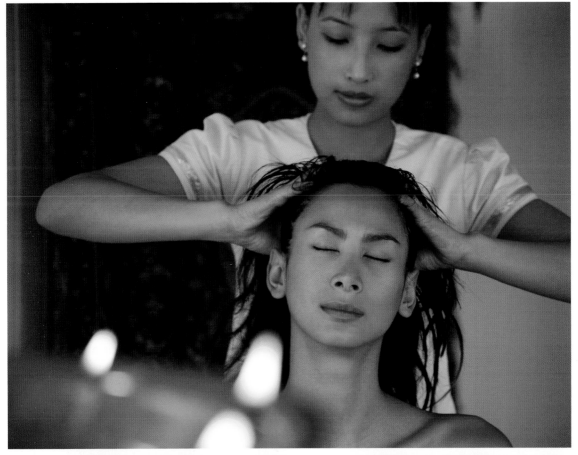

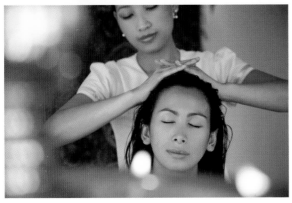

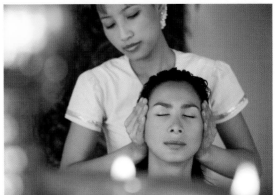

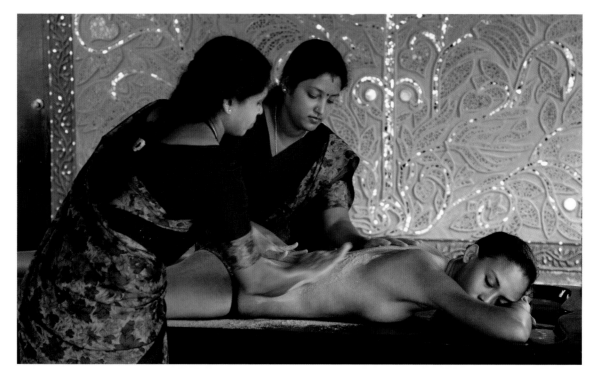

tinnitus, vertigo and depression are all reported to find it helpful. As the therapist works on the three higher *chakras*, the *vissuddha* (the base of the throat), *ajna* (the forehead) and *sahasrara* (the crown), mental and emotional stress is released. In addition, the localised massage improves the supply of glucose and blood to the brain, helps the circulation of cerebrospinal fluid and dissipates accumulated toxins. Benefits include improvements in memory, clarity of mind, eyesight and concentration.

Udwarthanam

A stimulating massage that uses dry powders (not oil), *udwarthanam* is vigorous, energising and not for the faint hearted. Coarse dry herbal powders,

chosen according to one's *dosha*, are rubbed into the skin in the opposite direction to hair growth with strong repeated movements. The friction of the powder during the massage creates heat on the body that increases circulation, helps break down cellulite, firms muscle tone and reduces fat by improving the metabolism of muscles. It is recommended for those who want to lose weight, as *udwarthanam* helps promote better digestion and reduces cholesterol levels and adipose tissue. It also removes toxins and exfoliates surface skin cells, leaving skin tingling, soothed and soft.

Most Ayurvedic massages tend to use long, flowing strokes moving away from the heart and going from bottom to top, but *udwarthanam* employs short, sharp superficial rubs that go in the opposite direction, away from the heart towards the extremities and from the top of the body downwards. This is the opposite of the *dosha* flow. In a clinical setting, *udwarthanam* is usually prescribed for 10–14 days for those with *ama twan* or slowness of flow in the channels, and as a means to reduce fat.

At Udaivilas where Dr Yogesh has trained all the therapists in the art of *udwarthanam*, one of three Ayurvedic powders or *choornam* are used: the popular *triphala choornam* or three fruit powder, a powder composed from *Terminalia chebula* (an antibacterial fruit) or *kota kula thadhi choornam* made from a variety of pulses and herbs. While the client has a cleansing footbath, the powder is briefly tested on the arm to check for allergies. Afterwards, the client is invited to lie face down on the bed while the cool, very fine powder is sprinkled on one leg, then one side of the back, then repeated on the other side. Before being rubbed in, the therapist does a small amount of acupressure massage on relevant parts of the body.

The massage is fairly invigorating, but may be a bit abrasive for those with sensitive skin. The idea is that the herbs in the powder enter the superficial bloodstream and nasally through inhalation. This

cleanses the internal system too. A front rub follows the back rub, after which the client is encouraged to spend 10 minutes in the steam room and further massage any residual powder into the skin. As sweating occurs, toxins are released through the skin's pores, and the skin is left feeling soft, smooth and rejuvenated. The treatment ends with a shower and choice of tea: ginger or chamomile.

Another place that practices *udwarthanam* is Soukya, a facility famous for its herb garden. Here, it is prescribed for guests who are obese and different powders are used for different patients. Powders may contain *vacha* (*Acorus calamus*) to alleviate

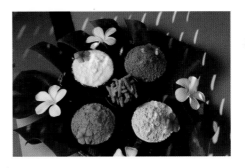

swelling, the Ayurvedic all-round wonder fruit Indian gooseberry (*Emblica officinalis*), green garam powder and/or basil. All the herbs are washed, cut into small pieces, dried and pulverised on site to make either a fine or coarse powder, which is then strewn onto the body and massaged in by two therapists simultaneously. According to Ayurvedic physician, Dr Ajitha, the powder helps to open up micro-channels in the body, to reduce the accumulation of fat, tauten muscles, reduce bad body odour and exfoliate dead surface skin cells.

Opposite: An *udwarthanam* session at Soukya employs two therapists and herbal powders made on site.

Right: Some of the ingredients used at an Udaivilas dry powder massage. Dr Yogesh explains the benefits: "The powders used contain what Ayurvedic doctors call *madagna* properties; these reduce fat and help to clear blockages in the *dosha* channels. In addition, the superficial rubbing is invigorating: it activates the blood circulation, increases the metabolism, removes surface dead cells and gives a tingling feeling on the skin."

The Herbal Pouch

In Ayurvedic practice, the herbal poultice is a time-honoured tradition of healing with heat. Packed with goodness, warmed pouches of herbs, plants, roots, and more, have been applied to sprained, sore or sad bodies for centuries. Classified as a *swedanam* (sweat therapy) in the Vedic texts, the herbal poultice is both detoxifying and healing. Specially selected ingredients are tied tightly in natural cloth, steamed for a few minutes, then dipped in medicated herbal oil and applied to the body. On application, the heat induces sweating, thereby helping to bring toxins to the surface of the skin; then, once the pores are open, skin absorbs the properties of the herbs for healing.

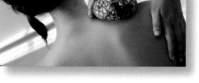

The *kizhi* (Malayalam word for "bundle") has proved so popular over the centuries, its fame has spread to other cultures too: Thailand's war-weary soldiers in Ayuthyan times used such poultices to soothe injuries after battle and both Malaysian and Indonesian herbal healing tomes record the use of such heated poultices as far back as the 13th and 14th centuries. In Indonesian *jamu* (herbal medicine) specially selected roots and spices are compressed into small balls, then dipped in water before being applied to swollen parts of the body for a soothing, curative effect. Called *param mustika*, they were (and still are) commonly used on muscle strains and sprains, neuralgic and rheumatic pains and cold feet and hands. They are especially useful for women following childbirth.

In Malaysia's Pangkor Laut and at some Maldivian spas, sand is used as a substitute for herbs: when dipped in warm, herbal oil, the pouches are extremely effective at maintaining their heat. Another favourite at Pangkor Laut is the modern version of a traditional recipe: containing steamed and warm fragrant lemongrass and aromatic pandan leaves, the *campur campur* or "blend of varieties" is highly stimulating.

Spas, wellness centres and salons throughout India offer different forms of the herbal pouch both as a stand-alone treatment or in conjunction with another therapy. The content, method of application and usage varies widely.

Patrapotlaswedanam

The Sanskrit name for this time-honoured Ayurvedic treatment is taken from *patra* meaning "leaves", *potla* translating as "pouch" and *swedanam, a* term used by Ayurvedic doctors for "fomentation" or "sweat therapy". Soukya, well known for its organic practices makes full use of plants grown on site for its *potla*. Leaves from the castor oil plant (*Ricinus communis*), rich in oil, are combined with *Datura alba* leaves (this plant is widely used by

Above and right: Sand, like clay, has the ability to retain heat or cold, so is an ideal filler for a heated compress. When dipped in warm, medicated oil, these bundles of goodness spread warmth and healing oils deep into tense or knotted muscles. At the Spa Village at Pangor Laut, a private island resort in Malaysia, pretty batik cottons are used to increase the pouch's appeal.

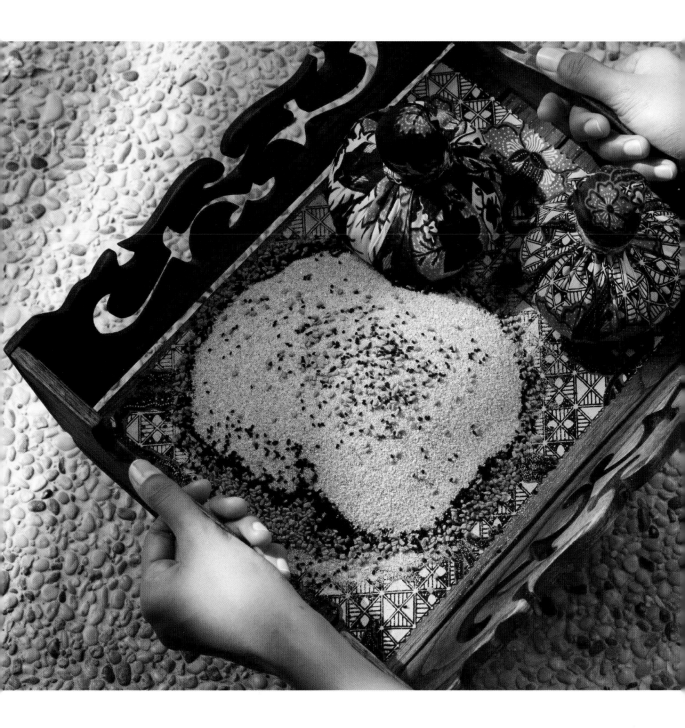

Ayurvedic and Siddha practitioners in oil-based preparations for dressings on wounds), skin tonifying *nirgundi* or *Vitex nigundo* leaves and leaves from the *moringo* or drumstick tree. The latter leaves are a known natural antibiotic. In fact, all these leaves have anti-inflammatory and pain-reducing properties, so are useful in arthritic and rheumatic conditions. To prepare the *potla*, they are washed, torn up and mixed with other kitchen condiments, then fried with medicated oil in a wok, before being knotted into beautiful linen pouches.

At Soukya, patients who have been prescribed this therapy will be on a course of seven to 21 days, and the pouch will be combined with other therapies. It may be given to people with sciatica, disc prolapse or lower back pain, and is usually administered after an external application of medicated oil. Two therapists are employed with four *potla*: one warms two of the pouches in medicated oil, while the other massages the other two on to affected areas. Movements include gentle thudding and rubbing away from the heart.

If you are lucky enough to experience Soukya's professional *patrapotlasweda*, be prepared for some internal detoxification as well as the speeding up of surface blood circulation and skin conditioning. The skin may turn a little pink, especially if the therapists concentrate on localised areas, but the overall feeling is nurturing and warming.

Navara Kizhi

Definitely worth a try is the intriguingly named Navara *kizhi*, a Keralan treatment offered at many spas and clinics throughout India. At Oberoi Spa at Udaivilas, Navara rice (a type of dehusked, red rice) is mixed with milk and a decoction of *bala* root (*Sida cordifolia*) and boiled for half an hour until it achieves a gruel-like consistency. It is then wrapped into a loosely-spun cotton cloth that allows the mixture to permeate and be applied to the body. The excess liquid is kept in reserve on a nearby warmer, so that the pouches may be periodically dipped and re-warmed.

Bala root is a powerful cell nourishing and cell regenerating herb, and is used in many Ayurvedic treatments to maintain youth and vitality. It means "youth" in Sanskrit, and is considered analgesic, diuretic and stimulating as well. When mixed with Navara rice and milk, the properties "go quite deep", according to Ayurvedic doctor, Dr Yogesh, who recommends the treatment to develop muscles and improve muscle tone. "The pouch nourishes the skin, alleviates *vata* problems, improves blood

Above and right: Straight from the organic garden, Soukya's leaves are washed and chopped, then mixed with crushed lime, shredded coconut and smashed garlic and fried in a wok with medicated oil chosen according to the patient's constitution. After frying for 10 to 15 minutes, the ingredients are transferred into soft cotton pouches, before being administered, wonderfully warmed in medicated oil, on problem areas.

46

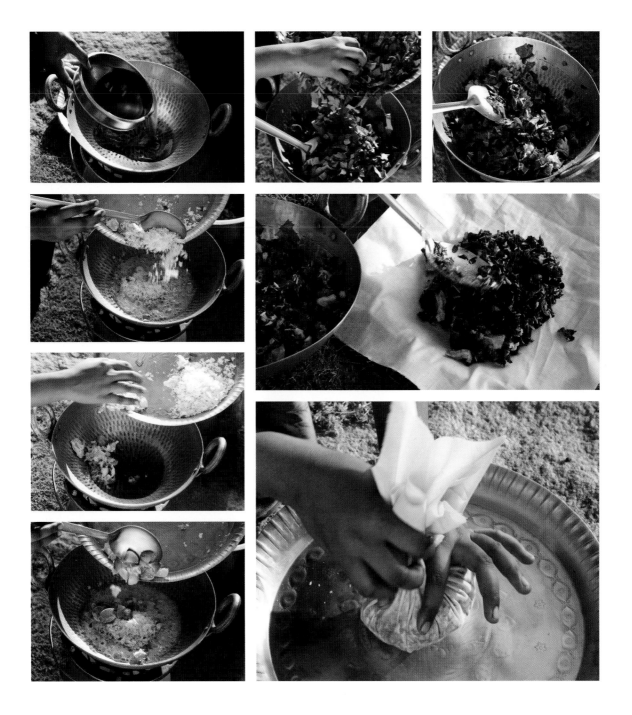

circulation, reduces stiffness and strengthens both the quantity and quality of the muscles," he says.

First, the client experiences a short massage with warmed oil, then the bundles are applied initially on the back, then on the front. Two methods are used: Sponging very quickly up and down to begin with, then, after the bundle cools, quick rubbing motions to allow the heat to penetrate into the skin. Dr Yogesh describes Navara *kizhi* as quite a dynamic treatment – it's great for sports injuries and the like – but doesn't recommend it for those who simply want to relax.

Adhbhut Potali Upchar

A more localised Rajasthani version of the herbal pouch can be experienced at Amanbagh, a resort that can arguably be called a healing spa in itself.

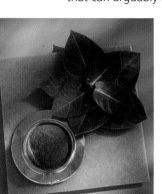

Everything about the hotel centres around the locale in which it finds itself: many of its spa treatments are based on local lore, it offers numerous expeditions to outlying villages and forts, and its staff is 50 percent local.

Amanbagh's herbal pouch treatment takes its inspiration from the surrounding country-side, once the playground of Maharajahs. Devised by their talented spa manager, as are many of the treatments, it is called *adhbhut potali upchar* in Hindi or "exotic bundle treatment". Spa Manager, Vijaya Lakshmi, describes it as "a detox herbal treatment that uses bundles of medicated herbal powders dipped in nurturing and warming oil and placed on the body".

Dashmool powder (*das* means "10", *mool* translates as "roots", a very popular Ayurvedic powder used in more than 40 percent of Ayurvedic preparations) is bought at the nearby market, and tied securely in immaculate linen pouches. These are dipped in warmed, medicated sesame oil before application. The sesame oil in which the bundles are dipped is first boiled with handpicked *aak* leaves (*Calotropis gigantea*), a plant in the milk-weed family that grows profusely around Amanbagh. Commonly known as swallow-wort, *aak* is useful in the treatment of paralysis, swellings and fever, and it is anti-inflammatory when applied externally. When combined with the properties of the 10 root powders, the pouches are anti-rheumatic, ease stiffness in the joints, and warm the skin.

At Amanbagh, clients may elect to have their *potali upchar* in the privacy of their room, deck or terrace or in a spacious, quiet spa room. Wherever the location, however, they have some control over the process. The therapist concentrates on joints and shoulder muscles mainly, but if there are any areas of stiffness or strain, the client is encouraged to share these areas of concern with the therapist. Warming and aromatic, the pouches can be immensely helpful for rheumatism and arthritis.

Spice Bundle Massage

Quan Spa at JW Marriot Mumbai offers a version of the herbal pouch that involves two spa therapists pressing steamed pouches infused with

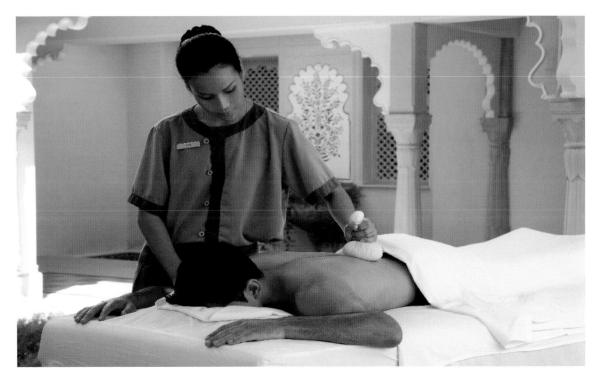

warm camphor oil on to the body, and combining this herbal heaven with some kneading massage. Recommended for easing joint stiffness, improving mobility and increasing flexibility, the pouches are filled with two Ayurvedic powders: *kola kula thadi choornam* and *kottam chukkadi choornam*. The latter is especially useful for those suffering from rheumatic conditions. Therapists tend to use thumping movements with the pouches – so be prepared for a fairly dynamic treatment. Dr Manauj, the spa manager, recommends Quan's poultice for chronic pain, and as an alternative to massage. He says that when the powders penetrate the skin, toxins are eliminated from the system and the body is invigorated. What better way to spend an hour?

Opposite: Dashmool powder and *aak* leaves at Amanbagh.

Below: At Udaivilas a therapist prepares the ingredients for the Navara *kizhi* therapy: a gruel of rice and milk is mixed with a *bala* root decoction, in preparation for dipping into medicated herbal oil and applying on the back *(see above).*

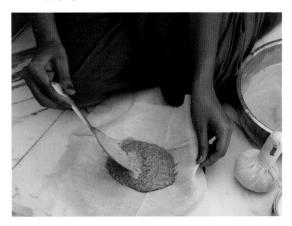

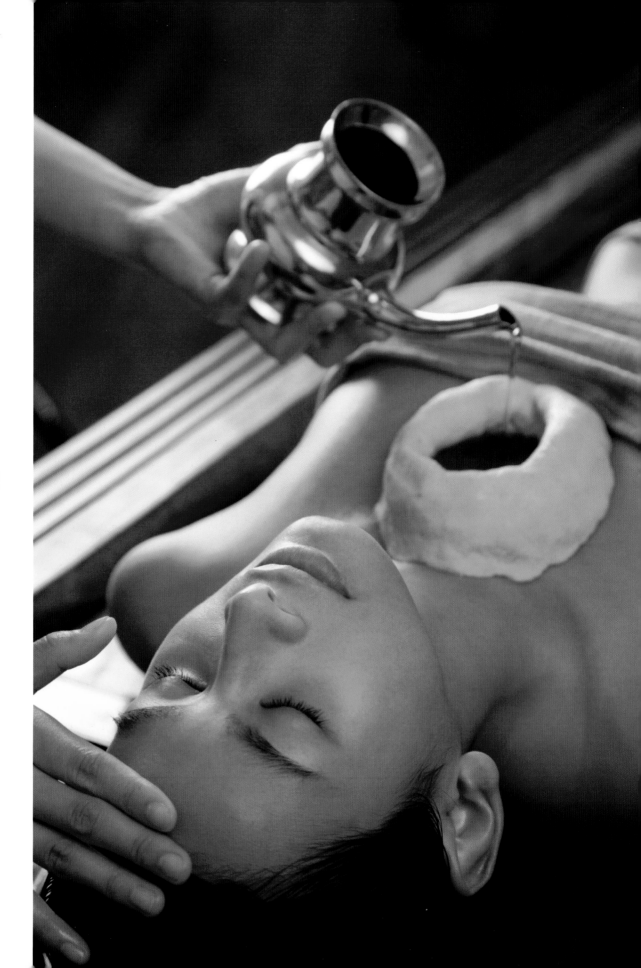

Vasthi Therapies

"Ayurveda is steadfast in insisting that medicine should always be centered on the person rather than on the disease. It believes that the twin goals of maintaining good health and deliverance of disease in ill health can be reached only if the doctor has a thorough understanding of the person."

— *Sukhir Kakar*

To most Westerners the subject of enemas is one to be avoided, at best; subjected to, at worst. This probably stems from an innate squeamishness, but, be that as it may, the insertion into the anus, urinary organs and genitals of various kinds of enemas such as medicated and non-medicated oils and milks, water and herbal decoctions is an integral part of Ayurvedic practice. This is because the "Science of Life" propounds that the status of the alimentary canal and other internal organs is of vital importance to one's overall health and wellbeing.

Vasthi (*basti*) is the word for a medicated enema, and in Ayurveda *vasthi* involves the introduction of herbal and medicinal concoctions in a liquid medium into and also *onto* the body. Sites where *vasthi* may be administered therefore also include external areas such as the eyes, lower back, head and chest region. It is believed that these medicinal *vasthis* remove wastes and toxins from the body (either internally or externally), balance the various functions of the *doshas*, provide nourishment and raise immunity.

Vasthi is most effective in the treatment of *vata* disorders (see page 20), although many enemas over a prescribed period of time are usually required. Different types of *vasthi* are prescribed for many vastly differing ailments, including chronic fever, sexual disorders, cold, kidney stones, heart pain, constipation, backache, sciatica and other pains in the joints. Many other *vata* disorders such as arthritis, rheumatism, gout, muscle spasms and headaches may also be treated with some of the differing *vasthis*.

In a clinic, *vasthi* is one of the five main procedures of the famous (or infamous) *panchakarma* therapy (see pages 62–63), but it may also be prescribed in conjunction with other therapies for any number of illnesses (see above). It falls into the category of therapies known as oleation therapies or *snehanam*. Externally, it may be used in localised areas for neck complaints (*greva vasthi*) or knee joint conditions (*janu vasthi*) for example.

In the Indian spa, a couple of *vasthi* therapies are offered for one-off "try-outs". These tend to be relaxing rather than therapeutic, and act as an informal introduction to Ayurveda. See if any of the following forms of *vasthi* appeal.

Above: At the Ayurvedic Penthouse at the Oriental Spa in Bangkok, a therapist prepares a dough of gram flour and water which is then placed on to the client's precordium (*left*). Once it is deemed watertight, warmed medicated oil (chosen according to the client's imbalances) is poured into the doughnut-shaped "container" to foment for 40 minutes or so.

51

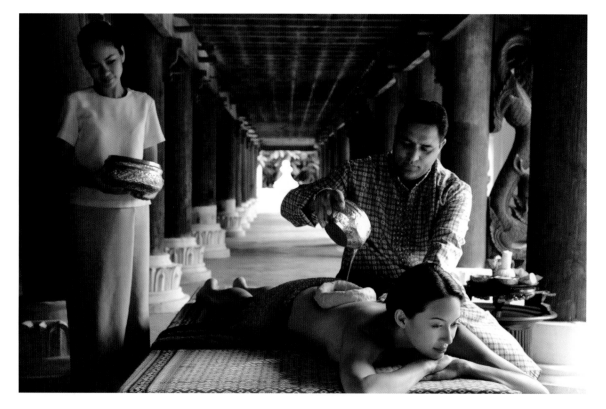

Hrid Vasthi

Concentrating on the heart area, *hrid* or *uro vasthi* is prescribed by Ayurvedic doctors for heart disease, asthma and respiratory diseases and muscular chest pain. Oil or ghee, enclosed within a "reservoir" of dough (a gram flour and water mix) on the chest, strengthens the heart muscle and increases stamina and vitality at a very essential level. This is also an effective therapy for emotional imbalances, as it relieves deep-seated anger, hurt and sadness.

Above: The beautiful surrounds of the Dheva Spa at the Mandarin Oriental Dhara Devi in Chiang Mai serve as a fitting environment for the somewhat homespun *kathi vasthi* therapy.

Kathi Vasthi

The *vasthi* treatment that concentrates on the sacro-lumbar region of the back (*kathi*) is more common. This is a curative treatment that is useful for lower back problems. In an Ayurvedic clinic, it may be part of a treatment for sacroiliac problems, prolapsed discs, lumbar spondylosis, osteoporosis, sciatica and chronic backache. It is also used for complaints that affect the abdomen, such as irritable bowel syndrome, endometriosis, urinary tract and menstrual disorders. It involves the pouring of warm medicated oil, as usual specific to the client, into an enclosed area on the lower back.

In spas *kathi vasthi* is used as a rejuvenative therapy to de-stress, relieve exhaustion or help with localised lower back pain. US doctors say that four out of five adults experience lower back pain at some time during their lives, and the causes are many: nerves may be damaged, muscles may be irritated, there may be injury to bones, ligaments, joints or discs, or it may be caused by a combination of the above. A mild manipulation or massage – or the application of lukewarm oil – in this area can be comforting in such instances.

Providing the *kathi vasthi* is administered by a qualified Ayurvedic doctor who has chosen the correct medicinal oil, a 20- to 60-minute session should not do any harm – and the gentle pouring of warm, soothing oil on the back can also nourish and strengthen the underlying tissues.

Siro Vasthi

Usually offered at an Ayurvedic clinic as part of a one- to three-week treatment for conditions such as facial paralysis, depression, insomnia, dryness of nostrils, mouth and throat illnesses and severe headaches, *siro vasthi* is sometimes available at Indian spas as a relaxing, stress-relieving and hair-conditioning therapy. *Siro vasthi* (*siro* means "head") involves the application of lukewarm herbal oils poured into a cap fitted on the head for 15 to 60 minutes. The oils are left to stagnate on the scalp for the time required; according to one's current imbalances and/or medical conditions, medicated herbs will have been added to the oil. An antioxidant medicated oil called *dhan wantharam* that contains 28 herbs and an earthy fragrance is often used as it has rich pain-relieving properties.

In the same way that vitamins, mineral or herbal tablets are used to keep alert, *siro vasthi* is used in Ayurvedic medicine to regulate brain functioning, as stimulation of the crown *chakra* relates to consciousness. It may also be used as a diagnostic tool by Ayurvedic doctors: by monitoring the pulse of the patient while the oil is kept on the head, the physician is able to locate where the medicine acts in the body, thereby determining possible disease.

53

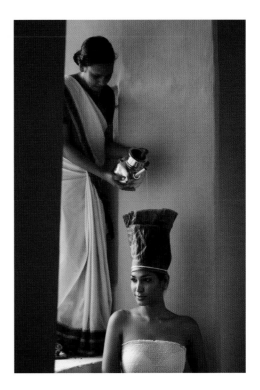

Above: A re-creation of the traditional *siro vasthi* treatment at Neemrana Fort Palace whereby a bandana of banana leaves fashioned in a tube replaces the leather or plastic cap used today.

Netra Tarpanam

In Ayurveda, the eyes are considered *pitta* ("fire") in nature, so they benefit from being kept cool. A drop of sesame oil in each eye is of general benefit to eyes, and sore or itchy eyes are treated with an eye bath of rose water or plain water no hotter than body temperature. The fifth-century Ayurvedic physician Vagbhata declared that the nerves in the soles of the feet are connected to the state of both eyes and ears – so Ayurvedic physicians often suggest oiling the soles of the feet with castor oil to remedy eye complaints. Honey, castor oil or *triphala* tea applications are also considered to be beneficial.

At an Ayurvedic clinic, a physician may prescribe *netra tarpanam* as an external eye care treatment to help with eye strain, dryness of eyes, poor sight and other eye-related conditions. It is believed to strengthen the muscles round the eyes, cool the eyes, oleate the area round the eyes and may even help with myopia. As an introduction to enhance the overall health of the eyes, in the areas of vision, strength of eye muscles, coolness, and more, it is also occasionally offered at an Indian spa.

The Oberoi Spas' *netra tarpanam* is similar in every way to the clinical procedure, the only difference being that the client will probably only receive it once. As with all Ayurvedic prescriptions, at least a two-week course is suggested, and during the period of treatment the patient should not expose the eyes to harsh light, use a computer, watch television or eat spicy food. In the spa setting, *netra tarpanam* serves more as a taste of the exotic, and an interesting and informative experience to boot.

The treatment uses the medium of ghee or *gritham*, a type of clarified butter essential in Indian cooking. "Ghee has what we call *samskarika anuvarthana* in Sanskrit," explains Udaivilas' resident Ayurvedic doctor, Dr Yogesh. "This means it has the specific quality of being able to absorb properties of herbal products and transfer them into the skin." He uses either *triphala gritham*, which is believed to be good for the eyesight, or *jeevanthyadhi gritham*, a ghee that helps develop immunity and purges the system. To keep the ghee in place over the eye socket, a dough of black or green gram flour paste (gram powder mixed with water) is made and secured around both eye cavities.

First of all the entire eye area is thoroughly cleansed with rose water to ensure it is clean and oil free, then the gram flour mix is fixed on the face. A small amount of ghee melted to room temperature is subsequently poured into the watertight enclosure, so that it fills the contained area and makes the eyelashes sink shut. The ghee is kept on the eyes for approximately 20 minutes, during which time the patient is encouraged to move the eyes around.

It is a somewhat fiddly process, and may not be to everyone's taste. Sometimes people experience a burning sensation when the medicated ghee is poured on, and having to hold still for a long time isn't easy for everyone. However "comforting and warming" was our prognosis. After the removal of ghee and dough and a cleanse with warm water, a gentle massage around the eye area completed the treatment.

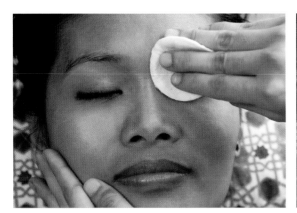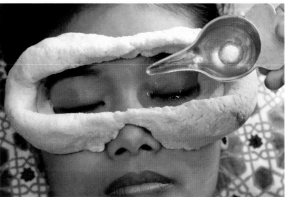

Ghee is used effectively in many different instances in Ayurveda. For *netra tarpanam*, a *vasthi* treatment, medicated ghee is poured into "reservoirs" enclosing the eye area. Eyes should be rolled around, opened and closed, to allow the ghee's properties to be fully absorbed.

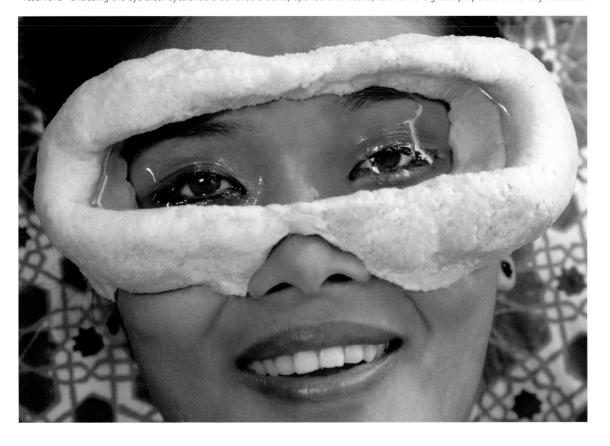
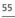

Sirodhara

Somewhat surprisingly, *sirodhara* is the most wide-spread Ayurvedic therapy offered at spas outside India. Why this is the case is unclear, as it is not prescribed for many ailments in a clinical environment. It invariably comes top of the Ayurvedic menu, and even spas without an Ayurvedic department offer bastardised versions. Many people have tried it, and even if they haven't, they will almost certainly have heard of it.

Coming from *siro* ("head") and *dhara* ("pouring of herbal liquids on specific body parts") *sirodhara* denotes the continuous pouring of herbal oils, milk, ghee or buttermilk over the "third eye", head and scalp. The patient lies on the back on a wooden treatment table, cocooned in warm towels, while a therapist trains a steady rhythmic stream of warm liquid from a perforated vessel made of clay, wood or metal on to the middle of the forehead. The table is made from one of seven therapeutic woods and is designed to catch the oil for recycling on the same client.

Oil stroking the sixth *chakra* (see page 122) has a balancing effect on the deepest recesses of the brain and is profoundly relaxing. In Ayurveda, it is a stimulating procedure for the nervous system and is prescribed for bringing down aggravated *vata* conditions such as insomnia, headache, insecurity, fear and nervous strain. Irritable *pitta* predominant people with overactive minds can experience a cooling, calming benefit from a session and *kapphas* often fall asleep. Used in conjunction with other

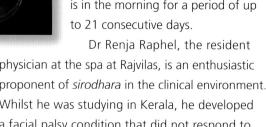

therapies, *sirodhara* has been practiced for thousands of years to treat many and varied conditions such as glandular problems, psychiatric disorders, skin diseases, hypertension, facial paralysis, ear, nose and throat disturbances, and more. During a session, the nervous system unwinds, busy brains become clear, and tired bodies are refreshed.

In a clinical environment, the choice of liquid and duration of treatment varies according to the individual. *Vata* patients are generally prescribed medicated herbal oil, while herbal milk, ghee or coconut oil are used for *pitta* types and *kapha* patients are often recommended buttermilk. Ancient texts denote 53 minutes for *vatas*, 43 minutes for *pittas* and 31 minutes for *kaphas*! It is suggested that the best time to receive *sirodhara* is in the morning for a period of up to 21 consecutive days.

Dr Renja Raphel, the resident physician at the spa at Rajvilas, is an enthusiastic proponent of *sirodhara* in the clinical environment. Whilst he was studying in Kerala, he developed a facial palsy condition that did not respond to

Above: The elevated wooden bed or *patti* is integral to Ayurvedic treatment. Preferably made from one piece of wood, this bed – from one of the four suites at the Ayurvedic Penthouse in Bangkok – is carved from a 100-year-old tree. In the *Charaka Samhita* seven woods are specified as being suitable for treatment beds: neem is one of the most popular.

Right: At Quan spa in Mumbai a *sirodhara* therapy takes place. "Sirodhara opens the third eye to absorb cosmic energy," the therapist reports. Guests are recommended to take a rest after the treatment, to allow the mind and body to re-centre.

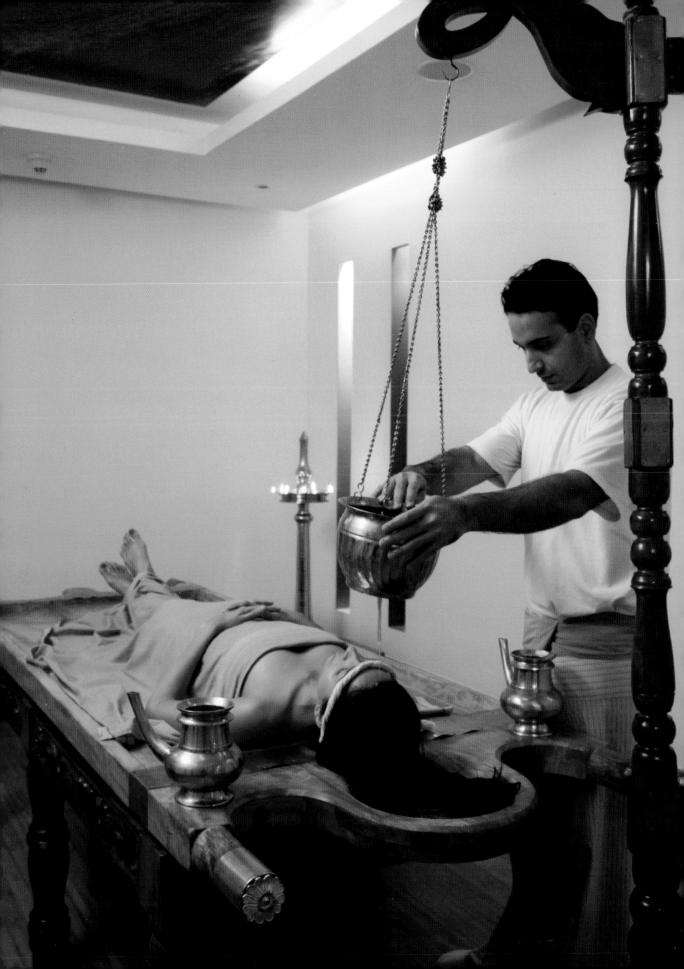

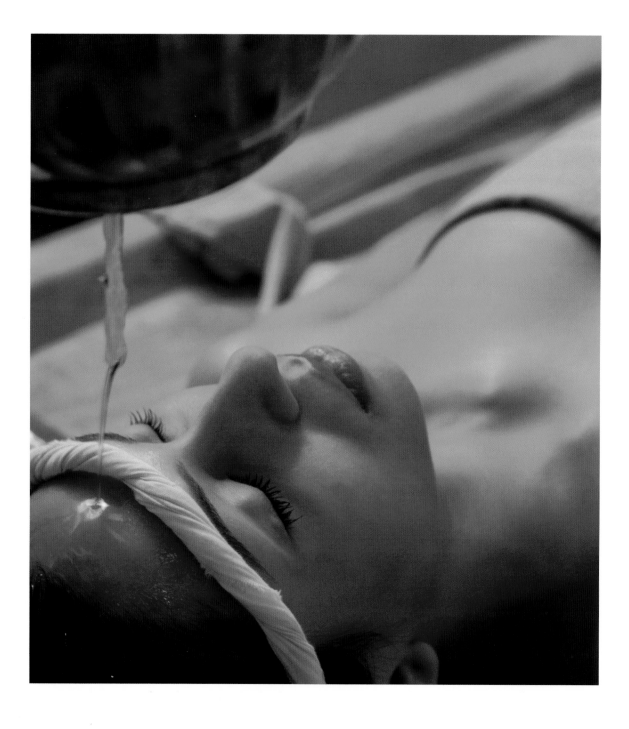

Western treatments, even after six weeks. His tutors advised that he should switch to an Ayurvedic doctor, so he enrolled in a three-week treatment programme that involved a strict diet, internal medicines, and two external treatments, one of which was *sirodhara*. "It was quite miraculous," he relates, "on the third day my eyelids began to blink for the first time in two months, and gradually as the treatment progressed, movement returned to my face." Within a month, he reports, it was as if the condition had never occurred.

Dr Raphel is less sure of *sirodhara*'s benefits in a spa environment, declaring that clients report wildly different experiences afterwards. Some become emotional or cry, he says, but 90 percent of people say it is soothing, comforting and relaxing. Medical studies back this up: they indicate that *sirodhara* induces a calm alpha brain-wave state which increases mental clarity and memory as well as improved stress and immune response.

A variation of *sirodhara* is *deha-dhara*, whereby two to four therapists pour a continuous flow of oil over the entire body. The Soukya *deha-dhara*, known as *dhanyamla dhara*, is particularly efficacious. *Dhanyamla* translates as a "decoction made from a fomentation of grains and herbs" and, each day, a decoction of herbs including *adjuven* and horse gram, mixed with a handful of Sali rice and lemon (all pacifiying *vata* ingredients), is prepared. Dr Ajitha explains that *deha-dhara* is "useful for arthritis as

Left: In Quan spa at JW Marriott Mumbai, oil at a *sirodhara* session is forced to flow back over the forehead with the fastening of a piece of cloth just below the "third eye".

the herbs reduce pain and swelling". It can also be helpful in treating rheumatic fever and obesity.

First the patient has an all-over oil application, then two therapists pour the warmed liquid with one hand on to the body and, with the other hand, gently massage it into the skin. The potency of the medicine is absorbed through the skin's pores, while the heat and massage act as a catalyst for healing properties to act on the sensory nerve endings. Water and toxins are expelled from the body and inflammation is reduced.

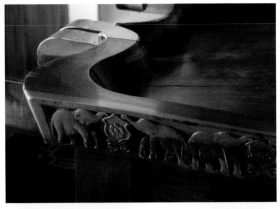

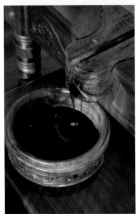
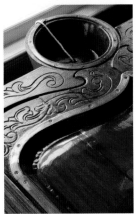

Spirit of Ayurveda

Devised by Dr Renja Raphel, the Keralan-trained Ayurvedic doctor at Rajvilas in Jaipur, this three-hour programme of indulgence is appropriately based on Rajasthani traditions. Jaipur is present-day Rajasthan's capital, and in times past its magnificent Pink City housed the Rajputana court of the Maharajah of Jaipur; as late as the 1940s over 400 women were still housed in the City Palace *zenana* and their beauty regimes invariably included 100 percent natural, Ayurvedic therapies.

A purifying footbath of crushed neem leaves begins the treatment. Traditionally, a footbath is offered to guests in an Indian home: both cleansing and welcoming, it signifies respect. At Rajvilas Spa, antiseptic neem leaves are crushed into a bowl of water and a two- to three-minute wash and massage set the tone for the ritual to come.

This takes the form of a *champi* or Indian head massage, a sand bundle therapy, a *sirodhara* and a soothing bath. All are designed to relax the body and calm and clear the mind.

In Ayurveda, it is believed that the entire nervous system starts from the brain, so the head is seen as the most important part of the body. As roots nourish the branches of a tree, the head nourishes all branches of the body. It is therefore appropriate that this ritual begins with the application of an Ayurvedic product called *bringadi* to the head. A blend of herbs processed in pure sesame oil and milk, it includes *neeli* (indigo), *bringraj* (false daisy) and *amla* (gooseberry) to promote hair growth, liquorice to act as an anti-fungal agent and balloon vine to prevent scalp

infection. For about 30 minutes, the therapist massages the oil into the scalp: Using rotating movements of the palm and fingertip pressure on certain points to stimulate nerve endings, it is deeply soothing. In addition, the oil nourishes hair roots and strengthens hair. It also helps with *vata* disorders, so is quite de-stressing.

The application of poultices filled with warm sulphur sand from Simla follows this promising start. The sand bundle is classified under *ushema swedana* therapies, which translates as "to warm up (bundles) to sweat". Sulphur sand, which can hold its temperature for a long time, is tied in small linen pouches, which are then dipped in warm medicated oil chosen according to one's *dosha* and pounded on the body. Accompanied by massage, the poultices are good for inflammatory conditions, stiffness of joints and aching muscles and also promote general wellbeing. The heat speeds up blood circulation and promotes sweating, which in turn helps eliminate toxins from the body.

Everyone's favourite, *sirodhara* (see pages 56–59), follows. Dr Raphel explains how this works: "Under clinical circumstances as part of a proper Ayurvedic programme, *sirodhara* is used to bring down aggravated *vata* conditions, but in the spa, it is simply a tool for relaxation." After this, a faintly leafy-scented purifying neem bath (see right), and a shower with *snarn choornam* made from garam powder, turmeric and fig bark to soak up any excess oil, completes the ritual. The powder exfoliates dead skin cells from the surface of the skin and leaves the body feeling soft, supple and cleansed.

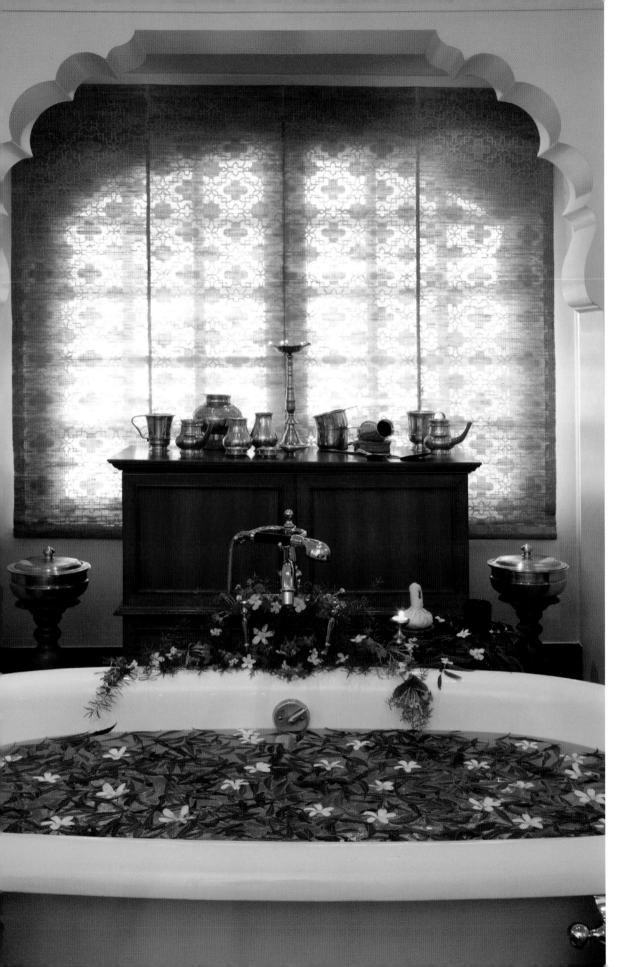

Panchakarma

"A purge properly carried out leads to clarity of intellect, power to the organs, elemental stability and glow to digestive fire and it delays aging."

— *from the* Ashtanga Hridaya

"To gain the maximum benefit, one should undertake a full course of *panchakarma* for 41 days," says Dr Baijuraj, the Ayurvedic physician at Kerala's Ayurmana. "Ideally it needs to be done in the monsoon season when herbs have been newly harvested and the skin is most receptive to oil – and it needs to be done with heart, body and soul."

Be that as it may, many people simply don't have 41 days to spare. Invert the numbers, and you can try the 14-day deep detox at Kalari Kovilakom. Here the *panchakarma* is offered as a stand alone revitalisation and detoxification treatment, even though it is really one part of a group of therapies belonging to a class of cleansing procedures called *shodhana*. One of this palace's specialties, it is offered in its pure form in two-, three- or four-week courses.

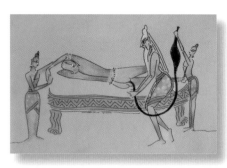

According to each patient, an individual programme of medication, diet, treatments and more is devised after an intensive consultation with one of the resident physicians. This is then closely monitored on a daily basis throughout. However, regardless of the personal *panchakarma* prescription, there are always three basic procedures: *Purvakarma* or "preparation", *pradhanakarma* or "treatments" and

paschatkarma, "post-treatment care". This is always the case with this five-pronged therapy as laid out in the classical texts – and doctors at Kalari Kovilakom are nothing if not thorough in their adherence to Ayurvedic authenticity.

The preparatory procedures take from three days to a week: They are designed to help the body discard toxins present in the stomach and tissues and help facilitate their movement to the alimentary canal. "This stage often includes special internal medicines and *snehanam* or oleation therapy and *swedanam* or sweat therapy," explains Dr Jayan, one of the physicians. "The latter may take the form of the application of warm oil over the body, a therapy known as *pizichil* or *kizhi*, the application of heated herbal pouches on the body. But, because each patient differs and has different *dosha* imbalances, the treatments always vary."

When the body and mind is deemed ready, *pradhanakarma* or the main treatment designed around each individual's needs, beings. As its name suggests (*panch* means "five" and *karma* translates as "action"), the process comprises five cleansing procedures designed to correct doshic imbalances. They are *vamanam* or induced vomiting, allegedly a painless, drug-induced emetic process; *virechanam* or induced purgation, whereby drugs that stimulate bowel movements are taken internally; *vasthi*, the use of medicated enemas inserted to alleviate excess *vata* (see pages 50–53); *nasyam* or nasal cleansing through the application of medical oils or powders; and, finally, *rakthamoksham* or blood letting, whereby impurities from the blood are extracted through leech therapy or other methods.

Clearly, this therapy is not for the faint-hearted, and the patient/doctor level of trust needs to be very high. This is why Kalari Kovilakom insists on a minimum stay of 14 days, so that doctors can truly assess and monitor a patient's needs. Dr Jayan explains that rarely are all five therapies prescribed simultaneously. "For *pita* imbalances, we prescribe purgation with oils or powders, *vata* imbalances go the herbal and oil enema route and *kapha* imbalances are always prescribed *vamanam*. Here patients drink two litres of milk or sugar cane juice mixed with special herbal medicines to induce vomiting after 45 minutes." He goes on to say that *nasyam* is included if there are any nasal, throat or brain problems and blood letting is useful for problems of the skin. Hence, a patient may be prescribed only one of the five processes; sometimes two or three, and in rare cases, five.

Naturally, the strict routine and caring staff at Kalari Kovilakom help to support guests on this somewhat gruesome journey; nevertheless, many first-timers describe both physical symptoms of discomfort and mental anguish. It is believed, however, that their special diet, medication, sessions of meditation and yoga, and the unchanging routine provide the support network needed for what can ultimately be a life-changing experience. Post-treatment, including after the guest leaves the premises, in the form of medication, contact with doctors, rest and diet is highly recommended.

Ayurveda, from time immemorial, has focused on anti-aging and rejuvenation programmes to prevent disease and to maintain an optimum healthy state. In today's world, curative therapies are increasingly replacing preventative ones – and *panchakarma* (both curative and preventative) is one of the more extreme examples on the Ayurvedic menu. Nevertheless, devotees with the stamina and the will swear by it, and if the venue is carefully chosen, it may be something to consider.

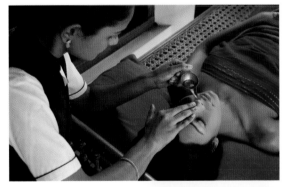

Opposite: A slightly tongue-in-cheek portrayal of the rectal *vasthi* process, one of the five cleansing actions in the *panchakarma* regime.

Above: A therapist administers medicated herbal oil into the nostrils during a *nasya* session at Ayurmana.

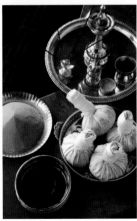

Right: Ayurvedic powders and oil used in the *panchakarma* treatment at Kalari Kovilakom. The *kizhi* pouches are for the preparation stage, while the tray with the oil lamp is used to bless the patient.

Ayurvedic Exercise and Body Conditioning

Ayurvedic texts indicate that there are two types of exercise that must be practiced for total well-being. The first is cardiovascular in nature, whereby the body undertakes aerobic exercise to stimulate muscle metabolism, increasing oxygenation to improve the function of the heart and circulatory system. The second is what physicians call *vyayama*, which means gaining energy by exercising. There are three specific forms of *vyayama*: Sun salutation (*surya manaskar*), yoga *asanas* and *pranayama* (see pages 108–113). These particular stretching and breathing exercises should be done in a slow and gentle manner, and serve to lower cardiovascular activity. They strengthen the internal organs in the abdominal cavity and chest to remove toxins.

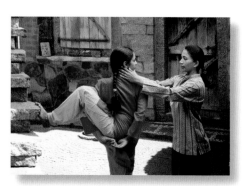

The *Charaka Samhita* says that exercise helps clear the channels of the body, cleanses the tissues via sweat and supplies the body with nutrients. It opens blockages to help the flow of *prana*, and, in addition to physical benefits, it helps on a mental and emotional level to reduce tension and anxiety, thereby promoting a sense of overall wellbeing. Ayurvedic physicians tend to favour gentle exercise, rather than anything too strenuous. As a general rule, *kapha* types can tolerate vigorous exercise like weight lifting and jogging, *pitta* types should partake in only moderate exercise and *vatas* are advised to stick to simple stretches and the like. In spas, gyms and clinics,

nowadays, most exercise sessions are monitored by personal trainers or resident doctors.

It is recommended that some people exercise more than others. For example, Indian classical dancers and martial arts practitioners need supremely strong, versatile and well-toned bodies to be effective. In addition, they must be mentally attuned and very disciplined, with a strong sense of self. Furthermore, they must be open to the Divine.

If this sounds like a tough call, it is. Most practitioners undergo years of training, with excruciating and long hours of exercise, practice and concentration. In the past, pupils were taught (often individually) by gurus in what is known as the guru-*shishya* tradition; education didn't just include the one particular activity, but involved a thorough grounding in the classical texts, as well as disciplines like yoga and *pranayama*. Nowadays, this tradition continues, but there are residential and non-residential dance, drama and martial arts' schools as well.

All the teachers we interviewed stressed the importance of maintaining fitness, conditioning the body, toning muscles, keeping concentration and trying to remain injury free. They all had different methods for keeping their pupils' bodies and minds stress-free with different preparatory exercises. Many of these drew freely from different disciplines: Pilates, yoga *asanas*, aerobic activities, Ayurveda,

64

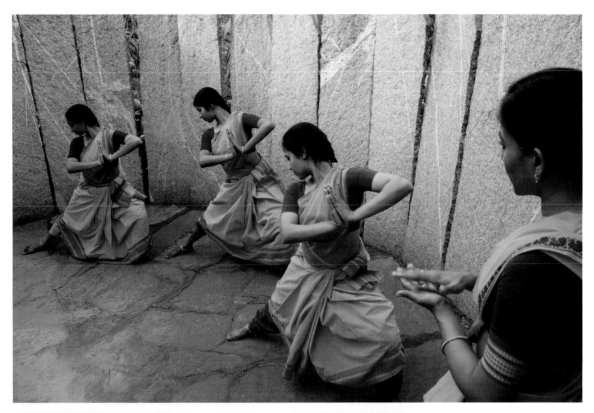

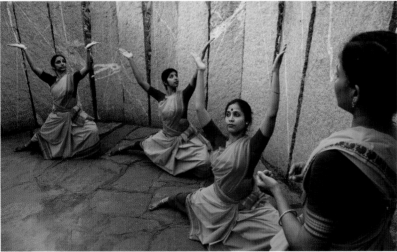

Above and left: Dancers need to be tough emotionally as well as physically, so regular body conditioning classes with stretches and lunges to build up core strength are conducted daily at Nrityagram, the dance school outside Bangalore. These exercises help the dancers to maintain certain postures, often for long periods.

Opposite: Repeated exercises on specific parts of the body are a part of every dancer's repertoire. Here a teacher takes a student through some individual stretching exercises to tone and stretch muscles, and achieve the perfect position for the *odissi* dance.

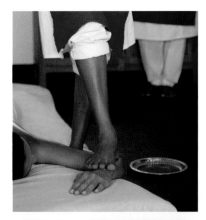

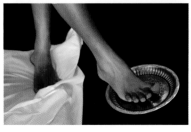

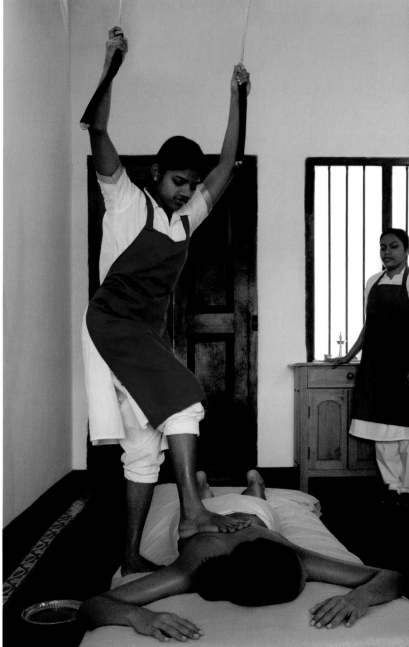

This page: Called *podha abhyangam* in Sanskrit and *chavitti thirummu* in Malayalam, this massage is conducted with the client lying on the floor and the masseuse maintaining balance with the aid of ropes hanging from the ceiling. Originally conducted solely for the benefit of martial arts' warriors, the massage has found its way into spas and Ayurvedic centres as it is effective in the treatment of rheumatism, arthritis, spondylitis, slipped disc, weakness of nerves, cramps and more. Here, a therapist at Kalari Kovilakom gives a client a full-body massage to improve muscle tone and flexibility and to stimulate the circulation of blood and lymph.

Opposite: Kalari payattu gurrukal Tomy Joseph uses vigorous oil massage techniques on the *marma* points of his pupil Siby Abraham. This massage opens up pranic channels, helps to maintain a compact physique and sheds fatigue.

kalari payattu (see pages 130–133) to name a few. All included basic warm-up routines, followed by stretching and lunging exercises to attain good posture, balance, alignment, coordination and strength. They also included methods for relaxation – of mind, body and spirit.

Warm-ups before dance or martial arts are an absolute necessity. Body conditioning to build up core strength is also a daily activity. "Every day our pupils do at least one hour of body conditioning," explains Bijayini Satpathy, a dance teacher at Nrityagram, "We often isolate certain body parts and work on expressing movement with them. In *odissi*, the upper body is fluid and graceful and moves in isolation to the lower body, so we need to practice many different movements and techniques. Hand *mudras* are practiced again and again, and every part of the body from lips and eyebrows to feet is exercised on a daily basis."

Tomy Joseph, *kalari payattu gurrukal* (master or teacher), also stressed the importance of conditioning the body to stay in shape. He said that expertise in *marma* massage (see pages 38–39) and *chavitti thirummu* techniques (see opposite) is mandatory for a *gurrukal*. Teachers routinely massage their pupils in this way to prepare the body for the stresses of the martial art. Furthermore, all *kalari payattu* sessions begin with a series of gentle exercises designed to awaken inner pranic energies. The session we photographed at Kalari Kovilakom was no exception: after saying a short prayer, the two participants warmed up by stretching arms, shoulders, legs and knees, then practised what is

known as *mayarakum* or special sparring, turning, twisting and jumping movements akin to dance. These involved quite jarring movements timed with breath exhalation and are designed for flexibility as well as strength.

Interestingly, the *Natya Shastra*, the ancient text of dance and acting that dates back to 400 BC, recommends *uzhchil* or massage to improve and enhance one's general health. *Chavitti thirummu* falls in the *uzhchil* category, as it involves the movement of energy in the body. By applying pressure and herbal oils with therapeutic value on the vital points, muscles and nerves, the body is primed for the fight and reflexes are sharpened.

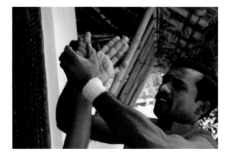

At the end of the day, exercise is a highly personal choice: aerobic or non-aerobic, vigorous or gentle, self-massage or massage by another. Trying out various activities and combining them with some relaxation in a spa and meditation at home opens minds and bodies to new possibilities. In an ideal Ayurvedic day, exercise should be done in the morning to help expel toxins that have accumulated overnight and should not exceed a level that suits the individual constitution.

67

Unani

Although many spa-goers may have heard of Ayurveda, they are probably not as familiar with another branch of medicine practised extensively in India. Unani, which originated in Greece with the philosopher-physician Hippocrates (460–377 BC), was formulated over time by various Islamic scholar physicians in what is now the Middle East. Noted Arab physicians such as Rhazes (850–925 AD) and Avicenna (aka Ibn Sina 980–1037 AD) further developed Unani medicine. Like Tibetan medicine, Unani was influenced by contemporary systems of traditional medicine in Egypt, Syria, Iraq, Persia, India, China, and other Near, Middle, and Far East countries. It became the authoritative basis for the study of medicine in the European Middle Ages and was instrumental in introducing professional standards of practice to medicine all over Europe.

Today, its influence is less far reaching, but it is still popular in some Arab countries and elsewhere – especially in the Indian subcontinent. It was introduced to India during the medieval period and was greatly boosted during the Moghul period. Over time, mass acceptance and continuous use led to many Unani hospitals, research centres and clinics being built. Its heyday in India lasted from the 13th to the 17th centuries, as the Delhi Sultans, the Khiljis, the Tughlaqs and the Moghul emperors provided patronage to Unani scholars.

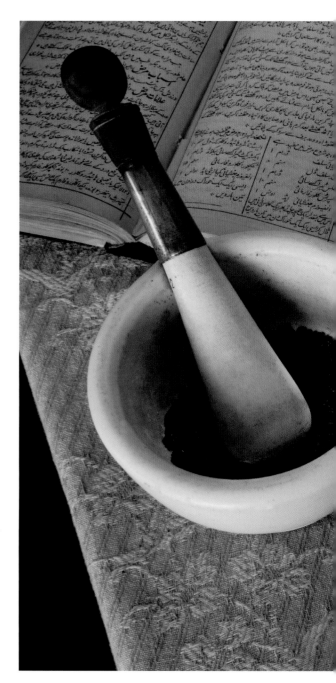

Unani medicines are always made from 100 percent natural ingredients and include plants, herbs and minerals. This *mufaras* (medicine) for excess palpitation of the heart contains musk, amber, silver, gold and *zafaran* leaf. The books are the *Makhzan-i-Hikmat* or *The Family Doctor and Hakeem: An Encyclopaedia of Domestic Medicine and Surgery*, Vols 1 and 2, by Dr H Ghulam Jilani.

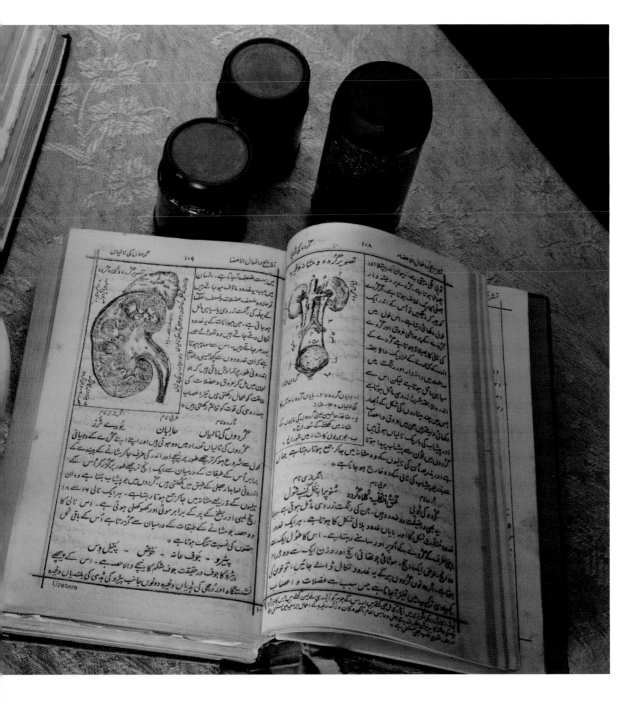

During this period, many drugs and herbs native to India were added to the existing apothecary of Unani remedies. Clinical trials and experimentation resulted in expansion, and even though Unani suffered setbacks during the colonial period, it had become entrenched in Indian life. Today, India has the largest number of educational, research and health care institutions of Unani medicine in the world with over 20,000 registered *hakims* or Unani practitioners and countless non-registered ones who practise on a hereditary basis.

Unani is recognised by the WHO or World Health Organization as a holistic traditional medical system. In 1977 when the WHO established its traditional medicine programme, it declared: "There is no doubt that this branch of medicine is making and will continue to make a very significant contribution to our efforts to achieve health for all."

The roots of the Unani system lie within the concept that medicine is a science by which the functioning of the human body can be discovered. Its goal was the preservation of health and the promotion of self-healing. In its infancy it was a rigorous system that eliminated superstition and harmful folk practices, and as developments and discoveries were made, it added to its repertoire of remedies and practices. Nowadays, Unani *hakims* combine herbal medical remedies with dietary advice, regimental therapy, psychological practices, surgery and spiritual discipline.

As with other holistic practices, a Unani *hakim* tends to look at the patient as a whole – mentally, physically, emotionally and spiritually – before

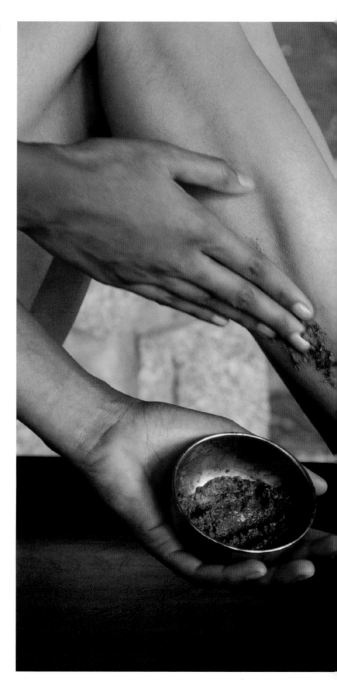

prescribing a course of treatment. Dr Mathai, from Soukya, an integrative medicinal retreat, explains: "Unani aims to promote positive health and prevent diseases and is based around six essentials: good air and water, a balanced diet, exercise and rest, psychic movement and rest, sleep and wakefulness, and evacuation and retention. Remedies are usually herbal, although ingredients of animal, marine and mineral origin are used. Humoural theory (the presence and balance of blood, phlegm, yellow bile and black bile) is at its heart, and the temperament of a person is accordingly expressed by Sanguine, Phlegmatic, Choleric and Melancholic. According to Unani theories, any changes in these humours bring about changes in the status of health of a human body."

The practice of Unani is widespread in clinics, hospitals and pharmacies in India, but is less well represented in spas. However, many herbal preparations are as likely to be Unani in origin as they are Ayurvedic, because historically the two overlap significantly. Unani herbology is well documented and spa treatments such as body

polishes, scrubs, wraps and facials often use ingredients from the Unani pharmacopoeia. Similarly, wellness clinics such as Soukya integrate elements of Unani knowledge in their unique formulations with successful results.

The overall aim of Unani is to restore the equilibrium of the body. Dr Mathai explains that Unani is particularly useful for ailments such as bronchial asthma, vitiligo, eczema, psoriasis and

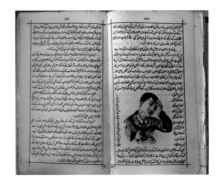

arthritis. This is good news for sufferers, as many such ailments do not have a cure in Western or allopathic medicine. Persistent psoriasis, for example, can be extremely debilitating.

Today's practitioners range the gamut from qualified doctors from government teaching hospitals and universities to local *hakims* who have inherited recipes and information from their fathers. Regardless of their qualifications, however, they possess a unique body of knowledge that encompasses herbal, nutritional and dietic medicine, psychological insights and spiritual discipline. The world has a great deal to learn from them – and this ancient natural healing system.

Left: Unani preparations are both internal and external and are always formulated from natural sources. This application is used on the skin to help with white pigmentation marks, a condition known as leucoderma. The application made at Soukya comprises a fairly thick paste, the main ingredient of which is *bakuchi* (*Psoralea corylifolia* seeds). The anti-fungal and anti-protozoal paste is applied on to the marks once a day and then exposed in direct sunlight for 20 to 45 minutes for at least a month. Afterward it should be washed off. Over time, the discoloration begins to fade.

Above: A copy of Unani *hakim* Sayed Riazuddin's *Makhzan-i-Hikmat*, in beautiful Urdu script, opened at a page that deals with advice and medication for migraine.

Siddha

Perhaps not so well known outside India as Ayurveda, Siddha is an ancient form of natural medicine that has been practiced in Tamil Nadu for centuries. Taking its name from the 18 Tamil *siddhars* (devotees of Shiva who obtained *siddhi* or "attainment") who formulated it, many of its practices and recipes have been handed down from father to son. Nowadays, however, there are government and private medical colleges training Siddha doctors.

The core fundamental principles of Siddha are encapsulated in several Tamil texts. Like all Hindu philosophers, the *siddhars* believed that all living things should seek oneness with God, so a productive long life was to be encouraged. Their basic premise was that the universe consists of two essential entities – matter and energy – that are found in five primordial elements: *munn* (solids), *neer* (fluids), *thee* (radiance), *vayu* (gas) and *aakasam* (ether). Each and every person is made up of these five elements in different combinations and proportions, and, as in Ayurveda, there is a *tridosha* system also. If these elements are maintained in equilibrium, the result is health; if there is disruption, the result is disease.

Alchemical ideas dominate Siddha medicine, with its *materia medica* consisting of herbs, roots, salts, metals and mineral compounds.

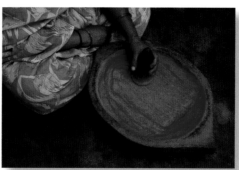

The 18 *siddhars* classified 4,448 diseases and prescribed medicines accordingly. Nevertheless, *bhasmas* (fine powders made from incinerated and purified metals and minerals, see pages 180–185) are at the forefront of their prescriptions. As with Ayurveda, other common preparations include *choornam* (powders), *kashayam* (decoctions), *lehyam* (confections), *gritham* (preparations made from ghee) and *tailam* (oils). Siddha specialities are *chunna* (metallic preparations that become alkaline after purification), *kattu* (preparations that are impervious to water and fire) and *mezhugu* (waxy preparations). The medicines are generally taken internally, although some are external too.

The Siddha system includes not only medicine and alchemy but also yoga and philosophy. Diet is an important part of Siddha, as doctors identify and associate different food types with different *doshas*, and the pursuit of longevity without illness and a useful, spiritual life is its

Opposite: Siddha doctors have been entrusted with a variety of methods to combat disease, some of which are extremely time-consuming and painstaking to make *(see above).* Here we see a number of minerals in raw, incinerated, semi-cooked and purified form at the practice of a doctor from the south of Tamil Nadu. Clockwise from top left: mercury, raw arsenic, iron in third stage of cooking, iron powder, processed and ground arsenic, raw sulphur, powdered arsenic, ground mercury, cooked mercury and cooked arsenic.

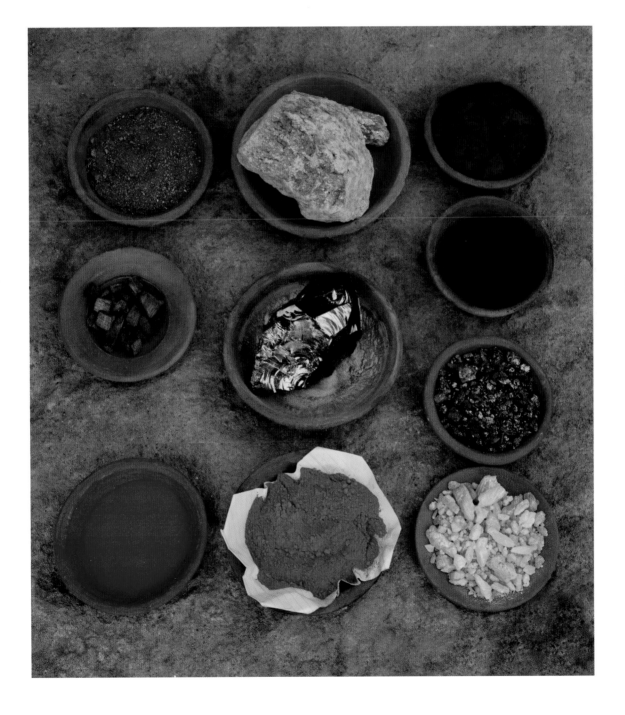

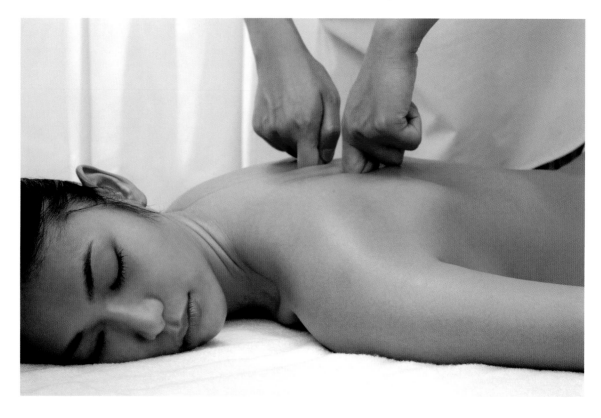

Above: This Siddha preparation from Soukya is a paste of crushed and powdered neem leaves and fresh, powdered turmeric. The plants are mixed with either water or herbal juice or oil, and the paste is applied externally. It has proved effective in the treatment of psoriasis.

74

ultimate aim. The spiritual aspect of healing, wellness and being at one with the Divine cannot be under-emphasised: it lies at the heart of the discipline of Siddha.

It is not often that visitors to India will come across Siddha practices outside Tamil Nadu, but sometimes you will find Siddha massage (a type of *marma* massage with herbal oil) and certain external applications in a spa or holistic centre. However, the practice is quite rare outside its state of origin, and, even there, is available only through specialist doctors who have inherited skills and recipes from their immediate families.

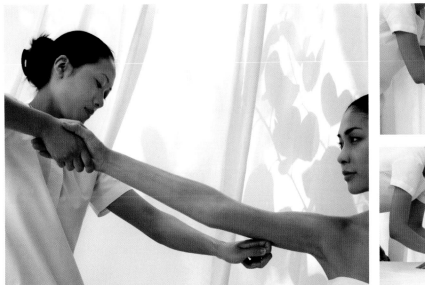
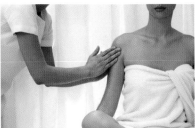
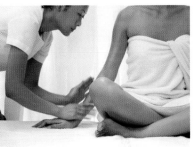

This page and opposite bottom: A type of *marma* massage prescribed mainly for rheumatics that dates from pre-Vedic times in Siddha culture uses medicated herbal oils. Here it is offered in Aura spas at Park Hotels, an unusual addition to any spa menu. "The 107 *marma* points are targeted to release stored emotions in order to restore mental, emotional and spiritual equilibrium," explains spa director, Megha Dinesh. "Each point is related to a particular concept: ie the knee is related to death, that's why so many old people get arthritis in such areas. Shoulder points store the emotions of responsibility; the sternum points are related to the heart, so people with hunched shoulders are loveless." Concentrating on certain areas for certain effects, this is a powerful treatment that can have long-lasting results.

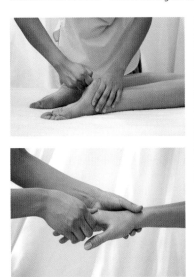
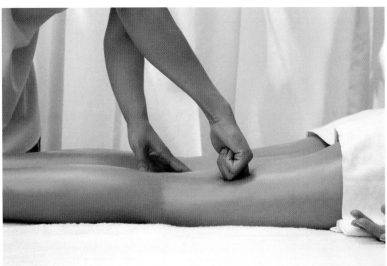

Tibetan Traditional Medicine

" Transcendent One compassionately acting
on behalf of living beings,
The mere hearing of whose name offers sanctuary
from the sufferings of inferior existences,
Spiritual Master of medicine, dispelling diseases
caused by the three poisons
Attachment, Aversion and Delusion."

– medicinal Buddhist Prayer

Tibetan medicine is an ancient and traditional system of medicine that has been practised for over 2,500 years and is still practised today both within Tibet and by Tibetans in exile. Called *Soba Rig-pa* or the "Science of Healing", it uses many natural ingredients including herbs, trees, rocks, resins, soils, precious metals and more. However, 95 percent of Tibetan medicine is based on herbs, and precious metals are used for the seven kinds of precious pill known as *rinchen rilpo*.

Soba Rig-pa's basic premise is that the body needs to be balanced to be well. When imbalance in what doctors call the three humours or *nyipa sum* (*rLung*, *mKhris-pa* and *Bad-kan*) occurs, a person falls ill; symptoms may be physical, mental, spiritual or a combination of all three. In brief, *rLung* is the subtle flow of energy in the body; *mKhris-pa* is the hot nature within the body or bile; and *Bad-kan* is concerned with the body's cold nature, ie phlegm. Attachment, Aversion and Delusion are considered long-term causes of imbalance, whereas in the short term, imbalances may be caused by time, temperature and season, the influence of spirits, improper diet and improper behaviour.

After diagnosis, Tibetan doctors offer four types of prescription: advice regarding diet, behavioural suggestions, a medical prescription, or surgery. As with other holistic systems of medicine, physical therapies are only part of a doctor's prescription. Based on the centuries-old Buddhist study of the mind, Tibetan medicine gives priority to factors of psychological and spiritual development in addition to the therapies prescribed.

Today, a limited number of spas are offering some Tibetan physical therapies that have been formulated over the centuries. The most common is the Tibetan hot stone massage which was probably introduced to Tibet from Mongols that settled in the Hor region around Lake Kokonor; in its pure form, it uses heated stones that have been "cooked" in the bellies of sheep. Other

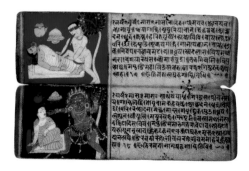

Right: In Mongolia, stones and minerals are commonly used both internally and externally for various ailments. The Mongolians believe that when hot stones are applied to specific points on the body, they help dispel blockages, enabling the smooth flow of *chi* or life force energy throughout the body. These stones have been carved with Sanskrit symbols by Buddhist monks and are used in the CHI spa hot stone massage at Shangri-La hotels.

Above: Unlike Indian texts, this ancient Tibetan medical text has colourful illustrations depicting both healing and illness.

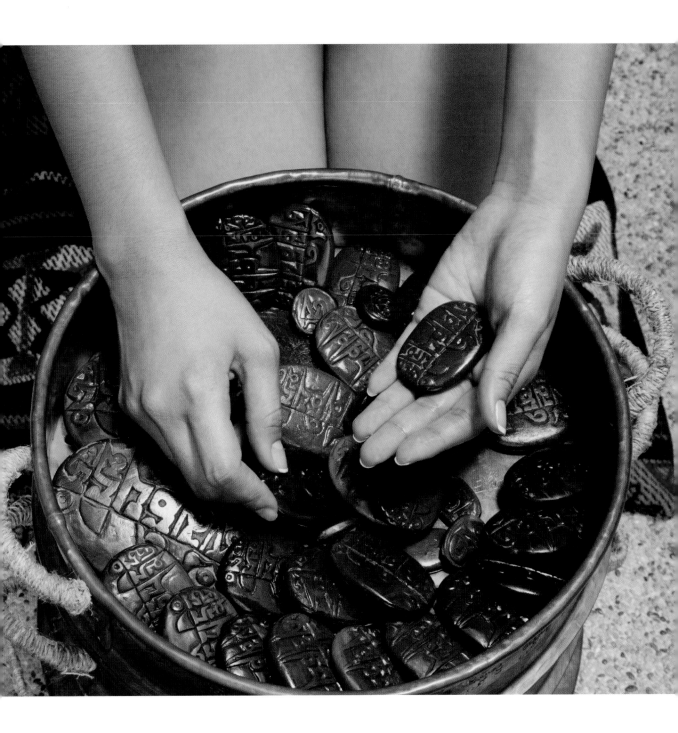

external therapies or *jampeche* include scrubs with salt, mud therapy, herbal wraps and moxibustion. We showcase two beautiful therapies formulated especially for CHI spas at Shangri-La hotels; found all over Asia, they are the closest you will get to an authentic Tibetan treatment outside a Tibetan clinic.

Healing Hot Stone Massage

Described in Tibet's medical bible, the *Gui Shi*, massage with stones has all but died out in Tibet today. As Tibetans are traditionally nomads, their therapies contain influences from many different sources, this profound practice being no exception. It combines the Mongolian concept of healing through heated stones; principles and techniques

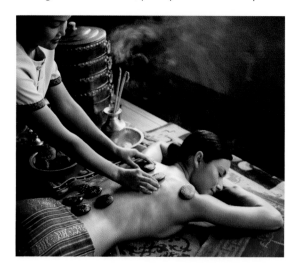

of Ayurveda that travelled up the Indian trade routes over Himalayan passes; pressure point techniques from Traditional Chinese Medicine; and Tibetan healing intent (imbuing the stones with awareness through visualisation).

The revival of this ancient hot stone treatment came about through the collaboration of Tibetan doctors, Sherab Tenzin Barma and Tsewang Ngudrup Rinpoche, with Tibetan Buddhist and Chinese acupuncturist masseuse, Joanna Claire. It involves the application of water-heated Himalayan river stones to key points on the body, giving a deep heat massage. The warmth from the stones relaxes muscles, allowing manipulation of a greater intensity than regular massage. Blood vessels expand, pushing blood and unwanted waste materials through the body. This has a sedative effect on the nervous system, at the same time strengthening it. On a physical level, it provides relief to sore muscles and fosters deep muscle manipulation, improves circulation and removes toxins from the body. On a mental level, it is nurturing and comforting.

Mountain Tsampa Rub

The second CHI spa treatment we showcase combines *tsampa* with ancient Tibetan massage techniques and transforms them into a powerful detoxifying and cleansing treatment. *Tsampa* is roast flour, most commonly barley, and is the staple foodstuff of Tibetans. Here, the flour is used as the postscript to the treatment.

Unlike acupressure or the Chinese style of massage, Tibetan massage works on the "wind" channels of the body – those that deal with the circulation of energy, blood and lymph. Massage techniques include stroking (long, longitudinal strokes or effleurage), rubbing with vigorous circular motions to create friction, and kneading. The aim is

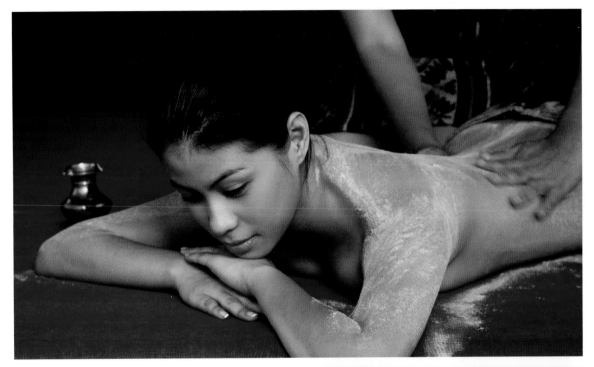

79

to increase lymphatic drainage and blood circulation in order to aid muscle nutrition, reduce stiffness in joints, improve flexibility and heighten body awareness.

The initial part of this treatment comprises an invigorating massage combined with powerful lymph draining herbal oils; particular focus is given to specific energy points on the body to help the oils penetrate into the skin and awaken *chi*. The second part of the treatment is considerably gentler and more relaxing. A blend of *tsampa* flour and lymph-draining herbs is applied all over the body to absorb excess oil and toxins that have come up to the surface of the skin. Rubbing the *tsampa* herb blend into the skin leaves the skin soft, gently exfoliated and free of inner toxins.

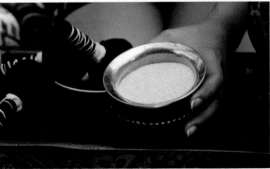

Opposite: CHI spas' hot stone massage utilises accoutrements sourced in Tibet and Nepal: blessed river stones, brass bowls and oils and large tiffin carriers for heating the stones.

Top: CHI spas' Mountain Tsampa Rub drains toxins accumulated in the lymph system, allowing for balanced movement of *chi*.

Above: Tibetan singing bowls, traditionally used in monasteries as aids for meditation, are rung before and after treatments at CHI spas. Another bowl contains *tsampa* flour.

Mud Therapy

In India, the application of mud therapy falls under the naturopathy umbrella, as it employs one of the Five Great Elements which consist of Earth, Water, Fire, Air and Ether. These are also known as the *Panch Maha Bhutas* (*panch* is "five", *maha* is "great", *bhuta* is "element"). Unsurprisingly, mud therapy utilises earth as its main healing ingredient. Mud absorbs, dissolves and eliminates toxins from beneath the skin's surface, opens the pores and improves peripheral blood circulation. As such, it is rejuvenating for the body and soothing for the skin.

Mud therapy is employed in the treatment of various ailments such as digestive disorders, skin diseases and more. The world-famous *Multani mitti* or "mud from Multan", an area now in Pakistan, was one of the earliest substances to be used as a beauty mask. This lime-rich clay was mixed with rice bran and milk or curd and used as a face pack to draw out toxins and polluting free radicals. Indeed, it is still used as such today.

Another formula for a facial clay pack is found in the 16th-century Moghul journal *Ain-I-Akbary*: Recorded as a mix of clay, cereal, milk and lime, it was used to bring toxins to the surface of the skin. Another astonishing use for the formula was found in 2002 when archaeologists recreated the mixture to remove black and yellow impurities from the walls of the 17th-century Taj Mahal. Brushed on in layers until it was an inch deep, the mixture was found to draw out polluting sulfates and carbonates. After 24 hours, the mud was washed off with water – and the translucence was restored to the marble.

Mud is good for skin, nails and hair. Because of its moisturising effect and high mineral content, it is a great nourisher and often acts as a conduit for healing ingredients to be absorbed into the system. It is reputed to help reduce arthritic pain caused by inflammation and soothes the pain associated with burns, insect and bee stings (bears roll in the mud when they have been stung). On application, mud causes blood vessels to dilate, increasing blood circulation near the skin's surface and reducing fluid retention. Ayurvedic texts record that mud draws out heat and excess *pitta* through the skin; it also says that *Multani mitti* can be used by all three *doshas*.

Today, humble muds and clays from all over the world are utilised in therapies for detoxification, rejuvenation and beauty. They are now considered as precious as rare herbs because of their unique abilities to remove impurities, relieve skin problems and help aches and pains. Be it a volcanic or desert mud, a kaolin clay or one of the mild kaolinites, they are naturally enriched with nutritious minerals.

At Soukya, the integrated wellness centre near Bangalore where naturopathic practice is combined with other medical and holistic systems to create individual therapeutic programmes, mud is used in three ways: as a localised application, as a pack or as a full mud bath. Mud is harvested from the many ant hills found on site; as the ants have taken the mud from deep underground, it's incredibly pure without any surface pollutants.

Right: An all-over body-blasting mud bath at Soukya improves metabolism and leaves skin fresh and clear afterwards. It is also internally detoxifying.

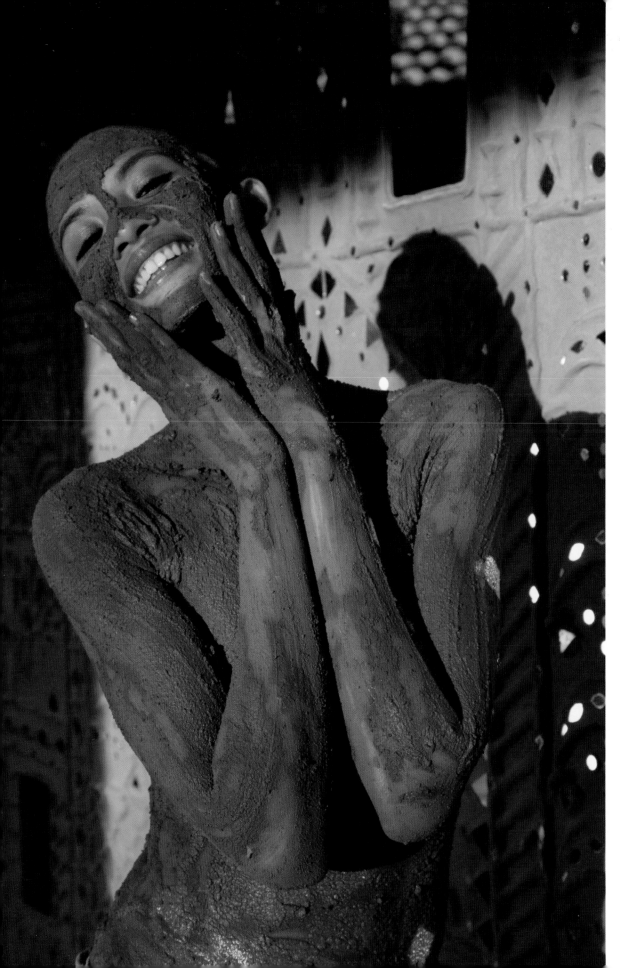

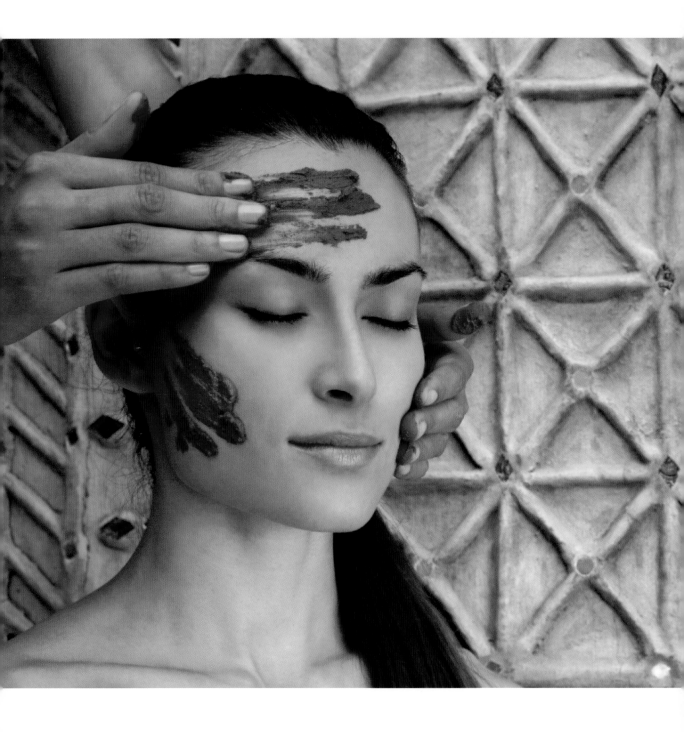

Therapists further prepare it by sieving it, washing it properly, and sterilising it by drying it in sunlight. It is then stored in airtight containers until it is used.

"Mud is healing in itself," explains resident naturopath Dr Usha Devi. "It has the property of retaining temperature for a long time, so depending on the ailment, can be applied either hot or cold." Hot mud is used for joint conditions such as arthritis and to reduce oedema or water retention in localised areas of the body. Cold mud helps in the treatment of skin diseases, such as psoriasis for example. Mud packs are beneficial for diabetic patients and people who are suffering from an internal organ problem.

Sometimes, depending on the condition, herbs may be added. Dr Usha says that disinfecting neem and turmeric may be added in local applications if there is a possibility of infection and castor oil may be added to an abdominal pack in liver conditions. It helps stimulate the circulation of blood towards the liver, thereby aiding detoxification.

Whichever mud therapy is assigned, the feeling is both nurturing and strengthening. The tightening experienced when the mud dries on the skin is pleasant – be it hot or cold – and as it is straight from nature, you can be sure it is doing good work. Face packs tend to be more cosmetic, while the body packs are therapeutic. The full mud bath is particularly invigorating: being slathered in soft, creamy mud, then having it washed off afterwards is a self-indulgent treat. The skin feels soft, smooth and tingly after the treatment – and there is no need for extra moisturising.

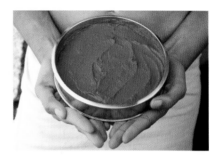

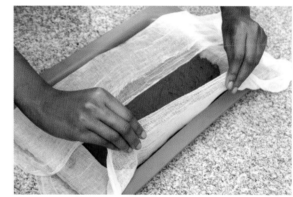

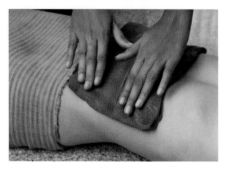

Above: At Soukya, mud packs are placed on the abdomen and left for 20 minutes. The pack improves digestion, strengthens the metabolism of the liver, prevents constipation and speeds up blood circulation to the internal organs.

Opposite: Used on the face, mud draws out toxins very quickly. It may also be used on the eyes, but only in a pack, to strengthen the optic nerve and muscles, relax the eyes and impart a cooling and de-stressing effect in the eye area.

Colour Therapy

Every visitor to India comes away marveling at the vibrancy of colours they've seen across the country. Whether it is a fantastic lime green turban wrapped regally around a Rajasthani head or a dazzling gold-and-silver palanquin, a plethora of powders stacked in conical multicolours in the market or a deep orange sunset – it is sure to impress. After all, colour is embedded in Indian life and probably has more significance here than anywhere else in the world.

Colours have a religious meaning and a special connotation. Each of the seven *chakras* is denoted by a different colour and the different castes are allocated different colours: Brahmins of the priestly caste traditionally wear white as they are meant to be pure; the Kshatriyas or warrior caste dress in fiery red; and the Shudras or artisans/agriculturalists don utilitarian blue. Festival colours are red and green; red is the colour worn at weddings as it signifies passion and energy; white is for mourning; and black stands for anger, darkness and negativity.

The ancient Indians, along with the Egyptians and Chinese, practiced the art of chromotherapy or healing with colours and light. A centuries-old concept, it involves the use of visible colours to cure various diseases. Charaka advocated the use of sunlight to treat a variety of ailments, while Avicenna (see page 88) took the theory further by allocating certain colours to certain conditions. He theorised that red stimulated blood circulation, blue or white cooled the blood, and yellow reduced muscular pain.

Today, chromotherapy is used in hospitals to treat seasonal depression, and trained therapists in spas and elsewhere use it to influence health through relaxation, rejuvenation or healing. Colour is applied to the body in different ways: through electromagnetic radiation, via gemstones on acu-points or different areas (see pages 182–185), through bath treatments or through coloured lenses, to achieve a variety of effects. In general, red is believed to stimulate physical and mental energies, yellow to stimulate the nerves, orange to stimulate the solar plexus and revitalise the lungs, blue to soothe and heal disorders such as colds, hay fever and liver problems, and indigo to counteract fever and skin problems.

In spas, chromotherapy may be combined with hydrotherapy through chromo-baths or showers where massage jets work with LED lights. Working on the premise that different colours have different vibrations and produce different moods and energy levels, the changing lights are often programmed to work in conjunction with a music system as well. Chromoenergetic massage and chromo-aromatherapy are other offerings.

Above: Holi or the "Festival of Colours" is a fun-filled Indian celebration of the arrival of spring. Although it is religious in origin, it is celebrated by people taking to the streets and throwing coloured powders and dyes at each other! Here a stall with a stock of vibrant-coloured powders waits for a buyer.

Opposite: CHI spas across Asia are known for their innovative chromotherapy treatments that combine powerful hydro-therapeutic effects with the balancing effects of colour. Their "colour bath" synchronises light, temperature and music.

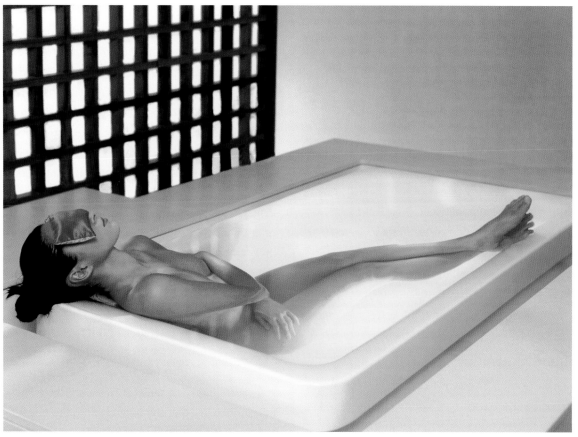

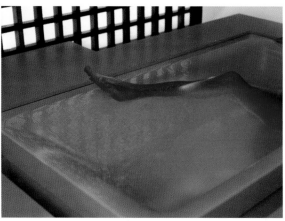

The Leela spa in Mumbai offers a treatment that combines colour and perfume. Developed in 1989 by French firm Altéarah, certain colours are teamed with certain essential oils that have the same "energetic wavelengths"; clients choose colours they feel affinity with and those colours' perfumes are applied to the body. A sequence of scents is believed to help rebalance a person's energies. The different perfumes may be inhaled, experienced as oils in burners, as bath salts or soaps – and the "treatment" is easily replicated at home.

Incense and Oils

Jasmine: induces euphoria, promotes relief of
nervous exhaustion
Eucalyptus: invigorating, clarifying, energising
Lemongrass: purifies the emotions, releases anxiety
Bergamot: refreshing, uplifting, anti-depressant

– incense scents as used by Oberoi Spas

A spa simply wouldn't be a spa if it didn't have an
oil burner or some incense smouldering somewhere
on the premises. The power of scent is well known,
with the connection between mood and smell a
given. We all know that certain fragrances make us
productive and active, while others calm or soothe
us, but as yet we do not fully understand the reasons
why. What is known is that scent triggers the
release of neuro-chemicals in the body; these send
messages to our brains to alter the way we feel.

History of Scent

The ancients have known this since time immemorial.
When certain branches or twigs were thrown on
to the fire, the aroma emitted from the smoke

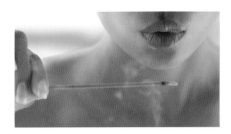

made people feel drowsy and peaceful. Hence, the
word "perfume" derived from the Latin "through
smoke" came into being. Similarly, holy or magic
smoke (incense) has been used in most major religious

rituals for centuries. The Egyptians were using
aromatics for embalming the dead, for medicine
and cosmetics since at least 3,000 BC and many of
their methods for making suppositories, pills and
purées are recorded in papyrus compilations. Later,
the Greeks and Romans utilised – and added to
– Egyptian practices.

In India, of course, floral oils and perfumed
waters have been used for millennia. Five-thousand-
year old perfume containers have been discovered
in India, and Vedic texts from around 2,000 BC talk
of aromatic herbal preparations and their effects
on both body and mind. In many instances, the
use of perfumes, incense (*agarabathi*) and oils was
purely cosmetic, but there are many overlaps with
health as well. For example, as Ayurvedic medicine
developed, it incorporated methods for incense
and oil preparation that included blends aimed
at harmonising all three *doshas*. Ayurvedic texts
state that a human's sense of smell influences the
more subtle levels of the body and has the power
to bring harmony and balance to mind, body and
spirit. And so certain plants were used for their
scents as well as their healing abilities.

Before the 10th century, perfumes were extracted
from plants by combining flowers with oils, by
mixing them with water, compounding them with
resins or gums and pressing them on a base of

Left and right: In human beings, the least used of the five senses
is the sense of smell, one that weakens as we grow older. In
India, however, scent or perfume is highly prized both as a
therapeutic and beautifying agent. As such, perfumes or *attars*
have been manufactured for centuries. Here we see an *attar*
(*right*) and a scented *agarabathi* on *left*.

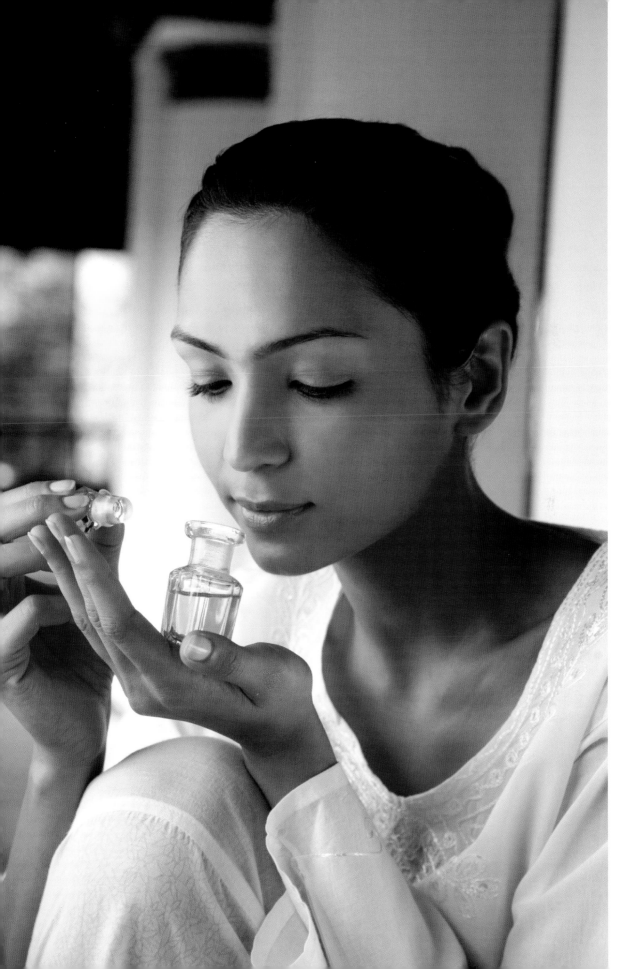

solidified fat. They were then made into floral oils, incense and perfumes. These inefficient methods came to an end with the discovery of the method of extracting essential oils from plants through steam distillation. This is accredited to the greatest of the Arab physicians, Ali Ibn Sina or Avicenna (980–1037 AD); apparently, in an experiment some 1,000 years ago, he added water to rose petals then distilled the mixture – and the rose water he collected was officially declared the first modern perfume.

Essential Oils and their Properties

Essential oils are the volatile substances that give plants and flowers their characteristic smell, preserve their moisture balance and protect them from insects. They are secreted by special glands and stored in tiny sacs found in the leaves, petals, berries, fruits, stems and barks of plants. Culled from the very essence of the plant, they number about 800. Different oils are obtained from different parts of the plant: For example, sandalwood comes from the wood, rose from the petals, cinnamon from the bark, clove from the clove itself, and so on.

Essential oils are highly concentrated and should only rarely be used in their undiluted form. They are very volatile, that is, they evaporate quickly on contact with the air, so they should be kept in opaque bottles away from direct sunlight. Chemically

complex, they often have antiseptic, anti-bacterial and anti-viral properties – and many have more than one therapeutic property. They may be inhaled, applied to the skin (where they are absorbed and enter the bloodstream very quickly) or dispersed in the air all around; depending on the oils used, a warm bath infused with essential oils or a massage with essential oils diluted in a carrier oil can be invigorating or soothing. Oils in creams or hot or cold compresses help with a variety of ailments; and burning oils, in the form of incense or oil burners, disperse scent to influence mood.

In India, the use of incense is widespread: Its main function is religious, with incense cones and

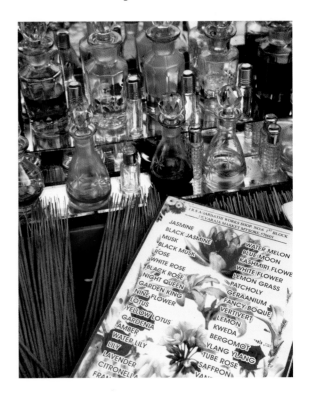

Right: In Mysore, scores of family-owned *agarabathi* (incense) and perfume production units exist, and, because the area is famous for its sandalwood, many are scented with this purifying substance. Not to be confused with essential oils, perfumes called *attars* in small clear glass bottles are also locally produced and widely available. A mix of essential oils with vegetable oils or alcohol, they smell beautiful, but are not therapeutic.

sticks being lit at *pujas* to deities in temples, wayside shrines and in the home. A *puja* is a multi-sensory experience, with chants of prayers, ringing of bells, symbolic bathing, embellishment and perfuming of the deity, burning of incense and lighting of lamps. Foods such as cooked rice, fruit, butter and jaggery are offered. Nowadays, incense is also a part of secular Indian life: Lit to perfume homes, deter mosquitoes and scent clothes and hair (see page 154), there are thousands of varieties to choose from.

Oils are no less popular in India. As well as being one of the world's biggest exporters of spices, India is also a huge producer of essential oils. The process is time consuming and intensive: 1,000 kilos of sandalwood, for example, will only yield 30 litres of sandalwood oil, hence the high prices. Unfortunately, many oils are diluted, severely reducing their efficacy, so, when buying essential oils or oil products, manufacturers need to be chosen with care. For details of aromatic products, see pages 316–321.

Popular Indian Oils

Below are some properties and suggested uses of some of India's more popular essential oils as shared with us by *agarabathi* and oil producer Aman Sharif in Mysore.

Sandalwood essential oil: Good for circulation of the blood, joint and muscle pain and tiredness, sandalwood essential oil is a blood purifier. Sixty to 80-year-olds should take a drink of hot milk with one drop of sandalwood oil before breakfast for 40 days. Massage with sandalwood essential oil and a base oil of almond oil (five teaspoons almond oil to two drops sandalwood essential oil) is effective.

White jasmine essential oil: Warming and relaxing to the body, it heightens sensual awareness and is a reputed aphrodisiac. Two drops in a bucket of warm water in the shower gives a very fresh scent. Indian women wear white jasmine oil in their hair to attract a husband!

Black jasmine essential oil: Two drops of this essential oil with a small amount of almond base oil is efficacious for skin diseases, such as eczema.

Green jasmine essential oil: This oil is excellent for relief of psoriasis. Mix two drops of green jasmine essential oil with the whisked egg white from one egg and apply on the affected area. Leave on for at least one hour, then remove with cool water. This treatment should be done daily in the morning for at least 40 days, according to Mr Sharif.

Lotus essential oil: One drop of lotus essential oil massaged into the temples is helpful for sufferers of migraine and those who are stressed or have high blood pressure.

Vetiver essential oil: A five-minute massage with a mixture of two drops vetiver essential oil and five drops almond essential oil on the affected area for 40 days is helpful in cases of varicose veins.

***Bala* essential oil:** Associated with the ancient Hindu Goddess of beauty and grace Parvati, *bala* is one of the plants commonly used in Indian beauty products. *Bala* essential oil mixed with a vegetable carrier oil such as coconut or sesame is a helpful preventative for hair loss.

89

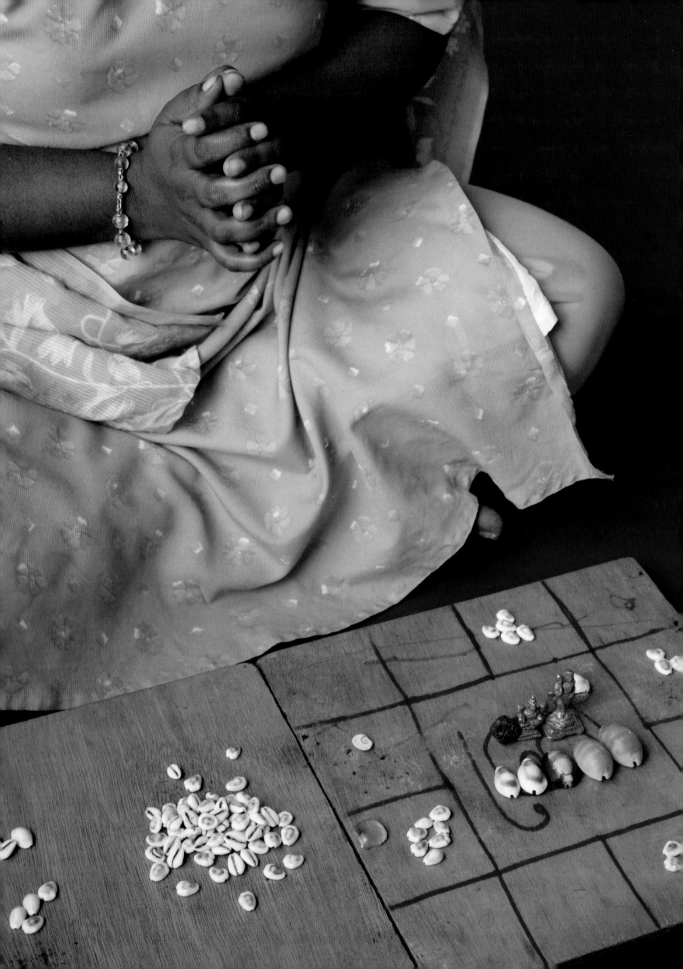

Vedic Astrology

Along with palmistry, numerology, face-reading, fortune-telling and other predictive arts, *jyotish* or astrology has a long history in India. Dating back to Vedic times, it has been used as a pseudo-scientific method of guiding people through life's choices for hundreds of years.

"All you need is your exact time and date of birth and geographical location – and we do the rest," says Pandit Manoj Joshi, a young astrologer priest at the Sri Durga *mandir* (temple) in one of New Delhi's more affluent suburbs. He goes on to explain that this information is used to ascertain planetary alignments at the time of a person's birth; from this, numerous mathematical calculations may be made about a person's future life. Pandit Joshi insists that *jyotish* is a scientific process that does not include superstition or dogma. "It is very straightforward," he says.

Unlike Western astrology which uses the tropical zodiac, Vedic astrology uses the sidereal zodiac, where the link between sign and sky constellation is more exact. For example, Aries runs from March 21 to April 20 in the tropical zodiac, but extends from April 14 to May 14 in the sidereal. Vedic astrology also takes into account the positions of planets (*graha*) except Uranus, Neptune and Pluto, the sun and moon, the lunar nodes (Rahu and Ketu) and certain sub-planets or *upgrahas*: each of these so-called heavenly bodies is believed to be able to impact human behaviour. In addition, each person falls within one of a category of twelve "houses"; again, each house is aligned to certain characteristics.

After an astrologer has determined a chart for a client, he can advise on propitious dates for any number of activities. Increasingly, today, astrologers use computer software for this, as it is less time-consuming and far more accurate than manual calculation.

Does this mean that one's life is pre-destined? Does it matter, for example, whether we act in a certain way or make a certain decision, if it's all mapped out in the stars anyway? "Absolutely," comes the rejoinder from Pandit Joshi, "because one has to take into account *karma* from past lives and actions in one's present life." If the astrological chart indicates that a certain month, day, or even hour, looks inauspicious, one can limit potential damage with good actions, propitiation, the performing of rituals of fire, the chanting of *mantras* or even the wearing of certain gemstones or metals close to the skin (see pages 182–184).

Pandit Joshi likens one's astrological chart to a signboard on a road. "It tells you there is a speed bump round the corner, but it is up to you whether you slow down or drive over it at ninety miles an

Left: More a fortune-teller than an astrologer, a *kori* (cowrie shell) divinator chants *mantras*, gives offerings and consults her board to give advice to a supplicant. Considered a Tantric *sadhana* or practice, such *tantriks* are a common sight in the countryside.

Above: The practice of telling one's fortune through palm-reading is a popular practice not only in India, but all over the world. Here we see a palmistry signboard from a temple in Myanmar.

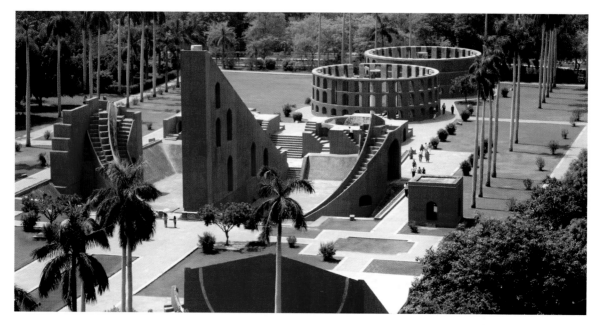

hour," he notes. In other words, we are not totally without power over our destinies.

On a day-to-day level, astrologers can offer reassurance in times of bad luck and guidelines for future behaviour, as well as advice on decisions to be taken. They may suggest a good date for a client to approach the boss for a pay rise (when the second House of Wealth looks good!) or when one should pluck up one's courage and embark on a trip (when the third House of Courage looks promising!). Naturally, an astrologer is consulted for opportune times and dates for weddings, funerals and life-changing events, and parents often seek an astrologer's advice as to which profession their children should be encouraged to follow.

The link between Vedic astrology and wellness is well documented, too. "Indians visit an astrologer in the same way that Westerners go to a doctor or therapist," says writer Namita Gokhale. When one needs an operation or course of medicine, the astrologer is as likely to be approached as the doctor: he may refer to the client's moon chart to see when he will be in a good frame of mind for surgery (as the moon is related to the mind); or he may advise when the planets are best positioned for an operation to be a success. Increasingly (if one is wealthy), he dictates when one should elect for a Caesarian section for the birth of a child.

Above: The Jantar Mantar in New Delhi, one of five observatories constructed in north-west India by Maharaja Jai Singh II of Jaipur from 1724 to 1730. All five were originally built to improve the accuracy of astrological charts.

Right: Part of a hand-painted astrological chart for a certain Manoj Joshi as formulated by Pandit Manoj Joshi, a young astrologer priest. It is written in Sanskrit and begins: "I pray to Lord Ganesha that this chart will be fine, accurate and useful…".

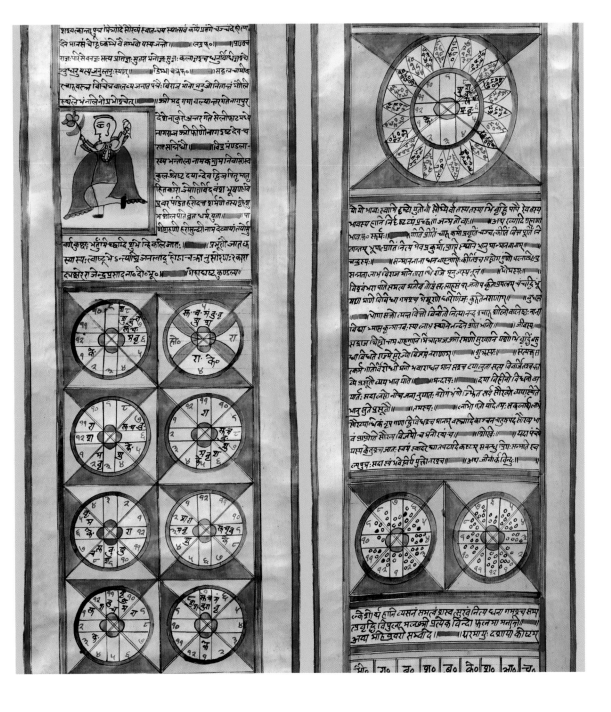

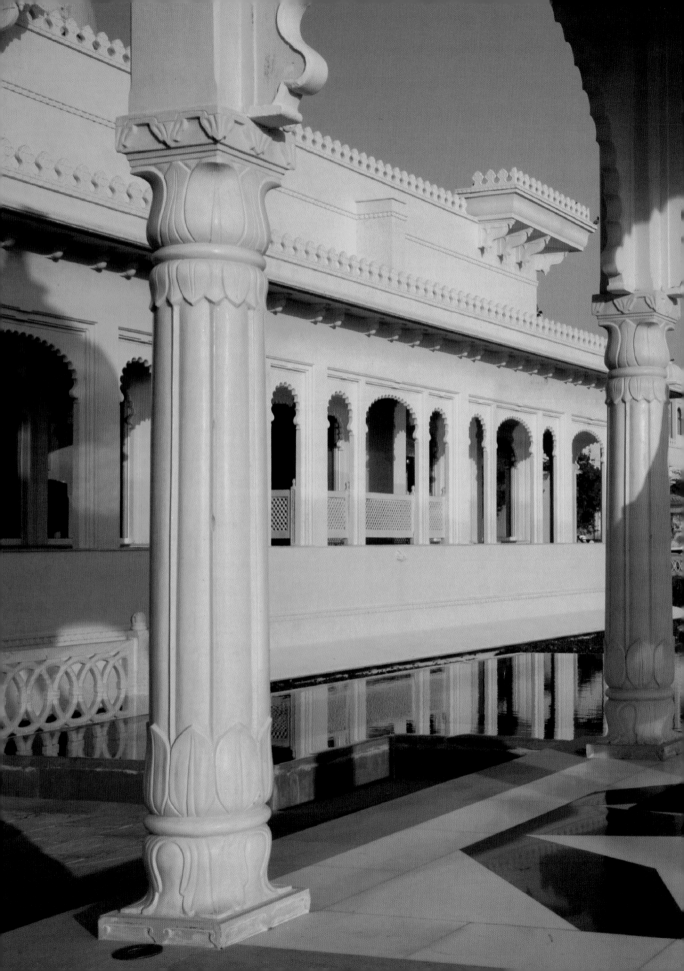

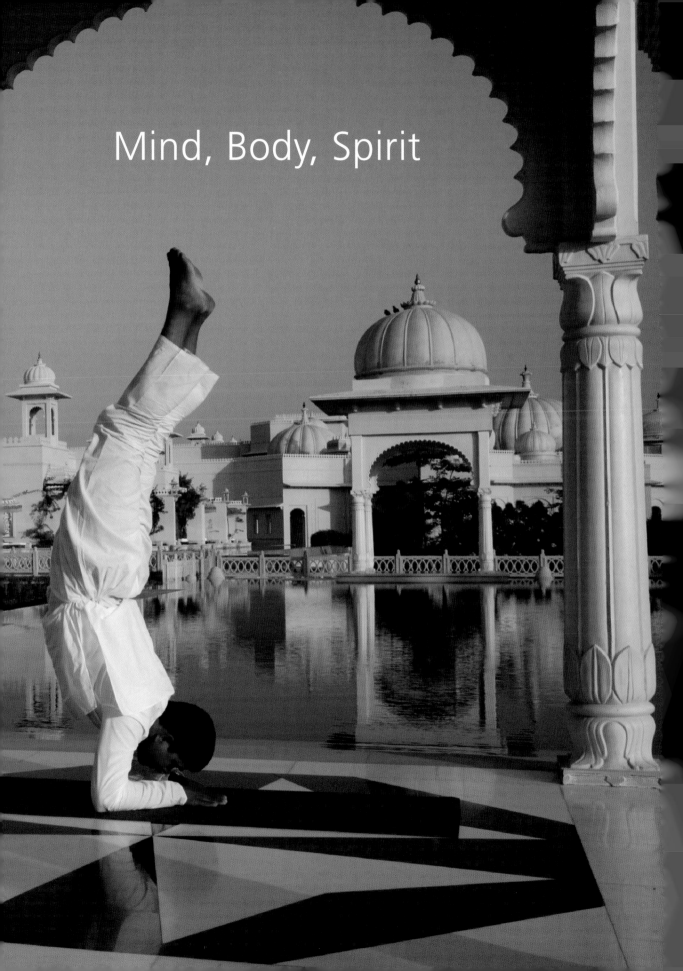

Mind, Body, Spirit

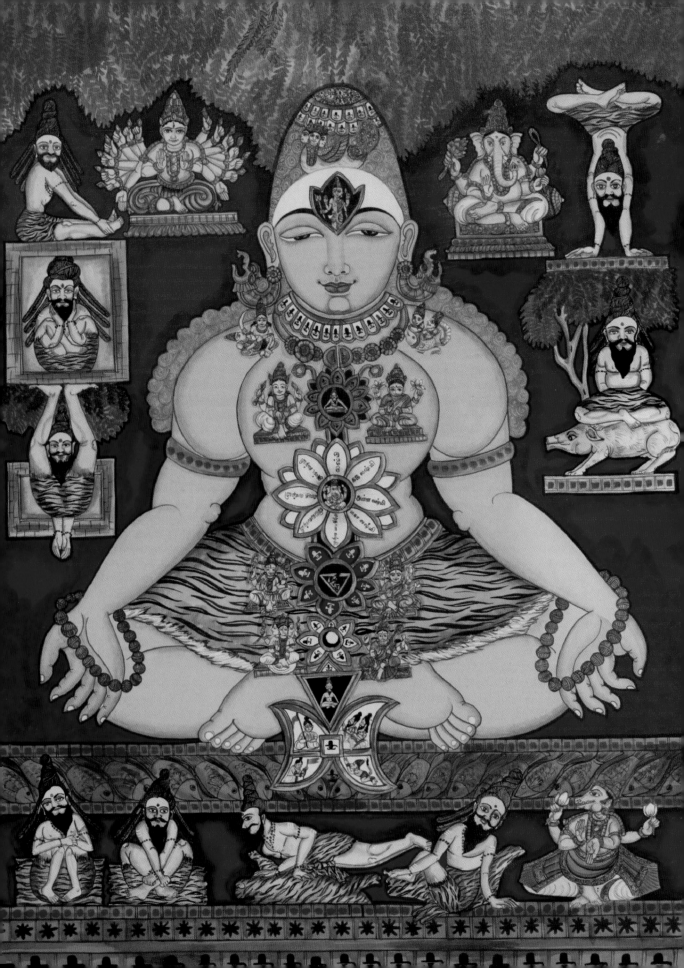

Yoga

It isn't known exactly when the ancient art of yoga began, but there is archaeological evidence of various yogic postures dating back to 3,000 BC. Many believe that it was Shiva who first brought yoga to the masses (see page 104), but the first written texts outlining the basic philosophy and practices of yoga probably date to 200 BC. Called the *Yoga Sutras*, they were written by a certain Patanjali, and are believed to combine all previous teachings into an organised system that continues to this day.

Patanjali states that yoga is a methodical practice, the ultimate aim of which is the attainment of perfection and merging with the Divine. Through the control of both physical and psychical elements, disciplined activity, spiritual exercises and the conquest of desire, one can attain salvation. He outlined an eight-limbed path *(ashtanga)* in order to reach this ultimate stage. It consists of the following:

Yama: Abstention, not doing bad things to other people. "The Don'ts".
Niyama: Observance, things you should do to yourself, ie cleansing *(kriya)*, celibacy, being happy/good. "The Dos".

Left: An inspirational illustration depicting some of the different *asanas* on the perimeter, and a lotus-posed devotee showing the positioning of the seven *chakras*.
Above: A Shaivite *sadhu* from Tanjore, Tamil Nadu, is shown in an 18th-century painting on glass.

Asana: Postures (umpteen numbers thereof).
Pranayama: Breath-control (with exercises).
Pratyahara: Withdrawal of the senses, controlling them and being aware of them.
Dharana: Fixed attention (concentration).
Dhyana: Contemplation (meditation).
Samadhi: Final stage (super-consciousness or equivalent of the Buddhist concept of Nirvana).

Today, there are many different styles of yoga, but all follow what are known as the Four Paths. These are the path of knowledge and wisdom *(jnana)*, the path of devotion *(bhakti)*, the path of action *(karma)* and the path of self-control *(raja)*. In general terms, yoga includes repetition of postures *(asanas)*, followed by resting poses, breathing exercises *(pranayama)* and meditation. *Hatha* yoga, a term often heard, is not actually a style of yoga but a generic term for the path that ultimately leads to self-control *(raja)*.

In addition to the main styles of yoga listed below, there are many other forms (mostly Western such as Bikram yoga and Power yoga) that are more recent additions to the practice. We will not be delving into them in this book.

Iyengar Yoga: The yoga teacher BKS Iyengar, born in 1918, started this style of yoga in Pune. The Iyengar concept includes work to achieve correct and accurate alignment and practising with an astute consciousness of how to build a

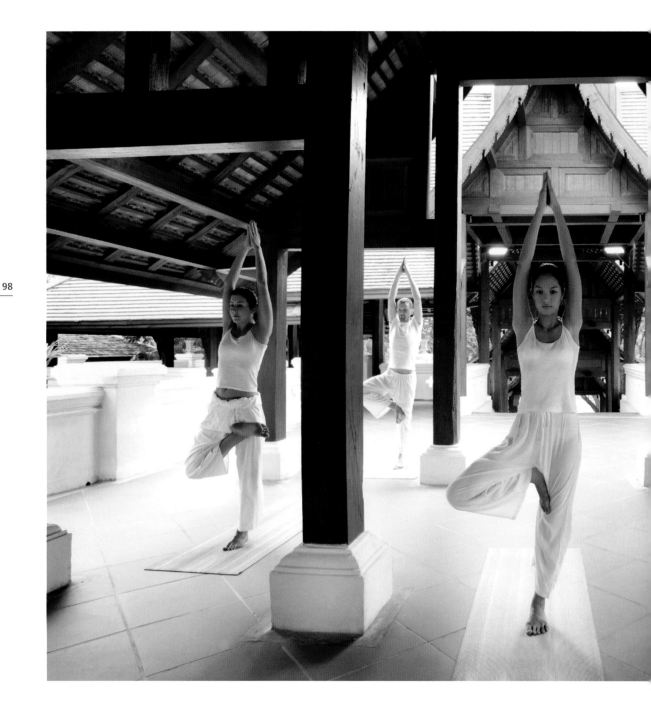

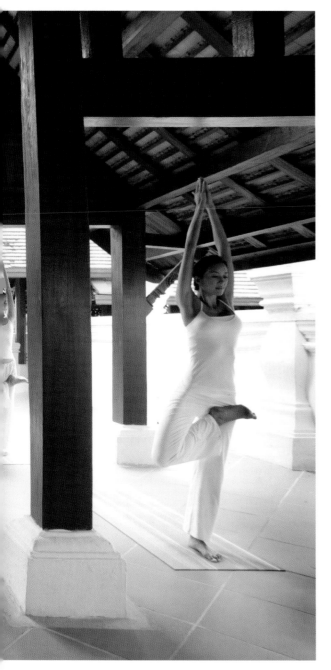

stronger *asana*. The aim is to make sure every pose is completely in line. Time is spent on getting the poses right, often using props such as straps, blocks of wood or blankets, then maintaining the postures for longer and longer lengths of time the more experienced one becomes. It focuses on strong standing postures.

Ananda Yoga: A classical style of *hatha* yoga, this style focuses on gentle postures designed to move the energy up to the brain and prepare the body for meditation. It is not at all aerobic: it looks inwards, but nonetheless places emphasis on proper body alignment and controlled breathing.

Ashtanga Yoga: This system involves synchronising the breath with a progressive series of postures. It was formulated by Sri K Pattabhi Jois, a yoga master based in Mysore. It concentrates on the flow from one pose to the next, on the breath (*ujjaipranayam*) and on strong, physical poses. During an *ashtanga* session, an intense internal heat and a powerful, purifying sweat is produced, so that both body and mind are exercised fully. The sweat acts as a detoxifier, resulting in improved circulation and a calmer mind. Each practitioner works on the progression of poses according to his or her own time and inclination.

Hatha yoga: Often called the original yoga style, *hatha* is a form of classic yoga practice that combines body, mind and breath with the goal of

99

Left: Soaring roofs supported by teak pillars form the basis of the open-sided, airy yoga *sala* at Mandarin Oriental Dhara Devi. A wide range of yoga, meditation and spiritual exercise classes to help promote stamina, peace of mind, energy and vitality are offered here.

self-improvement. Repetition of *asanas*, followed by a relaxation posture, help to purify mind, body and spirit.

Sivananda Yoga: This is a traditional type of yoga that focuses on connecting the body to the solar plexus where it is believed an enormous amount of energy is stored. Comprising repetition of *asanas* followed by resting poses, it also takes into account breathing, and advocates certain dietary restrictions, chanting and meditation.

Kundalini Yoga: The aim of this form of yoga is to awaken and reach one's spiritual potential. Using the metaphor of a serpent coiled at the body's bottom *chakra*, this yoga practice unwinds the serpent and helps it to rise up-wards in an attempt to reach the top *chakra*, the highest possible. *Kundalini* translates as "the curl of the hair of the Beloved", and concentrates on postures, chanting, meditation and breathing exercises.

Viniyoga: *Viniyoga* is a term used to describe the yoga taught by Sri T Krishnamacharya, a descendant of the 9th-century yogi Nathamuni. His son is the current lineage holder. *Viniyoga* concentrates on integrating different elements of yoga to develop a practice that is specific to an individual's needs. It respects the fact that as we age, we need to change our yoga practice. It aims to make yoga relevant to every situation, and concentrates on postures, breathing, meditation, ritual and prayer.

Benefits of Yoga

The Sanskrit word *yoga* means "union" or "joining", first between mind, body and spirit and ultimately with the Almighty. Whilst this is not within everyone's reach, yoga confers many less ambitious benefits also. There are many physiological, psychological and biochemical results that vary from simple things ("I can touch my toes again!") to increases in haemoglobin and lymphocyte count. In general, practitioners report increased flexibility, better lubrication of joints, massaging of internal organs, toned muscles and detoxification of the entire body. These physical improvements are joined by clarity of mind, relaxation, emotional stability and more.

As with many of the therapies discussed here, yoga works on the mental, spiritual and physical levels simultaneously. Devotees often report transformations in their lives once yoga is practiced regularly. Stress, anxiety, ill health, unhappiness and anger are replaced by peace, vibrant health, service and love towards all creation. Turn to pages 188, 236 and 248, for some inspired settings in which to practice this ancient art.

Above: Shiva, the lord of yoga, is depicted in this stylised painting in his Himalayan abode. It is entitled *Kailasphati Shankar*, referring to Mount Kailash under which he sits in meditative rapture.

Right: A painting depicts the Hindu *sapta rishis* or seven sages who are extolled in the *Vedas* and other Hindu literature. They are regarded as the patriarchs of the Vedic religion. The sage at centre bottom is in *urdhva-padmasana* or elevated lotus position.

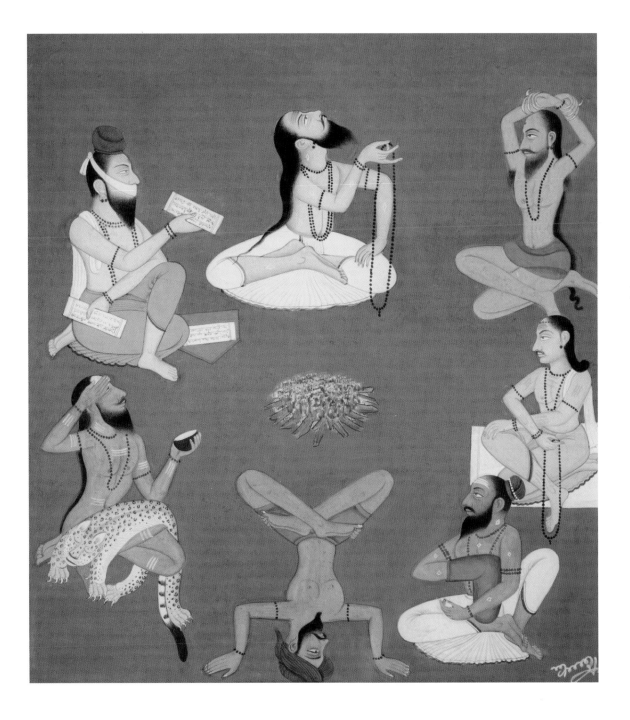

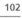

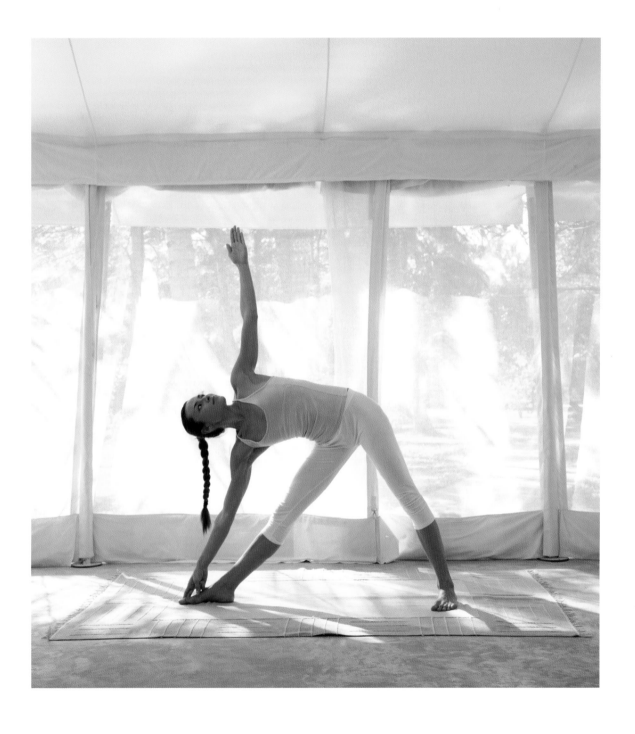

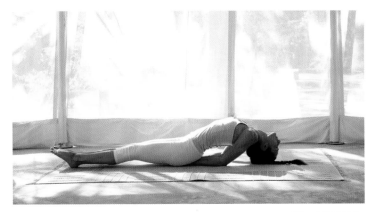

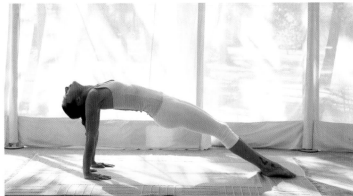

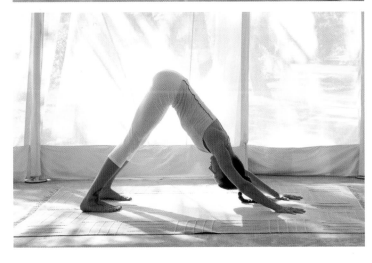

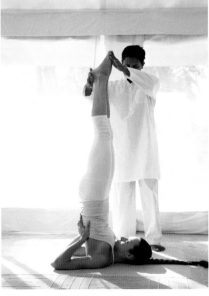

Our model and yoga teacher, Yana Odnopozov, demonstrates some of the different *asanas* in the yoga repertoire. *Asanas* are described by Patanjali as "steady and comfortable" in the second chapter of the *Sutras*. She is aided by Bharat Kumar Patra, one of the yoga teachers at Shreyas Retreat. Originally from Orissa, Bharat comes from a family of yoga practitioners. He took his Master's degree in Yogic Science at the Swami Vivekananda Yoga Anusamdhana Samsthan (SVYASA), a research institute aligned to the University of Bangalore.

Clockwise from far left: Trikonasana or "triangle pose": Maintained to strengthen knees and calf and thigh muscles, this *asana* is good for the spine, correcting any lateral distortions. *Matsyasana* or "fish posture": Helpful for neck and spine, this posture increases circulation of blood to the brain cells. *Sarvangasana* or "supported shoulder stand pose": This posture helps thyroid disorders, by increasing blood flow to the thyroid. *Adho mukha svanasana* or "downward facing dog": This is one of the postures in the Sun Salutation series of postures, probably familiar to most. *Purvatanasana* or "east extension posture": This posture strengthens the shoulders and wrist joints and gives a good stretch to the back.

Morning Yoga at Bhangarh

India chose her places of pilgrimages on the top of
hills and mountains, by the side of the holy rivers,
in the heart of forests and by the shores of the
ocean, which along with the sky, is our nearest
visible symbol of the vast, the boundless, the 'I'.

– *Rabindranath Tagore*

For many Hindus no day would be complete without
a visit to a temple or *mandir* ("doorway to the heart").
Some people visit the temple to perform a *puja*
("offering" or "prayers", literally "respect"), while
others go to give thanks or ask for blessings.
Different temples are dedicated to different gods.

Amanbagh guests have the option of a
temple visit with a yoga excursion to the nearby
uninhabited city of Bhangarh. It is difficult to
imagine a more inspiring setting. Practice takes
place on a raised platform in front of the beautifully
preserved 16th-century Rada Krishna temple, while
behind tower the ruins of the palace built by the
Jaipur royal family and the steep Aravali hills. Sun
salutations and thanks for the new day are the
theme of the *asanas* and the yoga guide tailors the
session to the ability of the group.

Aptly enough, the other temple in the complex
is dedicated to Lord Shiva, the Hindu god who is
credited with creating yoga. As related in the Hindu
scriptures, Shiva, after his epic argument with Brahma,
retreated to his Himalayan home at Mount Kailash
(see painting on page 100) to brood over the questions
that plagued his mind. Why was there suffering, misery
and frustration? What could be done to improve the
human situation? What was the meaning of existence?

He sought a way to control his mind, to make it see
the truth beyond the veils of illusion.

Eventually, the story goes, he found the way.
And that way was yoga: The means to connect
the individual's mind to the cosmos. Through its
practices – breathing, postures and clearing of the
mind – yoga helped Shiva see in a manner that
was pure, wise, dispassionate and uncoloured by
opinions, emotions and perceptions.

Yoga practice today continues to do just that:
A morning session at Bhangarh aims to raise
levels of consciousness, give practitioners a more
panoramic macro perspective and rid them of
delusions, ignorance, attachments and fear. Gentle

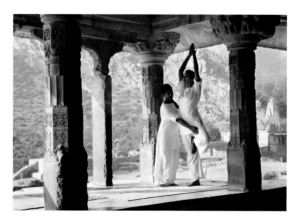

stretching, *asanas* that are not too taxing and an
encouraging teacher all contribute to the feeling
of wellbeing. Add to that the contemplative nature
of the site with its fresh air and unpolluted morning
light and the mind begins to still, the soul calms.
If yoga's aim is to make the practitioner serene,
aware and undisturbed by the turbulence of the
world, Bhangarh is the perfect place for it.

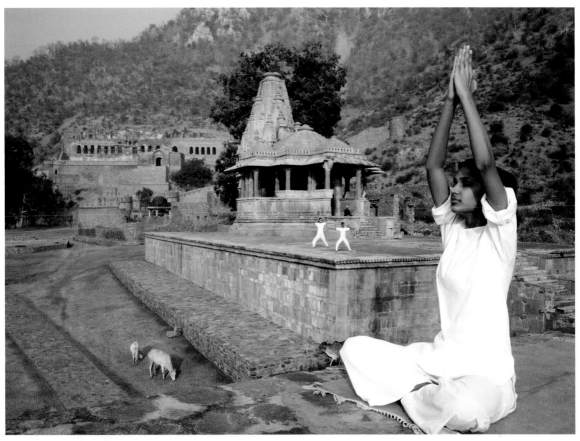

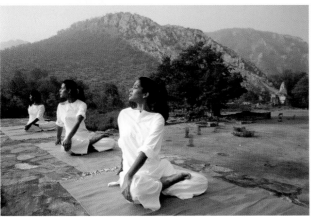

This page and opposite: Built in the 1500s by the Jaipur royal family, Bhangarh is an uninhabited city of temples (the Rada Krishna one is seen *above* and the Shiva one on *left* in background), bazaars, palaces, gardens and bathing pools. In the early morning, it is a quiet, contemplative spot – perfect for yoga. Amanbagh's yoga teacher takes clients through a series of postures designed to clear the mind and set people up for the new day. Seated twisting poses such as the one pictured on *left* help build up lower body strength, nourishing, lengthening and realigning the spine.

Amulya Uphar

Similar to Thai massage, but based on the stretching facilitated by yoga postures, Amanbagh's Amulya Uphar could be described as "lazy man's yoga". Translating as "Priceless Gift" from the Hindi, it is an oil-free treatment that takes place on a mattress on the floor, with the client wearing a loose *kurta* pyjama suit rather like the clothes given for Thai massage.

Yoga *asanas* were formulated to improve body flexibility, strengthen the muscles and open up blocks in *prana* flow. It is now known that they improve circulation of the blood and the functioning of specific organs as well. They even reduce fat build-up! By working on the meridian lines and main *marma* points and manipulating the client's body into different yoga positions, the therapist opens up the client's energy channels. This, in turn, stimulates blood circulation and movement of lymph and *prana* – in the same way that a session of yoga does.

First of all, clients are prepared for the body work with a foot wash with a hot towel to remove negative energy and a gentle touch on the solar plexus and crown *chakras* to let them know they are in safe hands. Lying on their back, they are requested to breathe normally before the massage begins. This always starts with the feet as it is here that the body weight rests: Using thumbs and palms on the meridian lines, reflex points are awakened on the soles, then the masseuse moves up the legs to stomach and hands, shoulders and head. After this, the client turns over and the therapist works on the legs, back, neck and head.

Amulya Uphar is quite a physical experience, with the therapist sometimes sitting on the client, and often pulling him or her into somewhat contorted positions. The cobra pose, for example, has the therapist kneeling on the pressure points of the client's thighs while holding both hands and pulling them backwards. At certain points the client may be requested to breathe in or out in order to facilitate the opening up of the body, but the skilled therapist – by listening to the body – knows how far it can be coaxed, stretched or twisted. Essentially, the body is being assisted into yoga *asanas* and stretches without having to make any effort itself!

This type of yogic stretching can be an amazingly de-stressing experience, with clients reporting deep relaxation, relief of tension and increased suppleness afterwards. It works best if clients give themselves up entirely to the therapist by relaxing completely. Such is the skill of the therapists at Amanbagh, this is easily done, and many guests go on to try the complimentary session of morning yoga the following day.

Above: A rangoli *made from lentils: At the Amanbagh spa the guest is welcomed to the therapy room with a* rangoli *pattern made from different powders, lentils or white chalk powder set on the massage mattress. All over India this home art is placed at the entrance to houses, either to welcome guests or to signify hospitality if the owner is absent. At the spa they are also placed beneath the head cradle of the massage beds.*

106

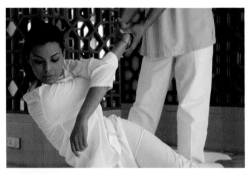

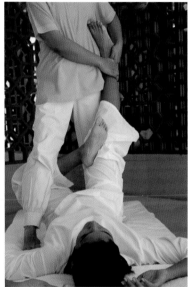

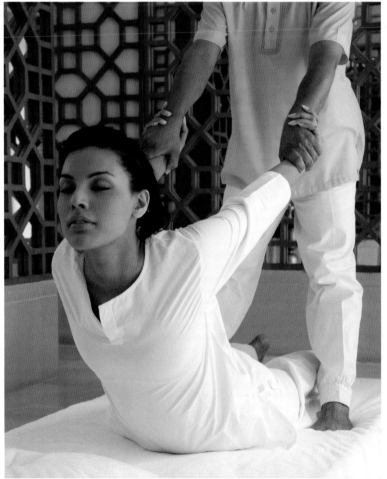

107

The Amanbagh therapist pulls, turns, manipulates and stretches a client's body to simulate certain yoga postures and stretches. All the while, she works along the energy lines, using acupressure, reflexology and internal organ massage. The aim is to clear blockages of *prana* and give the client a full bodywork to improve overall health and create a feeling of wellbeing.

Clockwise from top left: Twisting from the waist and stretching the arms frees up joints and muscles. A hamstring stretch is combined with acupressure massage on certain key points in foot and leg. The therapist pulls the client towards *dhanurasana* or the "bow pose" to stretch the shoulders and elongate the spine.

Pranayama

"Prana is a subtle invisible force. It is the life force that pervades the body . . . The body and the mind have no direct connection. They are connected through *prana* only and this *prana* is different from the breathing you have in your physical body."

– *Swami Chidananda Saraswati,
President of the Divine Life Society, Rishikesh*

Taken from the word *prana* meaning "vital energy" or "life force" and *ayama* that translates as "control" or "extension/expansion", *pranayama* comprises breathing exercises that help calm the mind, improve the condition of the abdominal and chest area and eliminate toxins from the body. Originally expounded by Patanjali, the ancient Hindu philosopher and yogi who wrote the *Yoga Sutras* (see page 97), it is all about expansion of the vital force in the body through regulated breathing processes.

Pranayama is usually practiced in conjunction with yoga and regular *pranayama* practitioners report that they are calm and balanced, their minds are focused and they have increased vitality and longevity. According to Patanjali, *pranayama* awakens the brain and the cerebrospinal nerve centres enabling people to reach their highest potential. Be this true or not, research suggests that it is beneficial in treating a range of stress-related disorders and it helps with respiratory diseases such as bronchitis and asthma.

All the exercises follow a sequence of inhalation (*puraka*), holding (*kumbhaka*) and exhalation (*rechaka*). The main focus is on correcting bad breathing habits and concentrating on the here and now. Inhalations should be deep, complete and focused, filling the lungs to capacity, while exhalations need to be slow, deep and uniform. Ideally, the latter should take twice as long as the inhalations, and, at the end of a *rechaka*, the lungs should be emptied to the maximum extent, their tissues contracting as much as possible. In the case of *kumbhaka* there is no question of speed or movement: it is simply stopping all breath by holding all the respiratory apparatus tight and still.

There are a number of different *pranayama* exercises and all should be practiced in a sitting posture. Choose from the half a dozen sitting positions laid down by Patanjali: the simplest, least strenuous one is *swastikasana* (sitting cross-legged with back straight and hands on knees), but more advanced yoga practitioners may prefer the lotus position (*padmasana*), the traditional recommendation for *pranayama*. We outline and illustrate a typical session offered at the beautiful yoga pavilion at Shreyas Retreat. It's a wonderful way to prepare for a meditation session.

If you want to recreate the exercises at home, remember to make the exhalation longer than the inhalation. Start your session with a prayer or a simple *om* chant, first making sure you are sitting comfortably, your spine is straight and your shoulders are relaxed. Don't push yourself too hard – and if you ever get out of breath, stop immediately.

Right: Rajasekaran, the yoga master at Kalari Kovilakom, practises *nadhi sodhana* or alternate nostril breathing with a client on one of the airy verandahs at the palace.

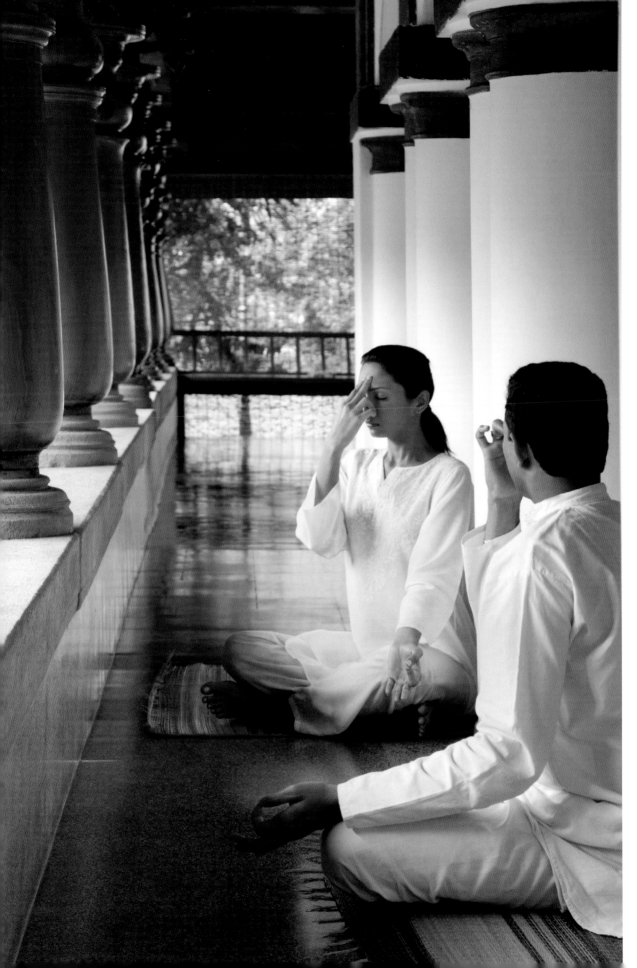

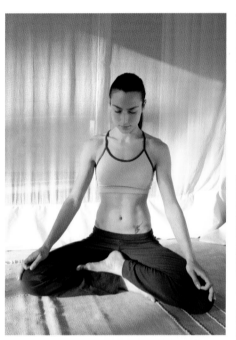

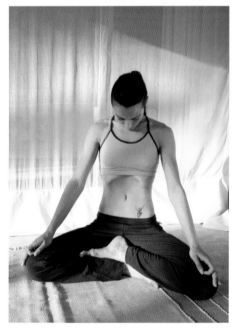

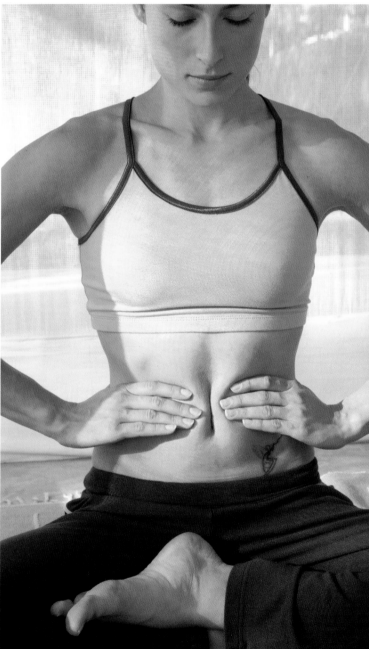

Pranayama at Shreyas Retreat

"Breathe in deeply, and on the exhalation, bring out an *om*," instructs Bharat, the retreat's yoga master, at the beginning of the *pranayama* session. After a couple of such introductory exhalations, Bharat asks practitioners to rub their hands together to stimulate the circulation, and give a gentle self-massage to the face and back of the neck (see below).

Before the breathing session starts properly, the process of *kapala bhati* takes place. *Kapal* is a Sanskrit word for "forehead", while *bhati* means "lighting" or "glowing". It is a *kirya* or cleansing process that is practiced in a meditative posture with spine and neck erect, and eyes closed. A session of rapid breathing, with active and forceful exhalation followed by passive inhalation, it has no *kumbhaka* or holding of breath stage. All the nerves reverberate during this exercise, you sweat profusely and on the exhalation, you should experience a flapping movement in the abdomen.

As *kapala bhati* is a very dynamic experience, it should only be done for about a minute, as this is enough time to give a massaging effect to the inner organs as well as balance and strengthen the nervous system. "It's particularly good for gastric problems, peptic ulcers and other similar ailments," explains Bharat. It also helps set up the entire body, not to mention lungs and respiratory tract, for the breathing exercises to follow.

Vhastrika is the first exercise: Translating as "bellows breath", it is a breathing technique used by yogis to build energy, tone the respiratory muscles and induce a feeling of alertness and mental clarity. As suggested by the name, the breath imitates the action of a bellows. Essentially a method of controlled hyper-ventilation, the practitioner is led through a series of inhalation/holding/exhalation sequences that focuses on the thoracic and chest region. Active inhalation with chest out and shoulders rising slightly is followed by holding, then active exhalation to bring the chest back in. These sequences help promote proper diaphragmatic breathing, oxygenate the blood and purge the lungs of residual carbon dioxide.

Alternate nostril breathing or *nadhi sodhana* follows. *Nadhi* is the word for "psychic passage", a specific pathway through which *prana* flows, and *sodhana* is "purification", so this sequence is designed to facilitate smooth flow of *prana*. It should not be practiced if the nasal passages are blocked; in fact, in any *pranayama* series, if the breath feels forced, stop immediately. In *nadhi sodhana*, the flow of

Above: At the beginning of a *pranayama* session at Shreyas Retreat, the practice of palming takes place. Originally a yoga practice, the hands are rubbed together to stimulate the circulation, and a gentle self-massage is given to the face and back of the neck.

Left: Vhastrika or "bellows breath" is a sequence of inhalation/holding/exhalation that should not be practiced for long periods of time as it is a form of controlled hyper-ventilation.

breath is controlled by either the thumb or the ring finger of the right hand in the *nasika* hand position or *mudra* (see below).

Bharat explains the process: "First of all, block the right nostril with the thumb, then slowly exhale through the left nostril. When the lungs feel completely empty, inhale slowly through the left nostril, then close the nostril with the ring finger. Now, exhale completely out of the right nostril, then inhale through the right nostril, and block again with the thumb." He explains that this is one round, and a few rounds should be practised one after the other. It is a good idea to mentally count

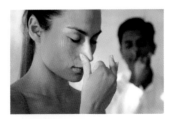

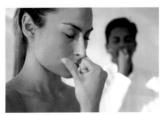

five seconds for each inhalation and six seconds for every exhalation. This process stimulates both sides of the brain and is recommended for insomnia and migraine, as well as for people with high blood pressure. It is also extremely calming and grounding. If you are in a stressful situation, a few rounds of *nadhi sodhana* may be just the ticket.

After this comes *uddiyana bandha* (*uddiyana* means a "jump upward", *bandha* is a "lock"). It involves the contraction of particular muscles in the body that are locked or held tightly in a certain position. There are four main *bandhas* associated with *pranayama*; the other three are *jalandhara bandha* (bending the neck forward and setting the chin below the throat), *mula bandha* (contraction of anal sphincters and pelvic floor) and *jilva bandha* (holding the tongue on the roof of the mouth).

In *uddiyana bandha*, the thoracic diaphragm is moved to an extreme upward position, held, then released. Practitioners sit in the lotus position with hands in the *chin mudra* (index finger touching the thumb and other three fingers relaxed), and focus on the lower abdominal section of the body. The sequence is as follows: Breathe in completely, contract the lowest *chakra* at the bottom of the spine, suck in the abdomen, lock in the chin with the chest, and hold the breath. Keep steady for as long as is comfortable, then release from the chin and abdomen, and exhale.

Bharat explains that *uddiyana bandha* takes quite a time to master. He stresses that novices should never exceed their individual capacity, as *pranayama* modifies normal breathing processes considerably thereby creating substantial internal pressures and stretches. After this, the session ends on a relaxing note with the practitioner in *shavasana*.

Above: Nadhi sodhana calms the mind, balances the mental state and stimulates both sides of the brain as both nostrils flow freely.
Right: Shavasana or "corpse posture" is traditionally the final posture in a *hatha* yoga session engendering deep relaxation.

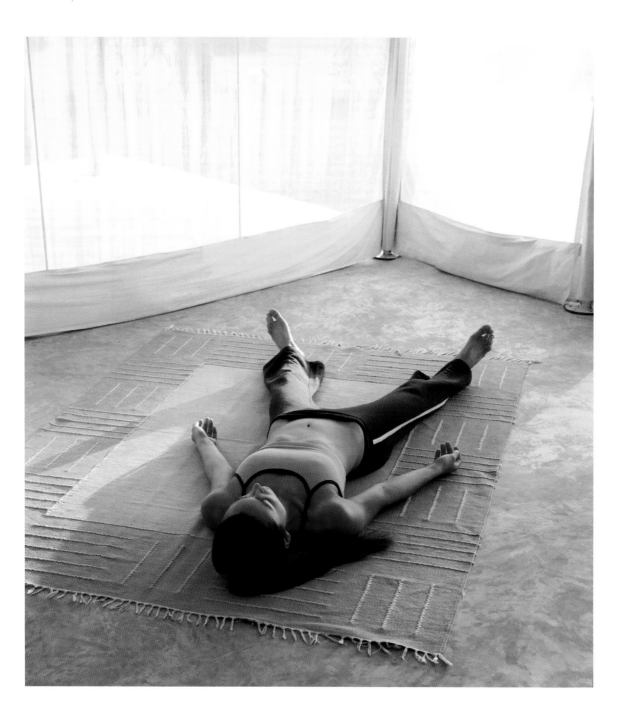

Meditation

In a world where stress, tension, lack of time and abundance of tasks predominates, the ancient practice of meditation is gaining ground. More and more doctors are prescribing meditation as a way to lower blood pressure, improve performance, prevent sleep disturbances and promote relaxation. After all, it is totally safe and simple: It needs no complicated machinery or drugs; it balances on a physical, emotional, mental and spiritual level; and can be of benefit to one and all.

As meditation is such a huge subject with multiple techniques and methods, only a brief summary is possible here. As with many of the mind, body, spirit practices covered in this book, we can only touch on its main tenets and history in India. Check the listings at the back of the book for reputable meditation centres and ashrams that offer more information.

Meditation and Hinduism

Rooted in many of the world's great religions, meditation has been used as a healing therapy for centuries. It originated in India with yoga which forms one of the six schools of Hindu philosophy. First mentioned in the *Puranas*, the *Vedas* and the *Upanishads*, it was later outlined by Patanjali (see page 97). Its aim is to still the mind, body and soul, alleviate suffering and promote healing. How this is done varies: *Japa* yoga advocates the repetition of a *mantra*, *hatha* yoga aims to raise spiritual energy, *raja* yoga works with breath, *surat shabd* yoga uses sound and light to meditate, and *bhakti* yoga or the "yoga of love and devotion" aims to concentrate practitioners' focus on a particular devotional subject.

Seen as a method of attaining physiological and spiritual mastery, meditation is central to Hinduism. The seven *rishis* or sages (see painting on page 101) were master meditators and today's *sadhus* (wandering mystics or holy men) employ meditation, along with asceticism, yoga, renunciation and celibacy with the ultimate aim of attaining enlightenment. However, one does not need to be a Hindu to practice Hindu meditation; many Hindu meditative techniques are secular in nature – and are open to all to try.

A popular choice for those serious about learning more about Hinduism and meditation is a visit to an ashram. Neither a temple nor a monastery, an ashram is more like a retreat. The idea is to lead a simple life, develop a positive attitude and come away with an understanding of selfless service. A 15-day visit is recommended as a minimum. The Bihar School of Yogashram offers a variety of ashram experiences including *sadhana* courses where yoga, *pranayama*, meditation, relaxation and concentration techniques are "taught" in a peaceful ashram environment. The school notes: "For meditation, as well as anything else, it is important to have the right

Opposite: A meditative pose is attained in the quiet sanctuary of Kalari Kovilakom in Kerala.

Above: Detail of hands and feet of the Buddha, 14th century, Sukothai Period, now housed in the Prasat Museum in Bangkok.

114

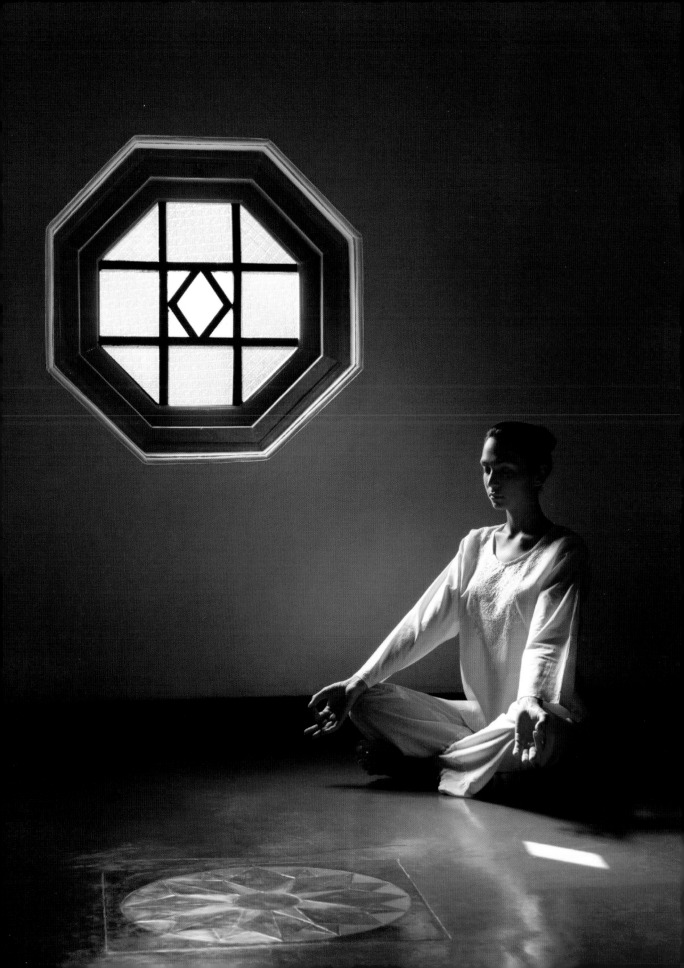

atmosphere . . . although theory and practices can be learnt in a yoga school, the training received in the ashram will influence the deeper layers of the mind."

Many people report that such a withdrawal from everyday life is a rich and rewarding experience. A supplicant who goes to a Keralan ashram at least once every two years notes: "Because the experience is so different from my usual routine, it allows my imagination to flourish, my body to relax and my spiritual side to come to the fore. It's always a good time to reflect and take stock of my life."

Meditation and Buddhism

Meditation is central to Buddhism. Indeed, around 500 BC, the Indian prince Siddharta Gautama rejected the material world and attained enlightenment through meditation beneath a bodhi tree. Theravada Buddhism advocates various meditative practices, but the two best known are Samadhi or concentrative meditation and Vipassana or mindfulness meditation.

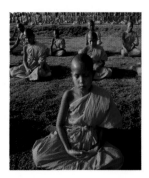

Both are considered part of the eightfold path that Buddhists must follow in order to achieve Nirvana.

At its most simple, concentrative meditation focuses attention on the breath, an image or a sound (*mantra*) in order to still the mind and allow a greater awareness and clarity to emerge. By concentrating on the continuous rhythm of inhalation and exhalation, the mind becomes absorbed in the rhythm, breathing becomes slower and deeper, and the mind becomes more tranquil and aware. Mindfulness meditation, on the other hand, seeks to open up the mind's awareness. The practitioner sits quietly, simply witnessing whatever goes through the mind, thereby obtaining a more calm, clear and non-reactive state of mind.

Again, both types of meditation are open to non-Buddhists. Of note are the 10-day residential courses offered by the Vipassana Research Institute. They are patronised by clients from around the globe. Pioneered by S N Goenka, an Indian who learnt the technique in Burma, the courses are non-sectarian, as is Buddhism itself. Completely free and funded by donations from previous attendees, they are silent retreats aimed at enabling people to "see things as they really are". A participant who attended a centre just outside Mumbai likened the experience to "major surgery of the mind", but declared the self-exploratory journey was both healing and fulfilling.

Meditation and Spas

Of course, other religions including Islam, Christianity, Jainism and Sikkhism advocate the use of meditation in one form or another as well. However, you are most likely to encounter Hindu and Buddhist meditation methods in India, especially in an Indian spa or retreat. Increasingly, such establishments are including yoga, *pranayama* and meditation sessions on their menus to complement the other range of therapies on offer.

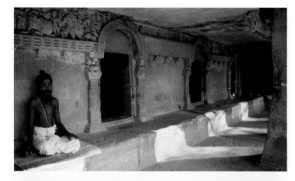

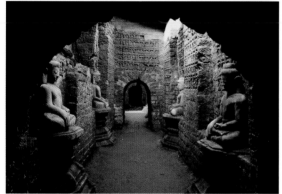

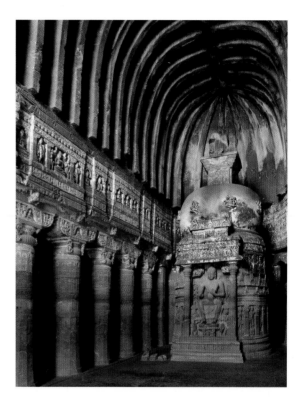

Visiting "masters" often run specialised courses, while residential teachers are also on hand. Shreyas and Ananda offer personalised meditation sessions guiding guests on a journey of inner contemplation to release tension and promote a positive outlook. As Ayurvedic doctors have to study meditation as part of their medical degree, Ayurvedic retreats routinely include meditation sessions. For example, Kalari Kovilakom guests are encouraged to start the day with a walking meditation known as *chandramanam*. Whilst walking, clients chant a *mantra*, prayer or *sankalpa* (affirmation) to open up their minds.

In addition to these traditional techniques, there is a plethora of what may be termed New Age

Opposite: Novice monks in "resting pose" during meditation.

Above, clockwise from top left: The ancient tradition of meditating in remote caves is illustrated by this Brahmin in Ranigumpha cave in Orissa, which dates from the 2nd century BC. Seventh-century Cave 26, one of 30 rock-cut caves at Ajanta that are popular pilgrimage sites today but housed monks in the past. Statues of the Buddha in the ruins of Mrauk-U, Arakan, Myanmar.

meditation techniques. Transcendental Meditation or TM, Deeksha, Global Meditation through *sahaja* yoga, movement meditations such as 5 Rhythms, Active or Dynamic meditation, Tantric meditation and more . . . all are offered at a variety of venues in India. If you are serious about improving your health and wellbeing through this ancient practice, the sky is the limit in India.

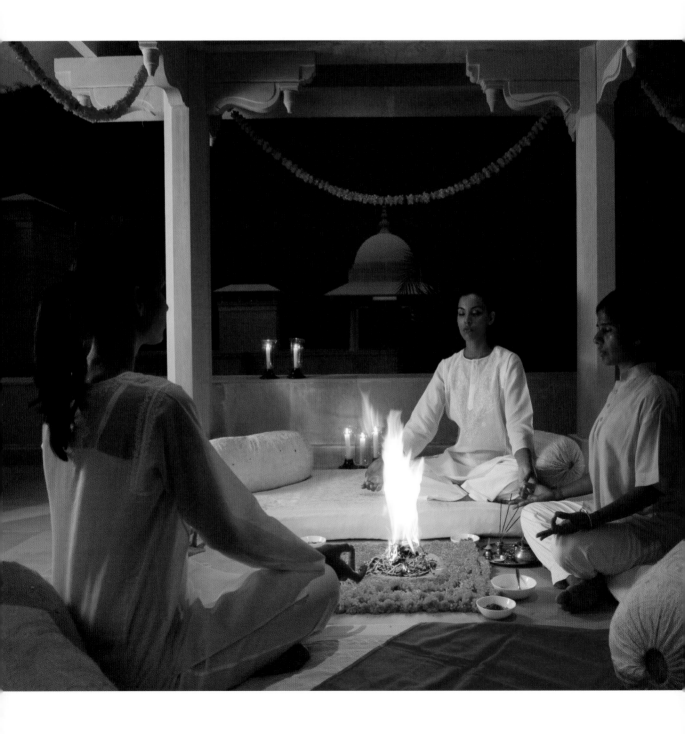

Meditation with Fire

Not until we see the richness of the Hindu mind and its essential spirituality can we understand India.
– *Lyn Yutang*

Designed to focus the mind through the continuous rhythm of *mantra* chanting along with fire offerings, the fire meditation at Amanbagh is both a tribute to Indian culture and a celebration of the unique locale of the property. Fire is considered the purest of the five elements in Hinduism: it is used at auspicious occasions, such as weddings and home-comings, and is associated with the solar plexus area.

As the sun is setting behind the Aravali hills, a fire begins to rise on the marigold bedecked meditation pavilion situated on the roof above Amanbagh's reception area. Guests, seated on low cushions on the floor, sit around a small central fire, dotted with candles and incense sticks (see left). First comes the *vedi* or the decoration of the fire, then guests are blessed with a *tika* dot of vermilion powder on the forehead. An *aarti* (or ritual) of incense begins the proceedings, then the fire itself is lit. At this point edible offerings are given up to the fire: rice, jaggery, sesame seeds and oatmeal.

Once the preliminaries are over, a meditation guide starts what is known as the *gayatri mantra*. Comprising 24 sounds that give homage to the mother of the tri-partite Hindu deity, the guide encourages guests to chant only five: *om*, *bhur*, *bhu*, *vah* and *swah*. Hindu philosophy advocates the use of sound, preferably in a low voice and a rhythmic manner, to facilitate concentration. In fact, many meditation techniques employ the repetitive chanting of simple sounds to clear the mind, open the heart and remove extraneous thoughts from the brain – and Amanbagh's mind-expanding ritual is no exception.

As a chanting rhythm is established and breathing becomes slower and deeper, the mind and consciousness becomes more aware. The fire flickers and hisses, and the light slowly seeps away from the sky; the surrounding hills give up their greens and browns for a deep dusky black. Night falls, and as the last sounds emit over the rooftop, the fire extinguishes itself. Guests gather up their things – and slowly slip away.

119

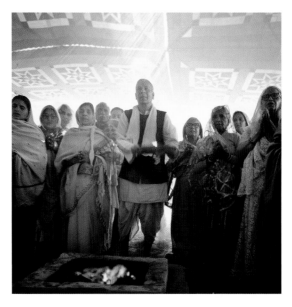

Right: Fire is used extensively in Hindu worship. In early Hindu mythology, Agni, the Hindu God of Fire, is depicted as one of the most important of the Vedic gods. His role in sacrifices and rituals was unparalleled: as fire consumes everything, he was seen as the mediator between heaven and earth. Here, a Jain priest conducts an *agni puja* (fire prayer).

Chakra Therapy

The term *chakra*, a Sanskrit word that literally means "wheel of light", refers to the seven basic energy centres in the body. In Indian philosophy, each of these centres correlates to major nerve ganglia branching out from the spinal column. In addition, the *chakras* also correlate to levels of consciousness, archetypal elements, developmental stages of life, colours, sounds, body functions and more. Some people reportedly see the *chakras*, describing them as spinning wheels of light and colour located along the backbone, going from the base of the spine to the crown of the head.

Each of the seven *chakras* has a physical, an emotional, a creative and a spiritual component (see listing overleaf). Colin Hall, spa manager at the Ananda, likens the spine to an elevator shaft of energy and the *chakras* as the various floors in the building of our body from which to view and experience life. When we rise from one floor to another within our consciousness, our perspective changes and expands.

"Based upon the area of consciousness that it influences, each *chakra* has its own purpose in the body," he explains. "In simple terms, we have a *chakra* for each issue that we commonly think about." He goes on to say that our thoughts have a direct relationship with our state of health. For example, love- and faith-based thoughts result in a smooth energy flow through the *chakras* and thus the physical body. Worry, obsession and fear-based thoughts affect the *chakra* that relates to the issues we are thinking about, thus causing a blockage or restriction in the flow of energy to that area.

Chakra therapists note that each *chakra* is found next to or near a hormonal gland in the body, so the *chakras* have the ability to push life energy or *prana* through the body to ensure vitality. These energy centres receive and radiate energy constantly, acting as storehouses and transmitters of universal energy as well. They say that it is necessary to balance the *chakras* from time to time to effectively regulate this flow.

According to yoga masters, disharmony on a physical, mental or spiritual level may be corrected by certain postures that concentrate the breath on the abdominal area. "*Pranayama* is especially active on the *chakras*," agrees Dr Sreenarayanan, also of Ananda, "and certain Ayurvedic treatments such as *sirodhara* can help open up flows of energy." In this therapy (see pages 56–59) he notes that medicated oils work on the pituitary gland, the gland responsible for certain growth functions; as a result, the body (and mind) is encouraged to open up and grow. Similarly, *chakradhara* or the pouring of medicated oils on to the *chakras* also effectively

Above: A figure in lotus position showing the location of the *chakras* from the base of the spine to the top of the head.

Right: Ayurvedic doctors recommend *chakradhara* after a period of *panchakarma*. "Once the body has undergone a detoxification process, it is ready for *chakra* balancing," says Ananda's Dr Sreenarayanan. "It is also good for patients with high cholesterol, diabetes and hypertension, as it helps reduce anxiety and stress."

120

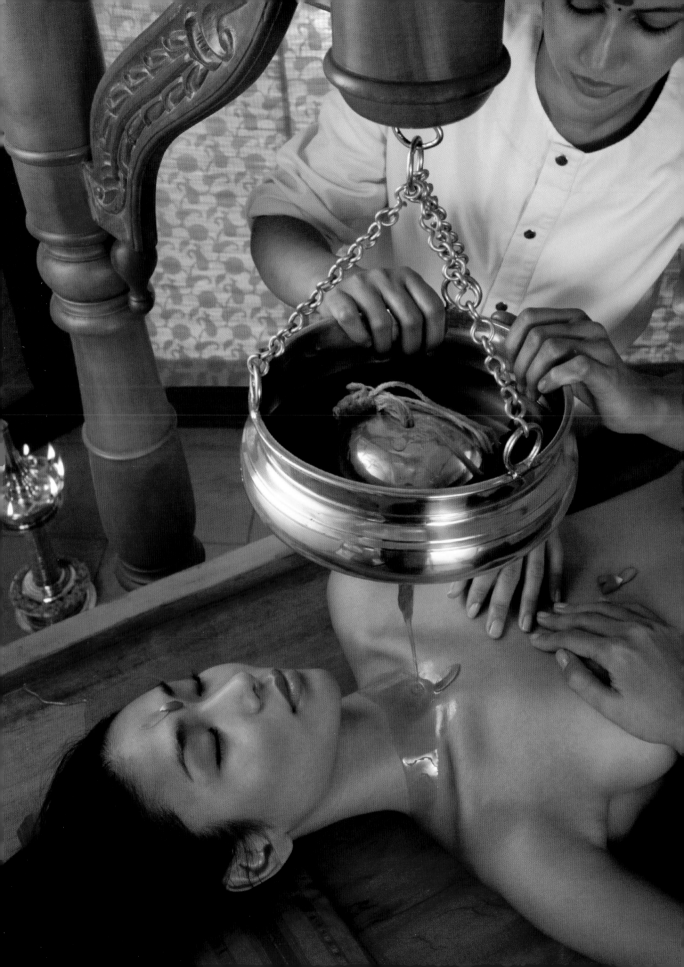

regulates the proper flow of the vital life. "It is particularly useful for people with improper lifestyle habits," explains Dr Sreenarayanan. "Their *chakras* are blocked as a result of stress, tension, bad diet, lack of exercise and so on. The therapy acts on the immune system, releasing energy flows, reducing anxiety and allowing the mind to become still and quiet." Another method for balancing the *chakras* is through stimulation of the *nadisuthra* points in *kalari* massage.

Furthermore, the *chakras* may be balanced by placing the hands gently over them, a few inches above the physical body. In this process, the recipient may be receptive to a flowing or warm sensation believed to be the transmission of universal energy.

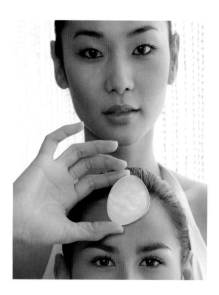

Known as Reiki, practitioners say it helps harmonise the body's biological and emotional systems. As universal energy is received, the "doors" for self-

healing are opened – helping with pain management and stress relief as well as with more spiritual goals. Reiki is offered at a number of spas in India, with the Ananda – in the Himalayas having a resident Reiki practitioner on hand.

The Seven Chakras

Chakra Seven: *Thought, universal identity, oriented to self-knowledge.* The crown *chakra* relates to consciousness as pure awareness. It is our connection to the greater world beyond, and, when developed, brings knowledge, wisdom, understanding, spiritual harmony and bliss.

Chakra Six: *Light, archetypal identity, oriented to self-reflection.* The brow *chakra* or third eye is related to the act of seeing, both physically and intuitively. As such, it opens our psychic faculties and gives us greater understanding of "the big picture".

Chakra Five: *Sound, creative identity, oriented to self-expression.* The throat *chakra* is related to communication and creativity. By experiencing the world symbolically through vibration (ie the vibration of sound representing language), a healthy fifth *chakra* results in expressiveness and erudition.

Chakra Four: *Air, social identity, oriented to self-acceptance.* The heart *chakra* is the middle *chakra* in the system of seven. It is related to love and is the integrator of opposites in the psyche: mind and body, male and female, persona and shadow, ego and unity. A healthy fourth *chakra* allows us to love deeply, feel compassion and experience a profound sense of peace and centeredness.

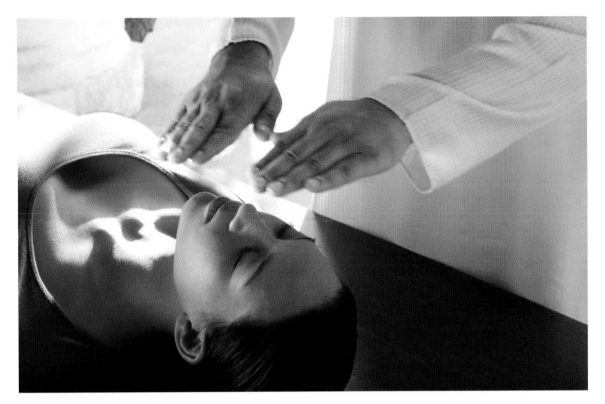

Chakra Three: *Fire, ego identity, oriented to self-definition.* Located in the solar plexus, this *chakra* is known as the power *chakra*. It rules our personal power, will and autonomy, as well as our metabolism. When healthy, it brings energy, effectiveness, spontaneity and non-dominating power.

Chakra Two: *Water, emotional identity, oriented to self-gratification.* Located in the abdomen, lower back and sexual organs, the second *chakra* connects us to others through feeling, desire, sensation and movement. Ideally this *chakra* brings us fluidity and grace, depth of feeling, sexual fulfillment and the ability to accept change.

Chakra One: *Earth, physical identity, oriented to self-preservation.* Located at the base of the spine, the first *chakra* forms our foundation. It is related to our survival instincts, our sense of grounding and to the physical plane. When healthy, this *chakra* brings health, prosperity, security and dynamic presence.

Opposite: Some of the world's principal oyster beds lie along the coasts of India, so references to mother-of-pearl and pearls are abundant in the Indian epics. They are potent when applied to the skin – as a powder or whole – especially on the *chakras*.

Above: Described by Ananda's Colin Hall as "calming and spiritual", Reiki comprises the laying of hands on, or above, the body's *chakras* and elsewhere to balance and heal. Here a Reiki master does his work at Mandarin Oriental Dhara Devi.

Classical Dance

Even though this book is primarily concerned with wellness and the various medicinal and therapeutic systems that have evolved in India over the centuries, it seemed important to include some of India's cultural practices that are associated with Indian wellness. All India's ancient systems emphasise the importance of the mental, the physical and the spiritual in their practices – and Indian dance (and associated practices such as music and martial arts) is no exception. It therefore seemed appropriate to touch on these ancient arts in some form or other.

In fact, Indian classical dance actually refers to a number of different forms of Hindu musical theatre. Its theory can be traced back to the *Natya Shastra* of Bharata Muni (400 BC) and it has been around for at least 2,500 years, probably longer. The Sangeet Natak Akademi currently confers classical status on eight forms: *bharatanatyam*, *kathak*, *kathakali*, *kuchipudi*, *manipuri*, *mohiniaattam*, *odissi* and *sattriya*. All include dance, story-telling, music and – most importantly – worship of the Divine.

Evolving in temples across the subcontinent, dance was originally performed by temple dancers in honour of the gods. Veneration of a god was conveyed by the dancing devotee with yearning expressions and feelings of loss and anguish when separated from him, as well as flirtatiousness and joy at his return. Dance's gradual move from sacred spaces to secular stages where elaborate performances were given at the various courts helped to further indelibly ingrain dance in Indian culture. Along with classical music, it is a powerful force.

The *Natya Shastra* is a common text for all Indian (and southeast Asian) dance forms. It contains descriptions of the different postures and *mudras* or hand movements, each depicting a particular meaning, and information about the construction of stages, makeup and orchestras. All dance forms are structured around the nine *rasas* or emotions:

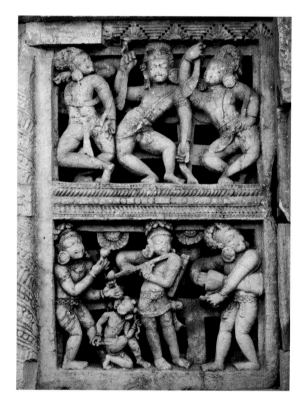

Above: The oldest of the Bhubaneswar temples in Orissa, the Parasurameswara temple dates to 650 AD. Dedicated to Lord Shiva, it is famous for its latticed windows; this one depicts musicians and dancers, notable for their sinuous, fluid forms.

Opposite: A *bharatanatyam* dancer from Tamil Nadu illustrates one of many *mudras* in the Pallava Dynasty Kailasanatha temple in the pilgrimage city of Kanchipuram. It is quite rare to find the performing arts practised in temples nowadays.

hasya (happiness), *krodha* (anger), *bhibatsa* (disgust), *bhaya* (fear), *viram* (courage), *karuna* (compassion), *adbhuta* (wonder) and *shanta* (serenity).

Indian classical dance is divided into *nritta* (rhythmic elements), *nritya* (a combination of expression and rhythm) and *natya* (drama). Most of its themes come from India's rich mythology and folk legends. As with many Indian practices, dance is also associated with wellness and wellbeing: by searching for truth and beauty, the performers are aiming for higher awareness. A brief summary of the different forms follows:

Bharatanatyam
Originating in Tamil Nadu, *bharatanatyam* is a 20th-century reconstruction of the ancient Tamil temple dance known as *cathir*. *Apsaras* or celestial dancers in *bharatanatyam* postures are found all over India in many Hindu temples. Developed in conjunction with the south Indian musical tradition of Carnatic music, it is today widely practised all over India.

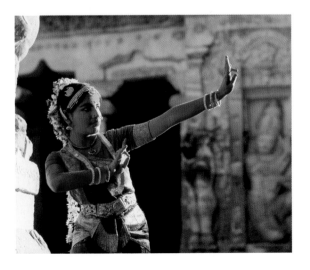

Mohiniaattam
Literally translating as "dance of the enchantress", *mohiniaattam* is a traditional Keralan dance. A drama in dance and verse, it was originally performed in temples; Lord Vishnu is usually the hero. The style is quite gentle, with approximately 40 different basic movements known as *atavukal*.

Kathakali
Kathakali is derived from *katha* meaning "story-telling" and *kali* translating as "play". Founded by the master Maharaj Binda Din, it is performed by two dancers; one who moves about and another who remains immobile the whole time. The latter expresses himself only with his face and hands. It is performed only by men.

On the physical side, the dancer must have perfect control of his body and limbs. This can only be achieved after at least 12 years of study and is facilitated by body conditioning, spiritual practices, massage and more. For the dancer who uses only facial expression, the control of the facial muscles is extraordinary: it is said that some masters of the art can laugh on one side of the face and cry on the other.

Odissi
Odissi hails from Orissa in eastern India. Originally performed solo by girls known as *devadasis* who received patronage from both king and temple, it is characterised by sinuous forms. It was revitalised in the 1950s – and three schools were formed: one followed the boy dancer tradition and was very acrobatic with strong hip movements. The second

125

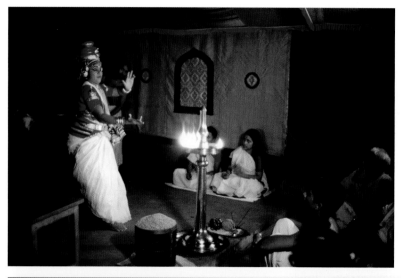

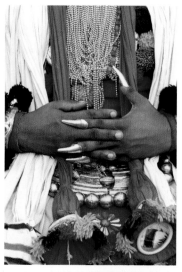

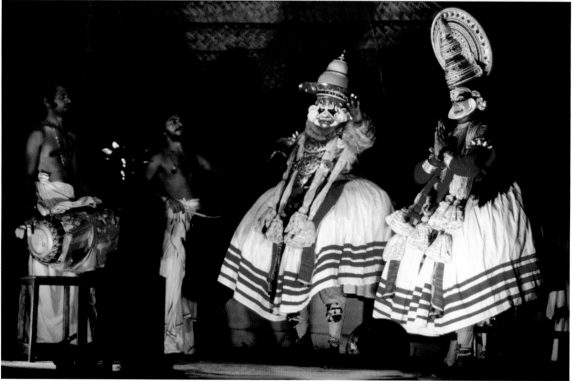

kept to the traditional, female style with the singing of songs and telling stories; while the third was a mix of the two. This latter type was further refined and developed and became the best known of the three. A typical *odissi* recital involves *mangalacharan* (invocation) to start, followed by *pallari* (pure dance) and *abhinaya* (interpretative verses), ending with *moksh* (a dance of liberation).

Kathak

Originating in north India, *kathak* is a narrative dance form, performances of which tend to follow a progression in tempo from slow to fast, ending with a dramatic climax. It originated in Hindu temples, but absorbed Persian influences from Moghul patronage in the 16th century. It is characterised by fast footwork and spins.

Kuchipudi

Originally performed by Brahmin boys in the village of Kuchelapuram, this dance form originated in Andhra Pradesh in southeast India. Talented performers were highly revered by the Deccan rulers. It acquired its 20th-century form when the dance was taken from the village to the stage by certain high-profile gurus. It is characterised by fast, rhythmic footwork and sculptural body movements.

Opposite top left: A perfomance of Vedic theatre, the earliest story-telling dance drama form, in Kerala.

Opposite top right and below: Kathakali performers take three to four hours to dress and make up their faces: Demons are characterised by red and black, *rajas* with red, and heroes and gods with green faces. Costumes are heavy and elaborate, and musicians provide trance-inducing drumming and singing.

Above right: Manipuri musicians in characteristic white costumes at a performance in Bengal.

Manipuri

A lyrical, graceful dance that originated in north-east India in Manipur state to adjacent Burma, *manipuri* is devotional in nature. Celebrating Radha and Krishna, it could very well have remained in the temples of the region were it not for Ravindranath Tagore, the Bengali poet, who fell in love with the dance and brought a number of *manipuri* dance teachers to the university he set up in Santiniketan

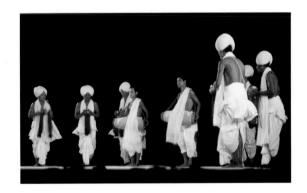

just north of Kolkata (Calcutta). Since it evolved in isolation in this remote mountainous region, it is very different from other Indian dance forms.

Sattriya

A 500-year-old classical dance form, *sattriya* originated in the remote Vaishnav monasteries of Assam, monasteries famous for their promotion of music, dance, drama and fine arts. *Sattriya* was first performed on a metropolitan stage in the second half of the 19th century, but it was only finally given due recognition as one of India's classical dance forms in 2001. Originally performed only by male monks, *sattriya* dancers are now both men and women. Its distinctive style is very physical.

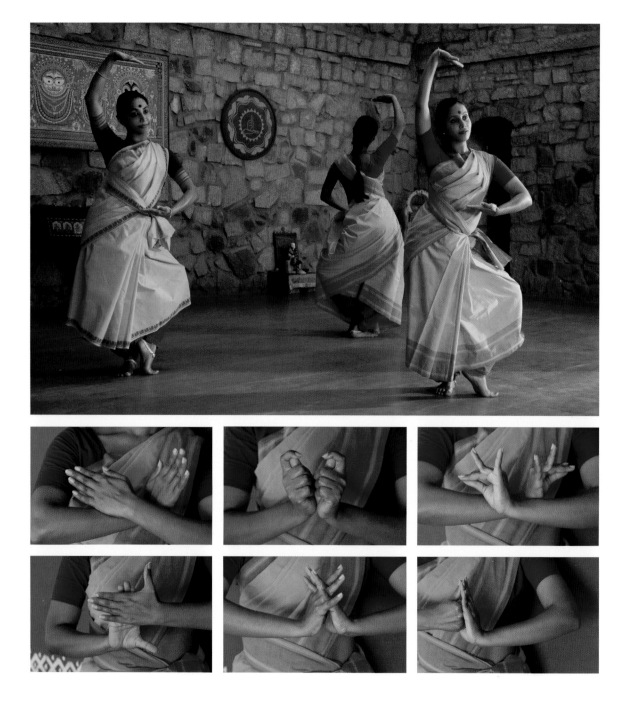

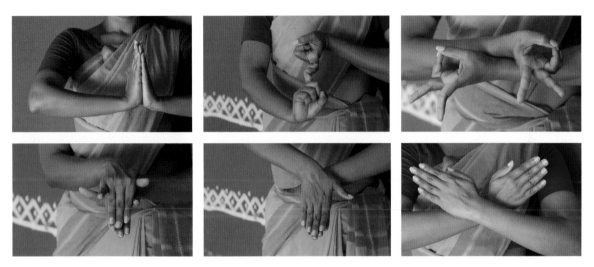

All the classical dance positions and movements are compiled and recorded in the *Natya Shastra* (400 BC): Hand positions, many based on physical imagery, are as important as other aspects, namely body positions, eye expressions and more. *Opposite top: Odissi* dance practice at Nrityagram. *Opposite below, clockwise from top left:* Swastika, two birds, two swans, *shankha* (conch), *karkata* (crab) and *chakra* (discus). *Above, clockwise from top left: Anjali* (greeting), knot, *kataka vardhana*, swastika, fish, snout of wild boar. *Below:* The *mudra* depicting the Shiva lingum, one of the holiest for Hindus.

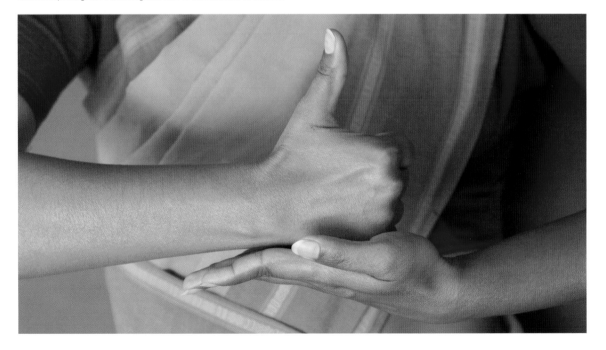

Kalari Payattu

A visit to "God's Own Country" (as Kerala is known) would not be complete without watching a highly skilled demonstration of the Keralan martial art of *kalari payattu*. Translating from Mahalayalam as "martial training inside a *kalari* or arena", it is a sheer joy to watch. Two combatants face each other – generally with swords and shields, long cane sticks or just bare hands – and perform a wheeling, dancing combat that involves high jumps, twists and death-defying sequences of agility and speed. Clad only in a loin-cloth, the practitioners of this art display strong self-discipline, moral integrity and spiritual awareness that is the result of arduous years of training. It is truly breathtaking in its beauty.

History of *Kalari Payattu*

Kalari payattu, the original martial art of Kerala, is believed to have been in existence from at least 1,500 BC, but its present form as practised today evolved during the ninth to the 12th centuries. It was first mentioned in the *Dhanur Veda*, the ancient Indian manual of warfare, where tales relate how the warrior sage Parasurama learned the lessons of this martial art from Lord Shiva. It is then believed that Parasurama taught these techniques to four Brahmin families to protect the divine land of Kerala; these families, in turn, passed its secrets to 21 masters who travelled to different parts of the country opening martial art schools.

Medieval Kerala comprised several small feudal principalities involved in frequent clashes, so the then kings recruited their soldiers from *kalari* schools.

Open to all castes and classes, *kalari* flourished as both a killing and a healing art. Traditionally, *kalari* fighters targeted their opponents' *marma* points to injure, but massage to these same or associated points, also stimulates healing. For example, if a warrior suffers a blow to the small intestine, the *marma* point on the back of the calf that corresponds directly with the upper intestine is massaged, to trigger a healing flow of energy to the area. Thus, masters or *gurukkal* of the art are experts in *kalari chikitsa*, a form of orthopaedic medicine, the science of *marmanam* or the art of the vital points, as well as the combat itself.

Kalari payattu suffered a setback at the end of the 18th century as the British banned the martial practice in 1793. *Kalari* schools were suppressed by law and the art was forced under-ground; only the truly dedicated dared to practise secretly at night. However, by the end of the 19th century, the dedicated efforts of the late *gurukkal* Sri Kottackal Kanaran and his disciple the late Sri CV Narayanan Nair revived this important part of Kerala's heritage: they gathered and systemised knowledge from the near-extinct schools, gave demonstrations, and instigated the opening of many new schools. Their efforts may be seen today at the C V N Kalari Sangham in Trivandrum, a training centre established in 1956.

Techniques and Training of *Kalari Payattu*

The martial art of *kalari payattu* may be divided into four different branches: *meythari* (physical methods of fighting); *kolthari* (fighting with wooden weapons);

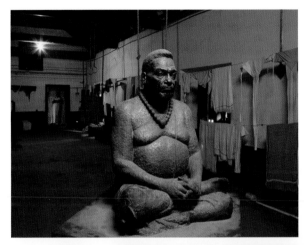

Opposite: A sword and shield is traditionally used in the more advanced combat techniques of *kalari payattu*.

Left: A statue of the sixth lord of the Poomully family, a large Brahmin family from north Kerala, stands in the *kalari* hall on the Pomully estate near Palakkad. Known as Arivinte Thampuran meaning "Lord of Knowledge", the late lord Poomuly Neelakantan Nambudiripad was a fountain of knowledge on the Vedic texts, yoga, Ayurveda and *kalari*. Revered as such, he instructed many disciples in the guru-*shishaya* tradition over the years; his statue serves to remind devotees of the skills they learned.

Below: Eighty-two-year-old *kalari* master from Poomully *mana*, Narayanan Nambudiri, has hung up his *kalari* equipment for a quiet retirement on the estate. Nevertheless, he still imparts advice to youngsters learning the art.

131

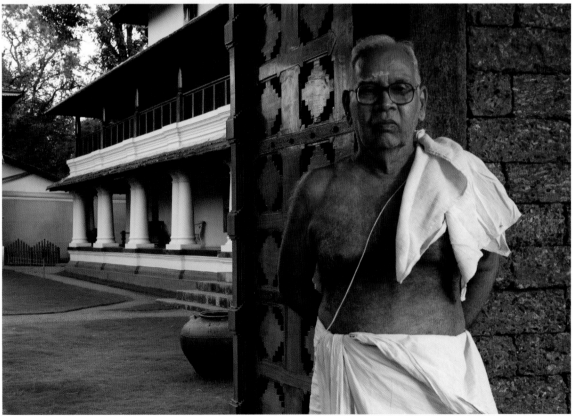

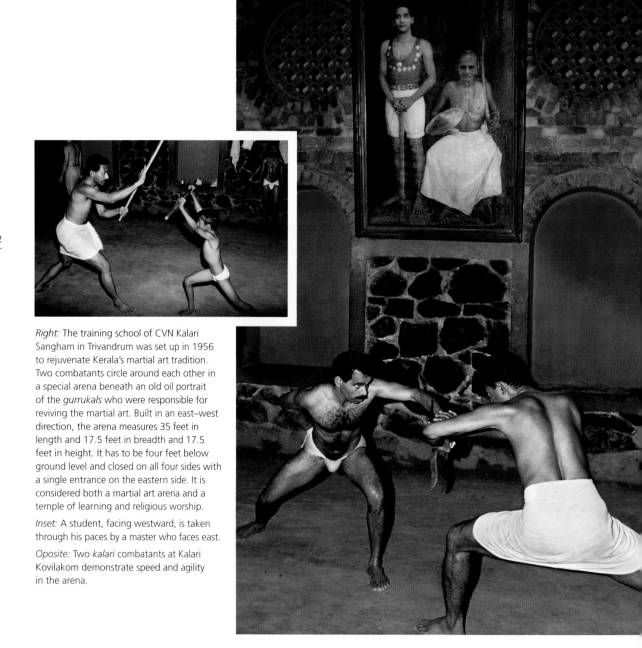

Right: The training school of CVN Kalari Sangham in Trivandrum was set up in 1956 to rejuvenate Kerala's martial art tradition. Two combatants circle around each other in a special arena beneath an old oil portrait of the *gurrukals* who were responsible for reviving the martial art. Built in an east–west direction, the arena measures 35 feet in length and 17.5 feet in breadth and 17.5 feet in height. It has to be four feet below ground level and closed on all four sides with a single entrance on the eastern side. It is considered both a martial art arena and a temple of learning and religious worship.

Inset: A student, facing westward, is taken through his paces by a master who faces east.

Opposite: Two *kalari* combatants at Kalari Kovilakom demonstrate speed and agility in the arena.

ankathari (fighting with weapons such as knives and swords; and *verum kai mura* (fighting with bare hands). Students, often as young as eight years old, begin with *meythari*, learning leg exercises, basic body postures and leaps. These scientifically prepared physical exercises and postures enhance the flexibility, firm footedness and self-confidence of the trainee. Once they are mastered, the trainee may advance to *kolthari*, whereby canes, cudgels and a special weapon in the shape of an elephant's trunk called an *ottakkol* are used. Certain sequences are practised again and again to enhance concentration and speed and ensure that the trainee has complete control over his weapon by making it an extension of his own body. Mastership of this stage only occurs after several years of intensive training.

The third phase, the *ankathari*, begins with the dagger and then moves on to the sword and shield, the weapons of the medieval Keralan soldier, as well as a number of other metal weapons. There are up to 12 different fighting methods using each weapon; these vary from highly accurate techniques of spear fighting to classical sequences with the mace and the dynamic *puliyankam* or "leopard fight" with the sword and spear, amongst others. One of the more famous is the *marapititcha kuntham*, a duel between a swordsman and a man armed with a spear.

During this stage, some advanced techniques of bare hand fighting may be taught; this is the final lesson in the curriculum containing some secret methods not revealed to beginners or outsiders for fear of misuse. Here, combatants learn how to fell an opponent by striking one or more of his *marma* points with his bare hands. Obviously *gurukkal* only reveal these techniques to disciples they feel totally confident in.

Techniques and Training of *Kalari Chikitsa*

Some of the healing techniques perfected by *gurukkal* are showcased on pages 66–67, but, in brief, they are techniques that have been formulated over time to care for wounded *kalari* practitioners. Comprising a number of different types of massage and various *kizhi* applications (see pages 44–49), they are instrumental in the cure of fractures, wounds and injuries to vital points. Most work on the principle of restoring energy flows of *prana* in the body; by releasing blockages, energy flow circulates to give life and animation to the physical body. This part of the curriculum is considered as important as the fighting techniques – as is the general demeanour of the *gurukkal*. He must be spiritually aware and strong in self-discipline, so that he may be a role model to his students.

133

Mud Wrestling

The Indo-Pakistani tradition of mud wrestling – although not nearly as popular as in its heyday some 50 years ago – is still a noteworthy inclusion in this book. As with some of the other mind/body/spirit practices, such as martial art and dance, mud wrestling is considered by Indians and Pakistanis (and Iranians, as much of its history comes from Persia) as much more than a sport or a profession.

As with *kalari payattu*, mud wrestling's origins lie in training for combat and self-defence, with matches often being fought to the death. The classical form of Indian wrestling known as *malla-yuddha* dates back to Vedic times with numerous legends describing wrestling bouts between gods and mortals from at least the 5th century BC onwards. Archaeological evidence suggests that the Hindu Aryan tradition of wrestling known as *kusthi* dates back to about 3,000 BC. Around the 17th century, it became integrated with a Persian form of wrestling (*pehlwani*) that was introduced to the subcontinent by the Moghuls; additional throws were added to the repertoire and Persian nomenclature became the norm. Over the years, it developed into a highly regulated sport with very particular rules, regulations, codes and standards.

Today, wrestlers are known as *pehlwan* from the Persian word *pahalavan* meaning "champion" or literally "a Parthian". A *pehlwan* is expected to be a man of high moral caliber, God-fearing and bound up in selflessness, humility and the greater good.

He follows a strictly disciplined routine that governs every aspect of his life. Rigorous training to build body strength and bulk and daily practice are part and parcel of a wrestler's life. He is expected to wake early, perform his ablutions, have an oil massage, then do weight-training and exercises that include press-ups and certain yoga *asanas*. After this, he enters the *akhara* or wrestling pit, turns to his coach (guru in Hindu wrestling, *khalifa* or *ustad* in the Moslem tradition) and asks his permission to wrestle with another *pehlwan* of his own age and physique. After lunch, a siesta is taken, then training recommences.

Diet is an important part of a *pehlwan's* routine. Buffalo milk, ghee and almonds were traditionally consumed in great quantities and, even nowadays, wrestlers are not supposed to take meat, alcohol or the digestive *paan*. By abstaining, they are able to discipline body and mind.

Training and fighting takes place in a standardised square earth-filled pit measuring approximately 20 by 20 feet (7 x 7 m) known as an *akhara*. A friend who remembers the art from her childhood relates: "Graceful movements, almost hypnotically spiritual,

Above and inset: The traditional Indo-Pakistani trophy awarded to champion wrestlers at a *dungal* or competition is known as a *gurz*. Varying in size, they are handmade, often of silver or gold, and are seen as a symbol of spirit, strength and skill.

Opposite: The wrestling *akharas* of Lahore still exist, although the sport is not as popular as it was in the past. Here a *pehlwan* grapples with a student (known as a *patha*). Such wrestlers are expected to practise morning and evening: the practice is tied up with such qualities as nobility, heroism and virtue.

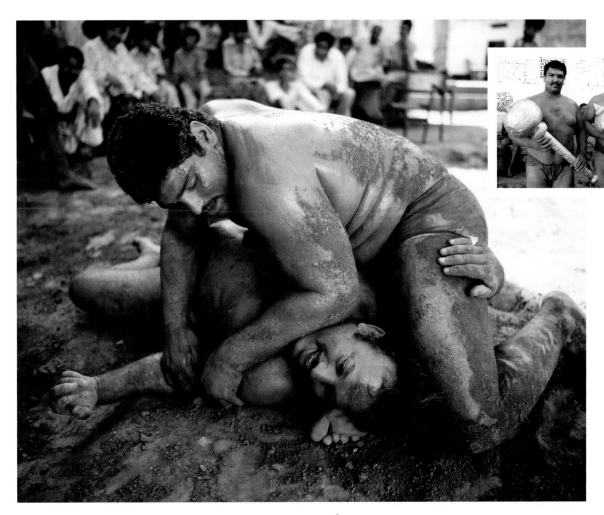

were accompanied by beating drums and poetry, but it was the silence and the beauty I recollect most about these powerful men and their skills."

Today, mud wrestling does not have such a popular following, and the *akhara* has more often than not given way to the mat and the ring. But the tradition continues to flourish mainly in the Punjab (in both India and Pakistan) and some academies for

pehlwani do still exist. Mostly charitable and privately owned, they are run along traditional guru-*shishaya* lines: Students are expected to devote their lives to clean living and hard exercise, and follow their teachers' example without question. In many ways, they are 21st-century equivalents of the spiritual disciple; by encountering tough physical and mental challenges, they become closer to the Divine.

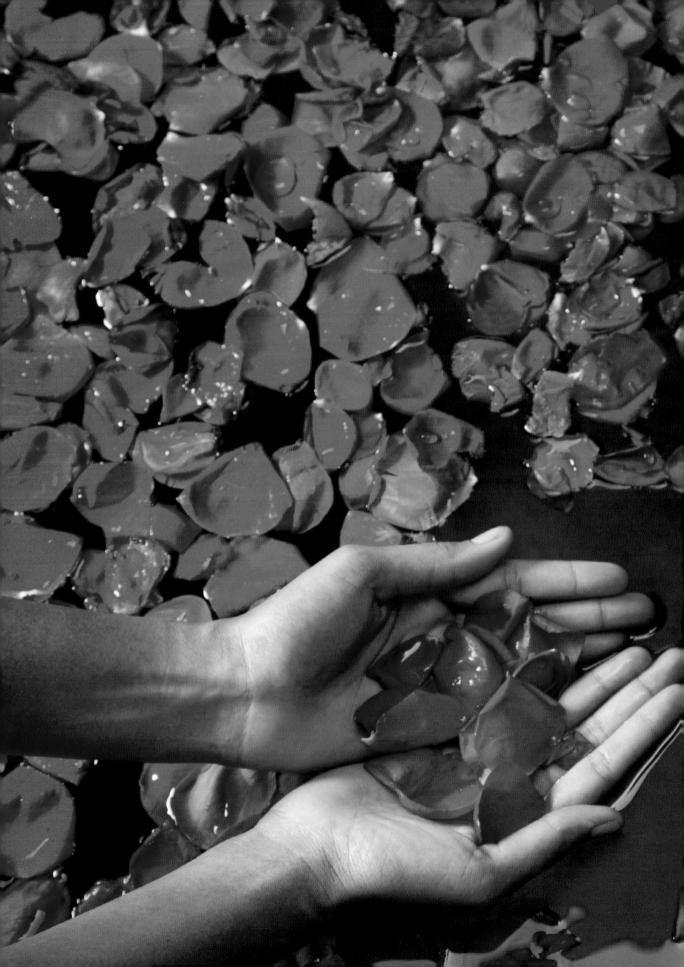

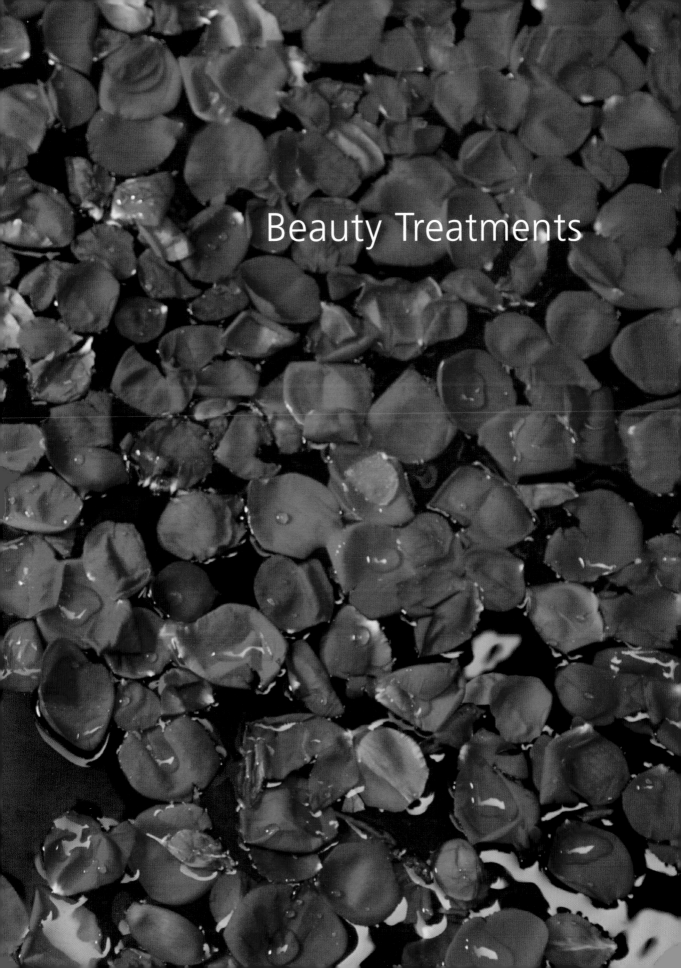

Beauty Treatments

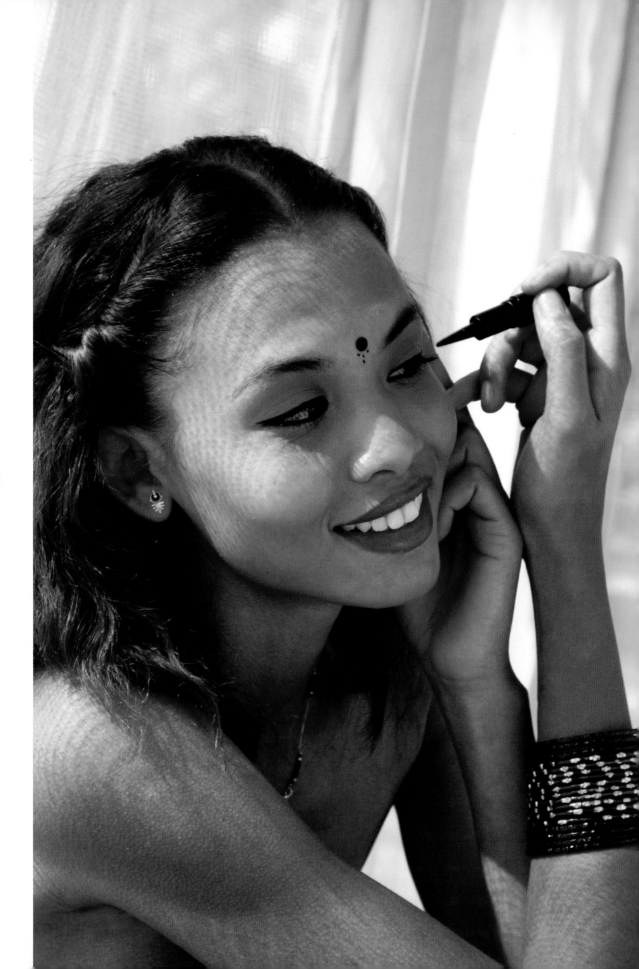

Traditional Facial Care

Indian women have been harnessing herbs and plants for skin and hair care for millenia. Numerous Sanskrit texts outline beauty treatments and evidence of natural cosmetics dates back to at least 3,000 BC in excavations of the Indus Valley civilisation in present-day Pakistan. Instructions for extracts of flowers, leaves, barks and herbs for both medicinal and cosmetic purposes are plentiful in the *Vedas* – and the flawless nature of Indian skin and hair is captured in countless paintings from the past.

Some of the more common Indian beauty products that have found a worldwide market include *kajal* or *kohl* eye-liner and *mehndi* (henna), as well as various perfumes and oils. *Kajal* was made famous by the Moghul Empress Nur Jehan; it is traditionally made from *triphala*, a three-part combination of *amla* (*Emblica officinalis*), *bibhitaki* (*Terminalia bellirica*) and *haritaki* (*Terminalia chebula*), almond, camphor and cabbage, all burnt in the oil of rose, and has been exported for decades. Oils of musk, sandalwood and rose have been traded along with Indian cotton and spices for centuries, and the Rajput combination of rose and milk for bathing is well documented. More recently, as people have become aware of the

Left: Kajal or *kohl* is used by Indians to define eyes, cool eyes and protect the wearer from evil. Thick and black, nowadays it is usually made from ground lead sulphide and comes in the form of a pencil.

Above: A Rajasthani miniature painting depicting a maid helping her mistress with her toilette (Mankot, *circa* 1720).

potential side effects of chemical and synthetic skin, hair and beauty products, Indian herbal recipes have become more popular in the global market.

Natural is the new buzzword, herbals are hip. The sages have always said this, and people around the world are beginning to listen. The brisk trade in herbal cosmetics and Ayurvedic creams, potions and lotions with their 100 percent natural tags is expanding from its exclusive domestic market to foreign shores. Indian homegrown remedies are no longer reserved for Indians alone.

The list of Indian manufacturers is too long to list here, but we have included some products we consider safe and excellent on pages 318–325. Particular mention must be made of Shahnaz Husain though. Herbalist, beautician and tireless promoter of the benefits of natural remedies, Husain is passionate about the power of India's herbal heritage. "The answer lies in turning back to Nature," she declares, "Treatments, cosmetics, plants and herbal extracts that have been lost in the mist of time are being revived once more, to be viewed in the light of modern scientific techniques." Husain's products, franchise of beauty salons and, more recently, foray into spas are testimony to the efficacy and safety of India's rich pharmacopoeia. If Selfridges and Bloomingdales believe in her, so should we.

In addition to manufacturing and selling products, India is beginning to capitalise on some

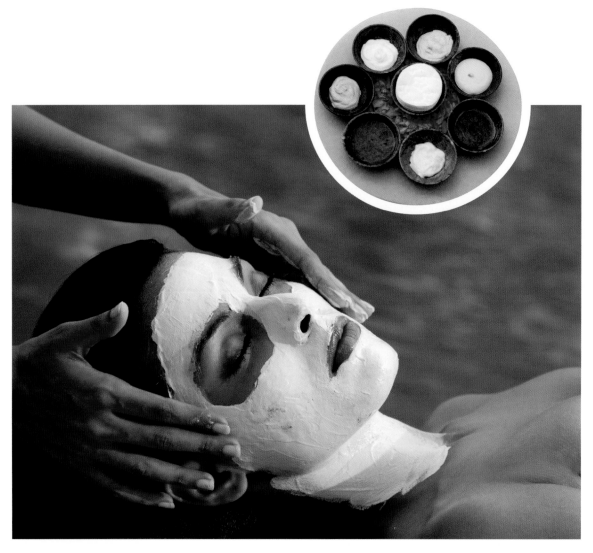

of its ancient beauty treatments too. Threading, the ancient art of facial hair extraction, is finding favour in London and New York day spas, and henna hair treatments are increasingly promoted in high-end hair salons. *Marma* massage on the vital energy points of the face is a therapy offered in many Asian spas and the Indian head massage is widely used as a "filler" whilst a client is resting with a face mask, for example. These, along with some of the more medicinal Ayurvedic treatments, are ones to watch out for.

We list some of India's most ravishing facial spa treatments in the following pages.

Shahi Nikhar

Aman Spa's "Royal Beauty" or Shahi Nikhar is a complete facial beauty treatment fit for a Maharani. A slight variation of the signature Aman facial that is offered around the globe, it is not particularly "Indian" but is worthy of inclusion because of the skill of the therapists who perform it. Products, from the 100 percent natural Aman range, are selected according to dry or normal skin and the sequence includes a cleanse, tone, scrub, massage, mask and moisturise. Between each section, a comforting hot towel is applied to the face to indicate a short hiatus in the rhythm.

Of particular note is the soothing, yet stimulating, facial massage with sweet almond oil: Nourishing for all skin types, almond oil has been used in India for centuries. Very gentle, it refines and moisturises skin, but also has a tightening effect. The massage begins with a flurry of soft strokes all over the face, and is followed by pressure point stimulation on the *marma* points on the face – around the eyes, below lips, above lips, either side of the nose, on forehead and temple and on the ear and earlobes. The pressure starts fairly soft, and increases in intensity through-out. The effect is extremely pleasant.

Kumarakom Mukhalepam

Ayurvedic facial treatments are offered at numerous spas throughout India, but the 100 percent natural sequence offered at Kumarakom Lake Resort is worthy of special mention because it combines plants, seeds, minerals and more in a thoroughly innovative manner. Known as *mukhalepam* (*mukha* is "face", *lepam* translates as "pack"), it conditions and nourishes skin, opens blocked pores, eliminates toxins and cleanses the face to improve skin texture.

Traditionally, Ayurvedic skincare recipes were designed according to the healing ingredients that women had to hand in their immediate vicinity. They took into account the condition or *vikruti* of a person's skin, and were made in the kitchen and

Opposite: The deeply nourishing mask in the Shahi Nikhar facial treatment at Amanbagh utilises honey, milk and rose for normal skins, and passionflower and geranium for dry skin. A mask is used to draw out pollutants from the skin's surface, as well as deep cleanse and refine the skin.

Opposite inset: Beauty on a plate: Amanbagh's selection of lotions for the *Shahi Nikhar* facial treatment are beautifully arranged on a marble plate with marigold flowers. Marigolds in India are often used for garlands and religious ceremonies: There is no special cultural or religious significance to the flower, but the vibrant colour is extremely appealing.

Below: The *Shahi Nikhar* pure rose moisturiser is perfect for normal skins: It is softening, anti-bacterial and stimulating and improves acne scars; it also has a beautiful scent. For dry skin, a cassia flower and chamomile moisturiser is used. Cassia is anti-oxidant, stimulating and warming, and chamomile is rejuvenating and soothing. Both moisturisers rehydrate the skin, and help to speed up the process of cell renewal.

141

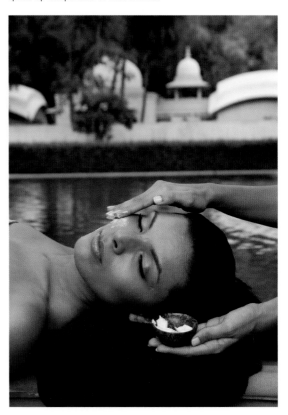

Right: Inexpensive, fast and neat, threading works well for facial hair and eyebrows. Using teeth and hands, the practitioner utilises a loop of thread to trap a series of unwanted hairs and pull them from the skin. As with normal plucking, results last from two to four weeks.

Opposite: Multani mitti, also known as Fuller's Earth, is available globally today. In fact, it is now synthetically manufactured and is composed mainly of silica, iron oxides, lime, magnesium and water. At Kumarakom Lake Resort, it is mixed with neem and sandal powder, carrot juice, egg white, orange juice, honey and a little cucumber juice to form a detoxifying face pack.

142

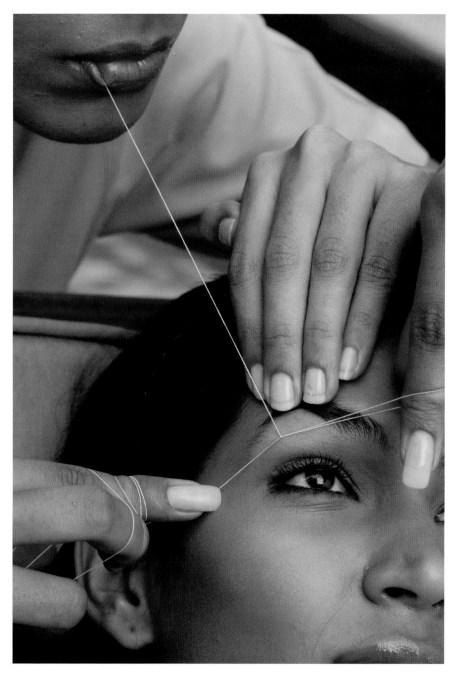

used immediately. Cleansing, nourishing and protecting are the three key components in Ayurvedic skin care and a full treatment is composed of eight steps: A thorough cleanse with an *ubtan* paste; an oleation massage on the reflex points and energy meridians on the face; a herbal steam or compress to bring out impurities; a gentle scrub to stimulate circulation and cleanse the pores; a mask or pack to deep cleanse, tauten and/or nourish skin; a toning/rejuvenating refresher to refine pores and tone the skin; a deep moisturiser to protect the skin from the elements and bacteria; and a gentle spray mist to assist absorption of the moisturiser and bring vitality to the complexion.

The Kumarakom ritual is excellent for dry, oily and combination skins and for people with different *doshas*. Made entirely from ingredients fresh from the market, it is good enough to eat. After the treatment, it is recommended that clients refrain from putting anything on the face for up to six hours. It comprises the following steps:

1. A mix of wheat powder and orange juice is applied to the skin to tighten it.

2. A natural cream made from pure aloe vera is massaged all over the face to cool the skin, help remove any blemishes and assist with sunburn.

3. Crushed cucumber is massaged on the facial area for ten minutes. Cucumber is a blood purifier; cooling and moisturising, it freshens the skin.

4. A gentle scrub, freshly made from orange peel and ground strawberry, guava and apple seeds, is applied in circular movements to exfoliate dead cells and stimulate circulation.

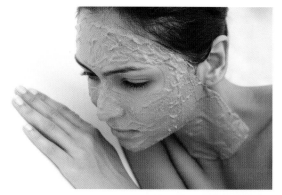

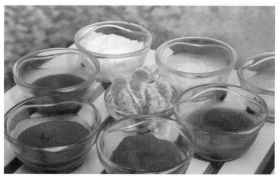

5. The skin is cleansed with hot water to help remove all traces of product without opening up the pores.

6. A polish of crushed papaya is massaged into the skin. Papain, the enzyme contained in papaya, softens and revitalises skin at a deep level.

7. A pack of *Multani mitti* powder mixed with neem and sandal powder, carrot juice, egg white, orange juice, honey and a little cucumber juice is applied all over face and neck, down to the décolletage. This dries very quickly and is left on for 20 minutes: during this time, the therapist may give the client a head massage while the ingredients work deep into the subcutaneous layer.

143

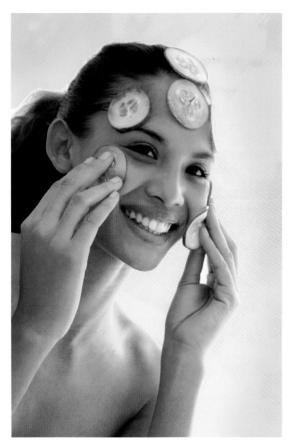

Above: Cucumbers (*kheera*) are plentiful in India, and often make the transition from the kitchen to the cosmetics' case. According to Ayurveda, they are best eaten in the morning, or second best at lunchtime, never at night. A cute little poem in India goes: "*Prabhat me kheera – heera hai; din me kheera – jeera hai; rat me kheera – peera hai*". This translates roughly as: "In the morning *kheera* are like diamonds (*heera*); in the afternoon *kheera* are like cumin (*jeera*); in the evening *kheera* are like pain (*peera*)." For cosmetic use, evenings are fine though!

Opposite: The energising facial treatment at Soukya: While the ingredients from Soukya's delicate warmed herbal pouches penetrate into the skin (*top*), a gentle massage increases peripheral circulation and oxygenates the facial cells. Turmeric, a staple in Indian cuisine, doubles up as a beauty product (*bottom*). When combined with *rawa* (wheat grains) and cleansing red sandal powder, it effectively exfoliates dead skin cells.

8. The ritual ends with the clay mix being washed off with cool water. There is no need for extra moisturising.

Soukya Ayurvedic Facial

According to Ayurvedic texts, the secret of beauty is *ojas* or the subtle quality of vigour or vitality that is the superfine essence of the seven *dhatus* or tissues of the body. If *ojas* is strong and healthy, one has a radiant inner self; this, in turn, manifests itself in one's outer physical appearance.

As with all the treatments at Soukya, its specially-formulated Ayurvedic facial works on both the inner and outer levels in order to develop *ojas*. It goes without saying that all sections are performed with Ayurvedic herbs chosen according to one's constitution and present state of health, combined with fresh fruits and vegetables selected according to skin types. Milk, curd, mint, honey, turmeric and sandal form its basis. The hand-picked ingredients supply much-needed vitamins and minerals to the skin, while packs even out colour tone, soothe and moisturise skin, and leave it soft and supple. Steam ensures that the ingredients are absorbed into the deepest layer of the skin, stimulating it and ensuring healthy new cell growth. The procedure is as follows:

1. Facial skin is cleansed with rosewater and massaged with honey. Honey is a humectant, both nourishing and moisturising, and can help soften scar tissue.

2. A freshly ground herbal mixture in which *chandana* (sandalwood) is the main ingredient is massaged on to the face to clean the skin.

antiseptic and antimicrobial properties work to remove any bacterial build-up.

3. A facial steam is given to open the pores and help dispel toxins from within.

4. A fresh scrub made primarily from *rawa* (wheat grains), turmeric and red sandal powder is used to exfoliate dead skin cells. Turmeric is a popular Indian scrub product, often used as a body scrub as well.

5. A small herbal pouch is warmed and used to massage the neck and face. This pouch contains the nourishing goodness of *lodhra* (*Sympiocos racemosa Roxb*), *yashtimadhu* (liquorice), *manjishta* (*Rubia tinctoriaa*), red sandal (*Santalum xanthocarpum*) and more, all boiled in milk for one hour. Astringent and cleansing both internally and externally, the warmth from the pouches helps send the herbal properties deep into the subcutaneous layers of the skin.

6. A pack, using the same herbal paste, is applied on face and neck and left on for 15 minutes.

7. A herbal skin toner made from a mixture of wild mint, rice and curd is applied. Mint is an antipruritic and curd helps the skin return back to its natural Ph balance. It is also moisturising.

8. The face undergoes a final cleanse, followed by a gentle skin moisturiser made from fresh aloe vera to leave skin cool and fresh.

The sequence takes about an hour. "The aroma of the fresh herbs helps rejuvenate the mind and the skin," Ayurvedic doctor, Dr Ajitha, explains "and the natural ingredients remove blemishes and scars, and soothe, soften and moisturise skin."

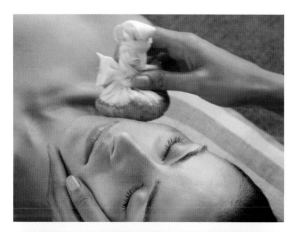

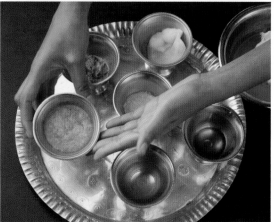

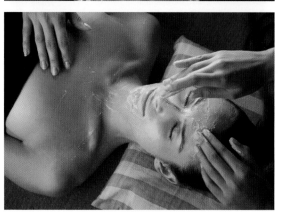

Aura Spas' fresh-from-the-garden Facials

Park Hotels are leaders in the hospitality field in India in more ways than one. Well known for its innovative, contemporary interiors and snappy service, it is now making waves on the spa scene with a line of day spas called Aura. With a tagline of "inner vitality, outer glow", the spas are guaranteed to combat stressful symptoms.

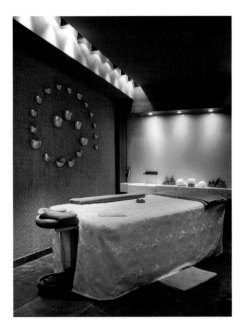

Designed to relax and refresh, each treatment is highly sensuous. Given either in your hotel room or one of the spa's relaxing treatment rooms (see above), you'll emerge feeling a hundred times better than when you arrived. If it's a facial boost you're after, you can't go wrong choosing one of the super-fresh, straight-from-nature facial treatments.

Harnessing the power of rare combinations of natural herbs, fruits, flowers and spices, each facial treatment is individually designed for different complexions. Those with dry skin would be well advised to try the saffron and almond facial: a gentle anti-aging treatment, it uses pure *rawa* (semolina) for exfoliation and then gives skin a beauty blast with a saffron and almond mask. Saffron is a useful ingredient for boosting skin longevity and almonds are high in Vitamin E, a crucial component in skin softening. The result is the minimising of fine lines, a tightening of the skin and a refreshed, clearer complexion.

The fresh apple facial, on the other hand, is recommended for oily to normal skins. Kashmiri women, renowned within India for their clear, fair complexions, have applied mashed apple and apricots, mixed with honey, to their faces for centuries. At Aura, slices of apple, rich in antioxidants and creamed with humectant honey, are rubbed on to the face to rehydrate and revitalise. With its fresh, fruity aroma and the gentle nurturing movements of well-trained therapists, this facial fires skin with an inner glow.

Left: With a colour palette of beiges and green and a homely use of organics in the decor, Aura spa in New Delhi gives guests the cream of the crop in facial therapies.

Right: Using ingredients once reserved for culinary purposes on the skin has gained popularity worldwide, especially with the growth in allergies and sensitivity to pollution. Of course, the ancients in India have known this all along: This aromatherapy facial from Aura spa New Delhi uses the healing powers of essential oils of lavender, tea tree and rose absolute with a base of grapeseed oil. It is effective in extracting impurities, nurturing new cells and maintaining the skin's natural pH balance. You'll be mentally relaxed with a gorgeous scent on the skin too.

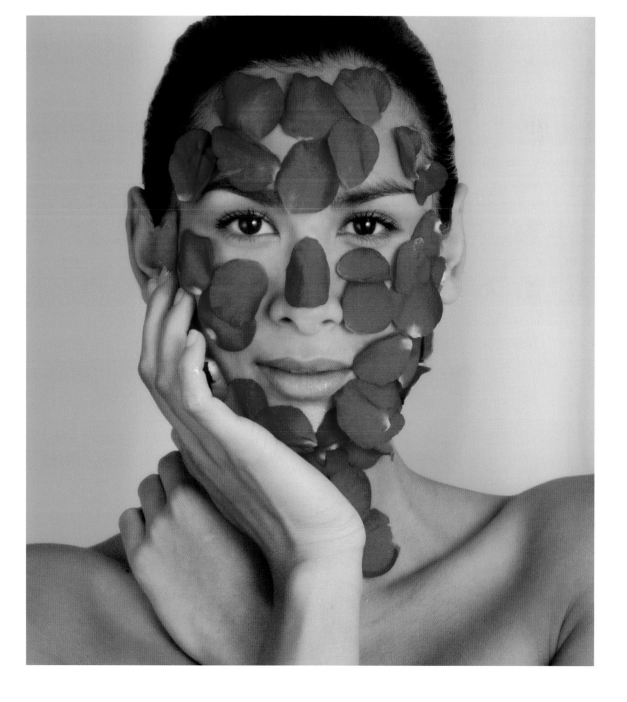

Hand Care

Ayurvedic texts emphasise the importance of self-care, declaring that the body has the means to heal itself. As such, there are numerous guidelines in the major medical treatises for maintenance of healthy skin, organs, digestive system and more. Ayurvedic practitioners are on hand to guide patients, giving them self-knowledge for healing, but ultimately people need to be responsible for their own health. If God really is to be found in the details (and it was not only Mies van der Rohe who believed this), self-care for every part of the system is *de rigeur*. Hand and nail care is no exception.

If *ojas* is strong and life force is flowing freely, a person looks dynamic, vigorous and well-cared for. A toxin-free internal system is reflected externally with glowing skin, bright eyes and healthy limbs. Similarly, such a person will be mentally assertive, emotionally caring and spiritually pure.

On the other hand, if there are internal health problems, they may be detectable externally. In many cases they are reflected in the state of one's finger nails. As nails are a by-product (*mala*) of bones (*asthi dhatu*), they often reflect problems within the body tissues (*dhatu*). For example, a liver condition called Wilson's Disease is easily spotted by the formation of exaggerated large whitish areas on the nails. White spots on the nails show a zinc or calcium deficiency, while brown lines running down the nail indicate possible inflammatory bowel disease. Brittle nails can warn of low iron or vitamin A, kidney malfunction or poor circulation.

Ayurvedic doctors suggest regular nail inspection, and daily or weekly hand and nail care. Hands are a vulnerable part of the body and are subject to premature ageing, so need daily attention. A hand massage is an excellent way to stimulate *marma* points and energy meridians, thus releasing toxins and invigorating *ojas*. As with the feet, certain points on the hands are associated with various organs and systems within the body, so a hand massage is not only locally stimulating. For example, pressing gently into the centre of the palm stimulates the kidney area, while a massage between the thumb and index finger helps with digestion.

Many spas in India offer hand massage, often as a prelude or to accompany another treatment. Comprising part of a *karashubakari* ("manicure" in Sanskrit), it can be very pleasant. Many of these manicures utilise homemade herbal pastes, scrubs and tonics and combine them with mainstream hand and nail care such as cutting and filing nails, cuticle care and the application of nail polish. Of particular note is the pampering manicure at the Indus Valley Ayurvedic Centre: in this sequence, milk (high in lactic acid) is used to soften hands; a disinfecting neem paste makes for a tingling purifier; herbal medicated oil according to one's *dosha* is the base for a vigorous hand massage; gelatine and lemon removes dead surface cells while lemon juice and sugar exfoliates; and a herbal pack made from *Multani mitti*, milk and rosewater tightens the skin. The entire procedure is offered in the bespoke beauty salon where the guest's comfort and relaxation are the primary concern. With a cup of hot herbal tea and views over India's healing heartlands, this is a ritual to relish.

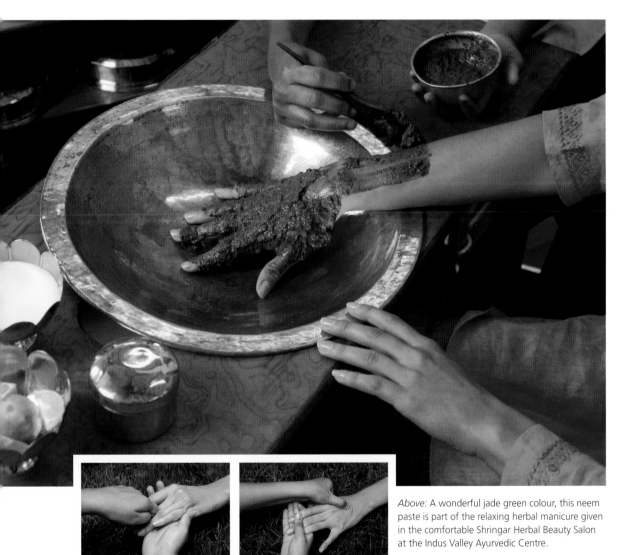

Above: A wonderful jade green colour, this neem paste is part of the relaxing herbal manicure given in the comfortable Shringar Herbal Beauty Salon at the Indus Valley Ayurvedic Centre.

Left: A particular technique of hand massage is employed by certain therapists at Aura spas at Park hotels. Designed to release emotions, it can be quite a powerful experience. The therapist pushes up from the tip of the finger to release energy – and the techniques are also employed elsewhere on the body.

Foot Care

In India, when entering a home, it is traditional to step across the threshold with the right foot first. Shoes are often taken off, as they are when entering a temple or mosque (here feet are often washed as well), and touching the feet of an elder is considered a mark of respect. As in other parts of Asia, feet are full of symbolism.

A footbath was traditionally offered to visitors after a long journey, and today, it often sets the tone at a spa. "At all our spas we offer a cleans-ing mint footbath and *marma* massage of feet, ankles and calves before therapy," explains Sangeeta Sharma of Sansha Spas. "It is both relaxing and calming, and sets the tone for the treatment to follow." In addition, it benefits more than the feet and legs: it revitalises the nervous system, improves circulation, tones muscles and provides a feeling of relaxation and general wellbeing.

According to Ayurvedic lore, an imbalance of *vata* lies at the heart of all foot problems. As is usual, physicians recommend prevention rather than cure, stressing that regular foot care, proper posture and sensible footwear also go a long way towards ameliorating existing problems. Hydrotherapy in the form of alternating hot and cold footbaths helps with aching feet and poor circulation, while regular foot hygiene and exercise allow you to put your best foot forward at all times.

Foot Massage

The *Charaka Samita* notes that the application of oil is the best remedy for tired or neglected feet. It is said to alleviate coarse and rough skin and reduce stiffness, fatigue and numbness. Furthermore, after a *padhabyangha* massage (foot massage with oil), localised veins and ligaments are strengthened and feet become firm and strong. In addition, vision is supposed to be enhanced, as nerves in the soles of the feet are associated with the eyes.

Padhabyangham tends to concentrate on the pressure points located on the soles of the feet as Ayurvedic doctors say that they are connected by energy channels to internal organs. Sesame or cooling coconut oil are favoured, and if the oil is

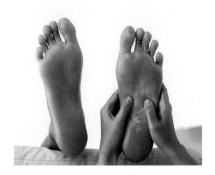

enlivened with essential oils such as peppermint, *tulsi* or black pepper, feet are also given a spicy, antiseptic and tension-relieving boost. It is said that a strong rotating, kneading foot massage before bed results in a tranquil night's sleep.

At many spas both in India and elsewhere, foot reflexology or foot massage is a staple on the menu. Often given whilst a client lies cocooned in a body wrap or as one part of a foot ritual, there is something wickedly sensual about having your feet nurtured in such a manner. Another option is to walk along an uneven path in bare feet (as recommended at Soukya and Kalari Kovilakom) or take a stroll in a Kneipp footbath. Developed by a 19th-century Bavarian priest who favoured long morning walks in grass wet with dew, this combines the benefits of the Asian reflexology path with its uneven stones underfoot and the healing powers of cold water.

At the Ananda spa, there is a wonderful marble circular foot bath in a relaxing setting: a couple of circumambulations around it sends messages from the trigger points on the soles of the feet through the meridian channels to the internal organs. Your body (and mind) will benefit, even if your feet feel a little painful.

Foot Scrubs

In the same way that soap was eschewed in favour of an *ubtan* scrub to cleanse and purify the body, Indian beauty therapists and physicians recommend the use of a scrub for cleaning the feet. Not only does this exfoliate dead skin cells, it helps prevent foot odour and the fungal and bacterial infections that are so prevalent in hot climates.

CHI spas offer a liberating Tibetan Foot Ritual that employs a pine-scented salt scrub enlivened with dried sage and juniper and tangy spikenard essential oil. For a very Indian sensation, try the Masala spice scrub at Taj spas: A surefire boost for the circulation, it also promotes deep cleansing. Another winner is the organic thyme and peppermint scrub at Quan spa at JW Marriott in Mumbai. When followed by a *marma* massage with *parijat* oil, it leaves the whole body profoundly relaxed.

Make your own exfoliating mixture of two parts coarse oatmeal, two parts chickpea flour (available at Indian grocery stores) and one part rosewater. Add warm water as needed to form a thick paste. Massage all over, then rinse off in a floral footbath.

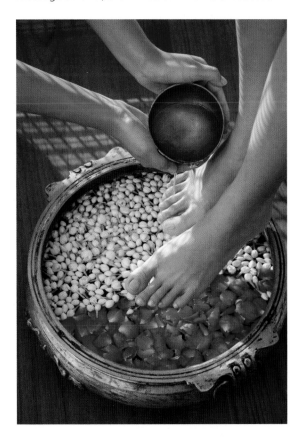

151

Opposite: "As the snake doesn't approach the eagle, so disease doesn't affect the person who massages his feet before sleeping" goes an old Indian saying. As such, foot massage to the *marma* points on the feet is a family activity, often given by children to elders. Invigorating and enlivening, it is good not only for the feet, but for the entire body.

Above: The floral footbath is a staple at Indian spas and salons, often offered at the beginning of a treatment. Jasmin and rose are perhaps the most scent-sual of combinations.

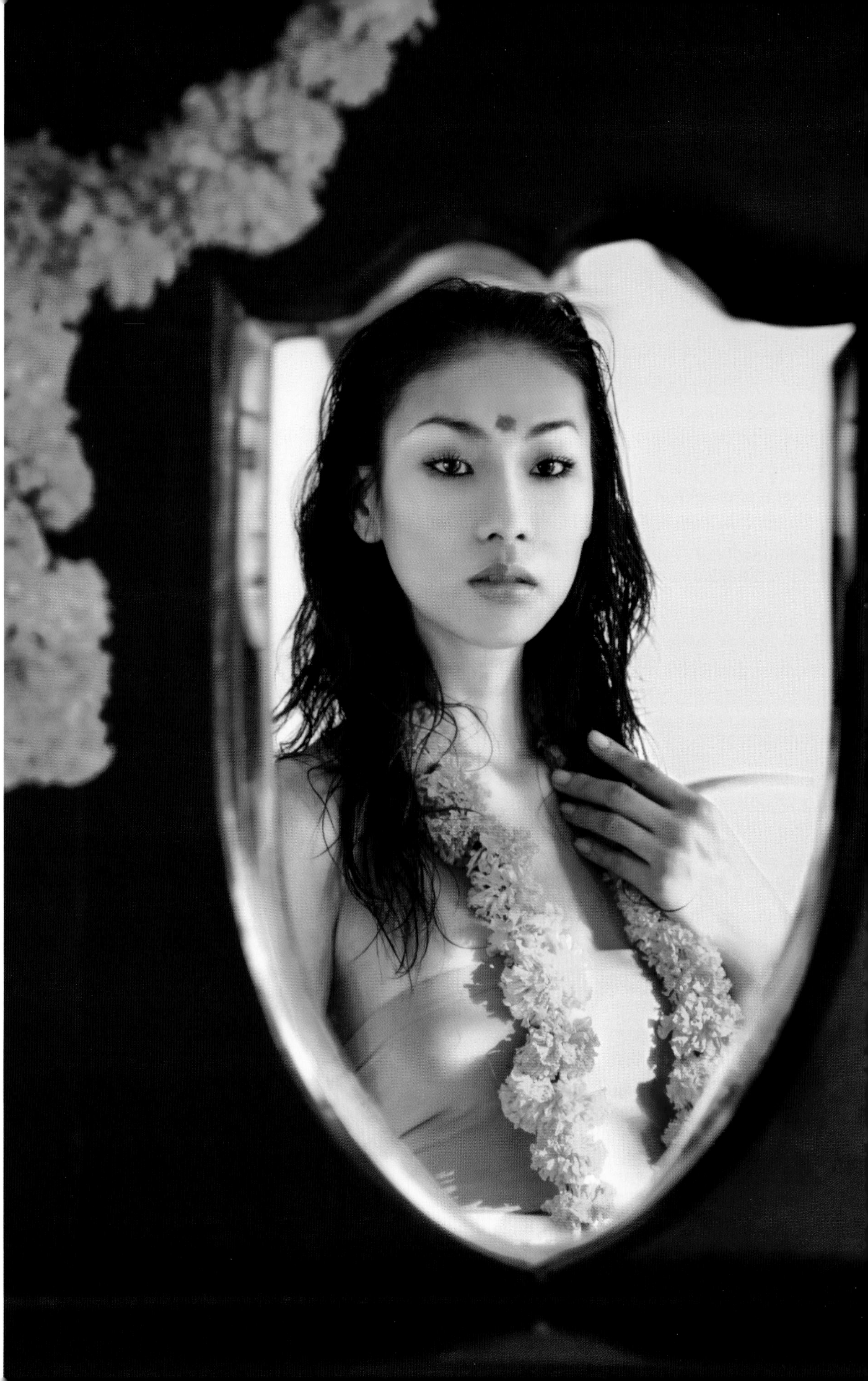

Hair Care

Indian women are renowned for their dark, thick and lustrous locks. Ancient texts contain numerous references to treatments, rinses, lotions, infusions and pastes for beautifying, strengthening and improving the health of hair, emphasising how Indians have always prized hair as an integral part of beauty. In Indian paintings, women are depicted with long hair or ornamented hairstyles, and the pantheon of Hindu goddesses is always depicted with elaborate head gear.

Indian brides take great pride in their hairstyles, with different regions favouring different styles. The Punjabi bride wears a red *parandi* (a silk tassel) in her hair, while Bengali and Maharashtran brides opt for buns decorated with white flowers. Further south in Tamil Nadu, white, orange and pink blossoms are woven around a central plait, while Keralan brides sport a veil of jasmine buds tied to form a net. In the *Kumarasambhavam*, the famous Sanskrit epic poem by the poet Kalidasa, the hair preparations for the goddess Parvati's wedding to Shiva are described in detail: First her maids dried and scented her hair with incense, then they

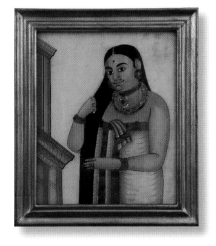

plaited it into a graceful braid, and finally decorated it with inlaid flowers and a garland of *madhuka* flowers woven with *durva* grass.

Scenting the hair with smoke or incense (*dhoop*) while it dries is a tradition that has been practised by Indian womenfolk for centuries. Burning charcoal, mixed with *sallaki* (a powder made from the gum of the *Boswellia serrata* tree), is placed on an earthen or brass tray and wafted beneath long tresses. The ancient equivalent of a hair dryer, it helps with drying after washing, imparts fragrance to the hair and prevents fungal infections, dandruff and other hair problems.

Shampoos were always traditionally made from herbal powders, both Ayurvedic and otherwise, and many are still in use today. Popular herbs for cleansing are the highly scented orris root powder, thickening arrowroot powder, *amla* or Indian gooseberry, neem and sandalwood for their antiseptic properties, and *reetha* or soap nut. *Shikakai*, literally "fruit for hair", is another traditional shampoo in the form of a paste: Made from *Acacia concinna* bark that contains high levels of saponins or foaming agents, it is a mild cleanser. Whilst the lather is rather weak, it has a naturally low pH, so does not strip hair of its natural oils. It also acts as a de-tangler and is a useful anti-dandruff tool.

153

Above: Indian women traditionally sport long tresses as this Keralan portrait on glass illustrates. Often depicting everyday, household activities, such paintings were probably introduced to India by the British in the 18th century. Subject matter included religious themes, portraiture, folk art, and more. Their intention was purely decorative.

Opposite: Finishing touches to tresses.

Another ancient custom for healthy hair and scalp often given on a daily basis is an Indian head massage (see pages 40–41). Less time-intensive is a quick application of hair oil: there are literally hundreds of such oils on the market and Indians believe that they help hair grow luxuriantly thick, soft and glossy. In addition, they are supposed to soothe and invigorate the sense organs and even remove wrinkles from the face! Popular hair oils

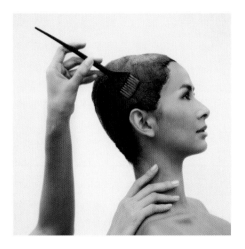

contain *bhringaraj*, *brahmi* and *amla*, often combined with other strengthening, conditioning and antiseptic herbs and plants.

A plant much used in Indian hair care is *mehndi* or henna (see pages 162–165). Antiseptic and nutritious, it is a popular hair conditioner and gives grey hair a red-orange tint. It has the ability to coat the hair shaft, thereby protecting and thickening hair. "One of India's age-old beauty secrets is a henna conditioner," says Shahnaz Husain. "Made from henna paste, mixed with lemon juice, egg and yoghurt, it cleanses and conditions hair, promotes new hair growth and restores good health to the scalp." She goes on to add that, unlike chemical detergents, it doesn't destroy the natural acid nature of the scalp or dry out the hair, and leaves hair shiny and supple. Essential oil of henna is also very cooling on the head.

A variety of hair cleansing and conditioning routines are available at Shahnaz Husain salons and day spas – and over-the-counter conditioners, rinses and tonics are available in her 100 percent herbal range. Of particular note is the fresh-from-the-fridge crushed banana, grated carrot and sliced cucumber combo, while the hot oil pack is nourishing, anti-bacterial and cleansing on the scalp. Many other spas in India offer the sublime head massage or *champi*, often as part of a face or body ritual. A wonderful treat for sensitive scalp and dehydrated and dry hair is the Ananda spa's aromatic hot oil treatment using pure essence of lavender, geranium and rosemary. For a four-pronged treat, head to the highly authentic spa at Neemrana Fort Palace for the heavenly *sirolepam* (see overleaf).

Left: Regenerating for the hair and stimulating for the scalp, a henna conditioning treatment is a staple at many Indian beauty salons. After application, the paste needs to rest on the head for at least half an hour, then should be washed off with lukewarm water. Hair is cleansed, fresh and vital after. This treatment is taken from the nail and hair salon, adjacent to the Aura spa in the Park New Delhi.

Right: The resin of the *Boswellia serrata* tree is harvested in a manner similar to rubber tapping; the gum is then ground into a powder and used in a charcoal burner to scent the hair. More commonly known as frankincense, the powder is also used in religious rites and perfumery.

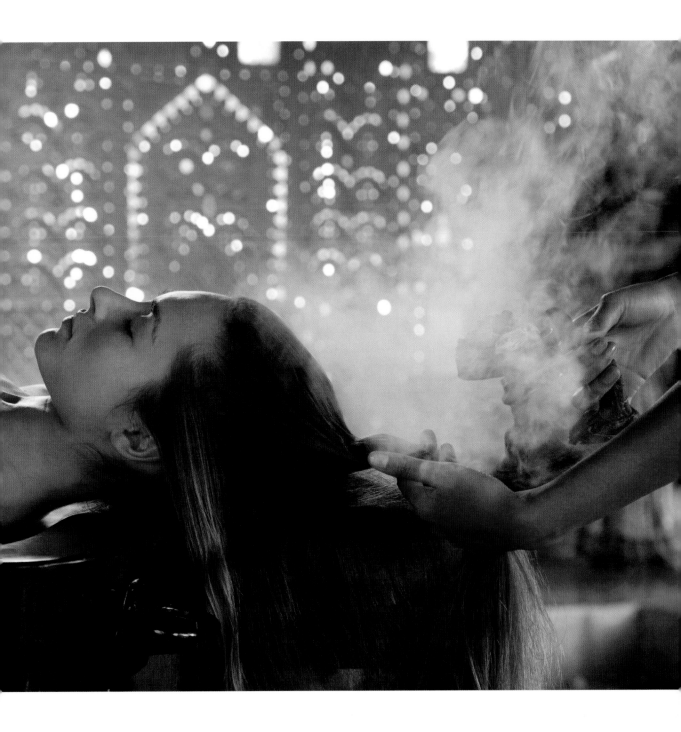

Sirolepam

Formulated by Sansha Spa therapists and using Sansha's 100 percent natural products, this is a four-part head, neck, face and shoulder massage along with a pack to stimulate hair growth and revitalise the brain. The massage is based on Ayurvedic head massage and *marma* point techniques, while the products are formulated with the best of both Eastern and Western herbs, plants and essences. Taken from the words, *siro* meaning "head" and *lepam* translating as "pack", the treatment is an authentic Indian salon staple. We take you through the therapeutic and relaxing ritual offered at the spa at Neemrana Fort Palace.

Head massage has been practised in India for more than 1,000 years if not longer, and is believed to have a strong effect on the three higher *chakras* of

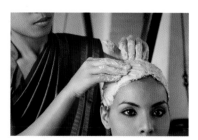

the seven. These are the crown, "third eye" and throat *chakras*, related to self-knowledge, self-reflection and self-expression respectively. As such, they can retain tension and stress if not opened effectively, so massaging the head, neck and shoulders can do much to affect our mind, body and spirit.

Traditionally an Indian head massage is done with oil, but Sansha's *sirolepa* treatment uses a coconut and jojoba cream formulation that is

cooling, moisturising and has anti-dandruff properties. Techniques include pressure point, root pull, spider walk and comb, all of which stimulate the scalp, aid localised blood circulation and ease tension. The head massage is followed by a face and neck massage that may also reach down to the shoulders. If the complexion is normal to dry, a deeply luxurious lotus, avocado and lemongrass cream is used; if it is oily, this is substituted for a saffron and wild turmeric formulation. Both are hydrating and nourishing.

It is hoped that the client will be in a state of deep relaxation by this point, so the application of the mud and yoghurt hair pack allows for a little rest time. Applied all over the hair, it has a thermal effect on the scalp, penetrating deep into the epidermal layer of the skin to help with such problems as insomnia, headache, depression, mental stress and the like. If you are lucky enough not to suffer from any of the above, it also helps to condition hair. Held in place by a piece of firmly secured cloth, the pack is left on for 15 minutes, before being shampoo-ed off with a coconut milk and apple hair cleanser. The latter is very gentle, so is suitable for all hair types.

Left: A mud and yoghurt pack is applied all over the head to penetrate deeply into the epidermal layer of the scalp.

Right: Traditionally hair packs were covered with banana leaf wraps. Here, leaves from a local tree hold the pack in place.

Opposite top: An Indian head massage usually includes the face, neck and shoulder areas in addition to the head. In Neemrana Fort Palace's *sirolepam*, the therapist uses an application of deeply penetrating Sansha Spa massage creams on these areas.

Opposite bottom: The origin of the English word shampoo comes from *champi*, the Hindi word for head massage. Being *champi*-ed works both on the surface (preserving the condition of hair) and within (relief of tension, spiritual awareness).

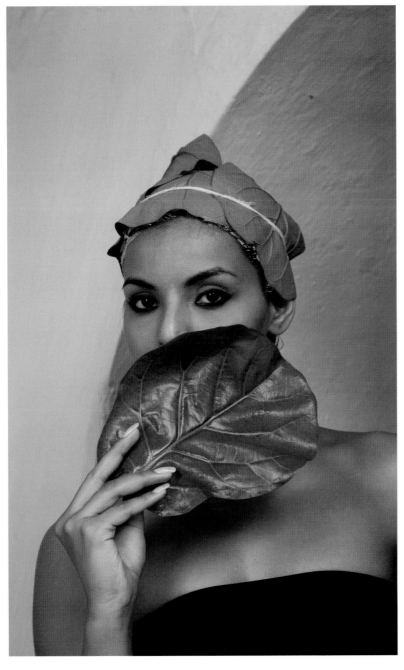

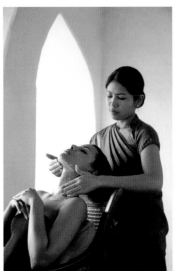

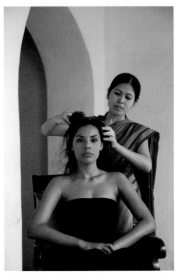

Shahi Angalepan

Oatmeal, herb powder scrub (*ubtan*), and jasmine oil,
Princess (bride) is sitting with dreams for *ubtan*,
Come on grandfather, see your beloved granddaughter,
Smiling face, eyes full of dreams,
Sitting like a princess for *ubtana*.

– *Old Rajasthani Folk Song*

Translating from Hindi as "Royal Experience", Amanbagh's re-creation of a typical Rajput beauty regime is thankfully no longer reserved for royalty. Hotel guests are invited to experience the medicinal and pampering effects of this indulgent two-and-a-half hour journey to bliss – and many swear by its long-lasting benefits.

Despite following quite a common sequence (scrub, steam, wrap, massage), it is the quality of the ingredients and the fidelity to local tradition that put this ritual ahead of the competition. Before Indian independence, when the princely states were at the height of their powers, certain ingredients were retained for the women of the Courts: Rose petals were out of the range of mere mortals, and saffron – rare, expensive and golden – was drunk with milk by pregnant Maharanis in the belief that any progeny would be born with a golden and light complexion. Whether this worked or not is anyone's guess, but certainly its cost would have been prohibitive to ordinary people. Indeed, the women's quarters or *zenana* of any Court was the domain of many beauty secrets, and these were carefully guarded.

Outside the palace gates, however, the villagers had their own, albeit less elaborate, beauty elixirs — and many of these may still be found in the countryside around Amanbagh's gates. Black clay is traditionally used in Rajasthan to nourish and tighten skin; it is applied externally on skin diseases and is also used to wash the hair. Garam flour and oatmeal, found in most kitchens, is used for the traditional *ubtan* scrub given to every Hindu bride, and blooms of hibiscus growing liberally in pots around village homes is used as a hair conditioner. All these everyday ingredients are used in the aromatic Shahi Angalepan.

The ritual begins with a body scrub that has been especially formulated by Amanbagh's spa manager as a tribute to the local vicinity. It helps to speed up blood circulation and prepare the skin for the wrap. Made from abrasive orange peel and oatmeal powder or garam flour, combined with rose and hibiscus petals, saffron and neem leaves bound together with water and a little bit of oil, it is wonderfully creamy.

Anti-allergic saffron, useful for removing pimples and soothing rashes, is known as *kesar* in Hindi. Applied to the temples it is used as a remedy for headache, and its fragrance is thought to have an aphrodisiac effect. Here, it is an effective, not to mention precious, skin cleanser. The scent of the rose is quite uplifting, while the orange zest is stimulating and astringent, the neem antiseptic and hibiscus soothing. The latter help to make skin soft and supple, while the garam or oatmeal rubs away dead surface cells, and, after a shower and steam, leaves the skin prepared to accept the wrap that follows.

Wraps are intensely detoxifying and can be a little debilitating, so clients are encouraged to drink some water afterwards. The Amanbagh wrap consists of a clay and water mix with hibiscus, rose and saffron, and it is applied all over the body directly after a ten-minute steam. Pores on the skin's surface open up in the steam, so the conditions are perfect for the application of a cool clay wrap. As the client lies, cocooned in clay and wrapped in a heavy towel, the therapist keeps contact with a gentle head massage for further relaxation.

As if this were not enough, the finale is a one-hour Maharani or Maharaja full body oil massage. Evoking the spirit of Rajasthan, with bergamot or patchouli with lime for men and mint and jasmine for women, the style of massage is dependent on the client's wishes. You won't want it to end.

Below: The cooling clay mask is applied all over the body. Around Amanbagh, clay plays a vital role in day-to-day life. Unbaked clay or *apakva* is used to make images of Hindu deities, and women use local clay in beauty and body treatments. Organic clay is one of the purest ingredients on earth: rich in minerals, it draws impurities and toxins from deep within the body.

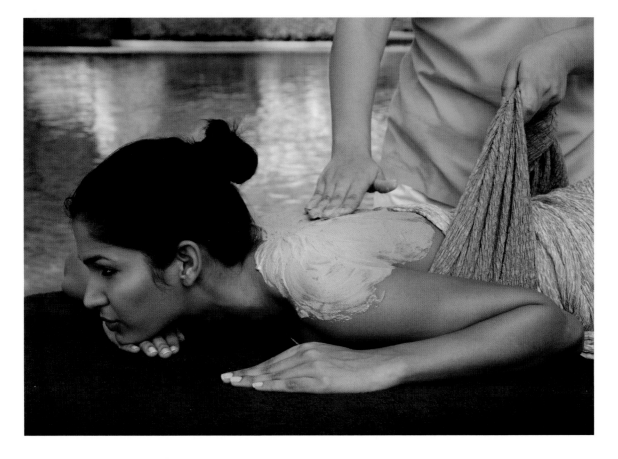

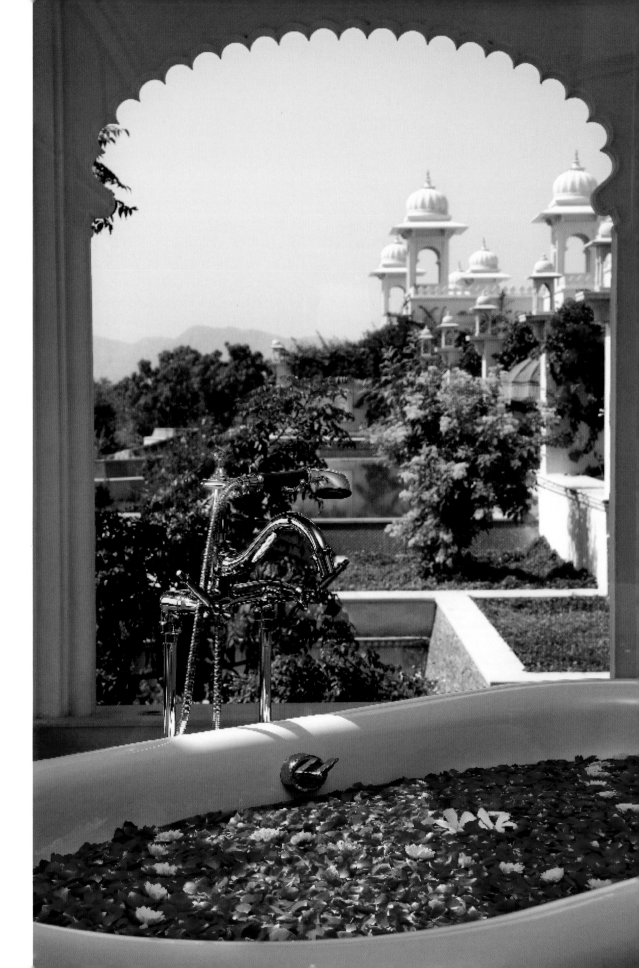

Magic of Mewar

The Maharanas of Mewar, who ruled Udaipur for over 1,200 years, are one of the oldest and most respected of the 36 Rajput clans. The only Rajputs to have held their own against the mighty Moghuls, the rulers of Mewar neither accepted Moghul sovereignty nor married their daughters into Moghul families. Their Maharanis (queens) were protected in strict purdah even up until Indian independence, and were revered as great beauties.

The Oberoi resort of Udaivilas pays tribute to the Mewar clan in more ways than one. Set on the shores of Lake Pichola directly opposite the granite-and-marble palaces, intricate temples, bathing ghats and royal pavilions of the city's founders, it is a celebration of Mewari craftsman-ship. Its aim is to treat guests like royalty and the spa does just that. Its palatial environment is just the place for the Magic of Mewar package, a glorious two-and-a-half hour indulgence that would have had past Maharanis clamouring for more.

The treatment starts with a body scrub of turmeric, sandalwood, green gram flour and yoghurt (see above) to exfoliate and smooth the skin. Turmeric rubs are used extensively in India and are believed to cleanse skin and leave it smooth and shiny with a golden glow. Combined with the soothing, anti-septic properties of sandalwood and moisturising, enzyme-rich yoghurt, the scrub is a great exfoliator.

This is followed by a full body massage. On offer are a number of different choices: Thai, Balinese, Hawaiian, stress-relieving and more. The signature Oberoi massage uses palms and fingertips to apply pressure with continuous strokes that rhythmically flow to stimulate blood circulation, ease tension and iron out muscle knots. It is soothing and conditioning and flows well after the slightly abrasive scrub.

Next comes an Ayur face massage, a therapy derived from Ayurveda to cleanse, energise and de-stress. First, the face is cleansed with rosewater, then the therapist conducts a short dry massage, lifting and pinching the muscles in the face, to stimulate blood circulation on the surface. This is followed by a *marma* massage concentrating on the ten vital energy points on the face: The point in the middle of the forehead, two points on the outside top of the eyes, two on the outside bottom, either side of the nostrils, below and behind the ears, and at the central point below the lips. Different complexions are allocated different oils: *Kumkumadi tailam* (an ancient Ayurvedic recipe with 16 precious ingredients) is used on acne-prone skin as it reduces coloration and blemishes, while oily skins are massaged with a sandalwood facial oil.

The final step in the procedure is a wonderfully relaxing bath with a view to die for. Many opt for the highly perfumed milk and rose petal combination (see opposite). This is a fitting finale, as the Doodh Talai stepwell (*doodh* means "milk"; *talai* is "pond"), which Maharanis in the past filled with milk for a cleansing royal bath, is across the lake within the client's field of vision. What better way to end a ritual imbued with all the magic of Mewar?

161

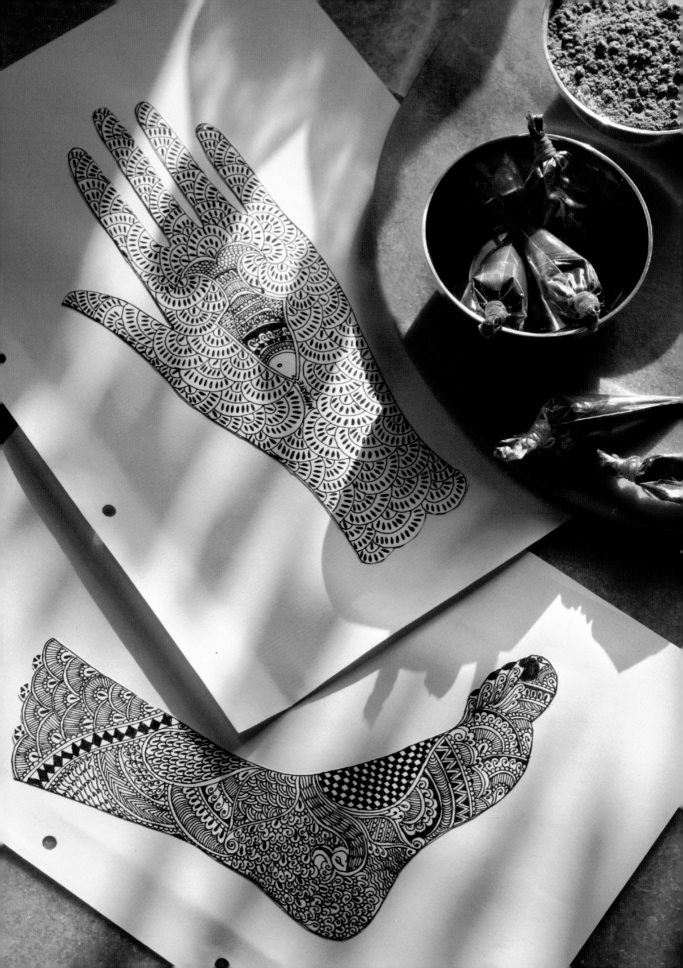

The Art of Mehndi

Thy henna lies soaking in a fine red bowl.
The love juice of henna is a lovely tint.
O Lady, who has painted thy hands?
The love juice of henna is a lovely tint.
O lady, put thy hand on my heart.
The love juice of henna is a lovely tint.

– A Rajasthani folk song (sung while
mehndi *is applied to a bride's palms)*

The application of *mehndi* (henna) as a colourant on hair, hands and nails is a time-honoured tradition across the Middle East and south Asia. With its origins in ancient Egypt, *mehndi* was most likely first used as a cooling device. Coming from the *Lawsonia inermis* shrub, it is known as *madayantika* in Sanskrit.

The small leaves, when crushed into a powder and mixed with water and a little bit of sugar, make a dark green paste that turns orange when it comes in contact with skin. The paste is applied to the skin using a plastic cone or a paintbrush, but sometimes a small metal-tipped jacquard (or jac) bottle is used. Hands and feet are the main areas painted, because skin colour is darkest here. This is because these areas contain high levels of keratin, a substance that binds well with the colourant of henna.

After the *mehndi* is painted on, the area may be wrapped in tissue or plastic to lock in body heat, thereby creating a more intense colour on the skin. The wrap is kept on for a minimum of six hours, and then removed. The final colour is reddish brown and can last from two weeks to a few months depending on the quality of the paste.

Mehndi leaves have anti-irritant, deodorant and antiseptic properties, and are used by Ayurvedic physicians for skin irritations. The paste is also used as an antidote against heat and sunstroke and, in the past, a poultice made from the leaves was applied to bring down high fevers. Today, henna may be applied to the body during the intense heat of the day, and people embarking on a long walk often apply it on the soles of feet. Orange-dyed feet are a common sight in India. Because of its cooling properties, *mehndi* leaves and flowers are made into lotions and ointments that are used externally for boils, burns, bruises and skin inflammations.

163

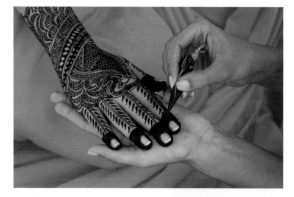

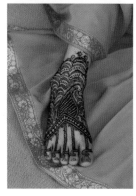

Opposite: Mehndi powder is readily available in markets all over India. Different henna patterns indicate different geographical locations and cultural associations.

Above and right: The spa manager at Amanbagh, who learnt the art of *mehndi* application from her grandmother, applies henna paste through a cone similar to the type of apparatus used for icing a cake.

164

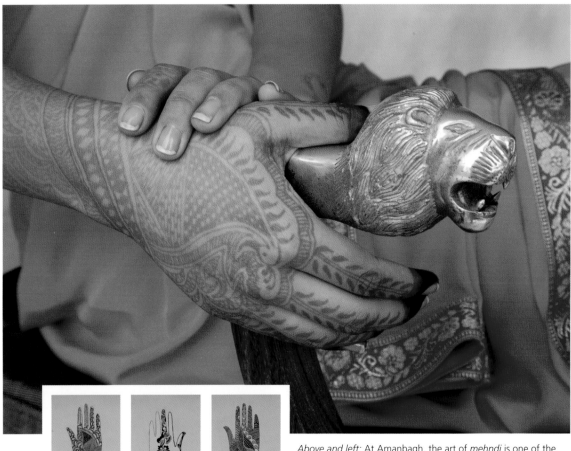

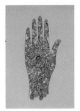 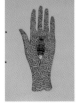 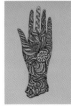

Above and left: At Amanbagh, the art of *mehndi* is one of the items on the spa menu. If a guest wants a pattern on the arm, back or wherever, it can be done.

Historically, there are numerous references to this versatile plant. The prophet Mohammed used *mendhi* for healing and he also dyed his hair and beard with it. It is recorded in the *Qu'ran* that his wife and daughters used henna for decoration on occasions such as Eid celebrations and weddings. Some Muslim girls are named after the *mehndi* plant. Its small intensely fragrant white flowers make a wonderfully strong-smelling perfume that is favoured by both men and women.

Over time, henna developed into a beauty aid, and the application of *mehndi* in intricate patterns on palms and feet is still an integral part of both Muslim and Hindu marriage ceremonies. It is considered a sign of love – the darker the coloration, the greater the love of the groom for the bride!

In her compelling autobiography set in a bygone era, *A Princess Remembers*, the Maharani of Jaipur, Gayatri Devi, writes about the preparations for her wedding to the Maharajah of Jaipur in the 1930s: "The adornment of a bride is a ceremony in itself and I was prepared for my wedding by a shoal of chattering married ladies while my own friends looked on giving me smiles of encouragement. In the bustle and confusion, somehow my insteps got painted with henna, my sari and my jewels were put on and one by one the ivory bangles of a Rajputana bride were slipped onto my wrists. Finally, my forehead was decorated with sandalwood paste and I was ready."

Sometimes, the *mehndi* decoration is applied with the name of the husband-to-be hidden in the pattern; if the groom can't find it, he has to pay a forfeit! Often applied with the singing of songs, there are multiple patterns, most of which have cultural associations. In Rajasthan, where most of the photos on these pages are taken, patterns typically have lines of v-shaped leaves, peacock feather patterning, the *bhandhej* (tie-dye) pattern, little acacia leaves and the *laheria* design (this literally translates as "waves of the sea" and is

found in geometric or floral patterns on brightly coloured Rajasthani saris). Other areas utilise motifs and designs associated with their own locales.

It isn't only at marriages that women decorate their hands and feet with *mehndi*. Many other festivals offer an excuse for girls to dress up and adorn themselves, and, increasingly, variations of traditional patterns may be applied as tattoo-type insignias on other parts of the body. Many visitors to India try a henna decoration at least once. Because it is a safe, painless and non-permanent alternative form of body ornamentation that is gaining favour in the West, nowadays you'll find henna artists in popular tourist destinations such as beach resorts and markets.

165

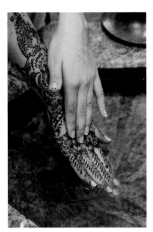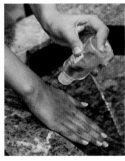

Above: After application, henna paste needs to be left on the body for a minimum of six hours, then the paste is rubbed off and the area oiled. A traditional method of making *mehndi* colour darker is to burn a clove and put the burnt ash followed by some lime juice on the pattern. A lemon juice and sugar mix may be applied afterwards to preserve the design.

Sunburn Soother

Education about sun-tanning and after sun care has mushroomed in the past decade, not least because of the increase in skin cancers that are proven to be a direct result of over-exposure to the sun. However careful we are, though, we have all been sun-burned at one time or another. We forget to reapply our SPF after a dip in the ocean, or go sightseeing without the anti-sun cream. We wash our faces, then forget the SPF moisturiser. Or we simply fall asleep in the sun on holiday.

Whatever the reason, it's useful to know that help is to be had from simple ingredients on hand in the kitchen and garden. The moisture from the blades of the versatile aloe vera plant contain aloectin B, an immune system stimulant; this works on burned skin to help with scars and soreness. Vitamin E and Vitamin C are antioxidant, so they speed up skin repair. An application of cool black tea on sunburn soothes skin as the tannins contained within tea are calming. Similarly a bath with half a cup of baking soda boosts healing – and soothes sore skin. Another useful plant is St John's Wort: it contains cooling properties that may help tone down some of the heat in the skin as it soothes damaged nerve endings.

You'll be surprised by how many ingredients in your fridge can help. Yoghurt, curd and milk are known to have soothing qualities for sunburned skin, as their fat and lactic acids have cooling properties. Cucumber is another useful product: Full of moisture,

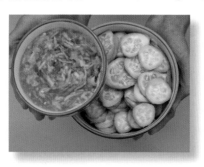

it is cooling and calming. Similarly, cool water mixed with lemon juice disinfects skin and promotes healing.

The bathroom can yield some hidden gems too: Calendula, bergamot, peppermint and lavender essential oils have an anti-inflammatory effect, and a bath of Epsom salts is an effective pain reliever.

At Aura spa in the Park Hotel Chennai, a four-pronged treatment has been specially designed to soothe sunburned skin. It uses the cooling properties of cucumber, along with creamy yoghurt and curd, rose, lavender, or jasmine essential oil and purifying mint, lemongrass, lemon and peppermint essential oil.

Starting with a cucumber wrap, and followed by an Esalen massage (a type of unique bodywork massage that is based on long, slow *t'ai chi* strokes to awaken awareness) and a cucumber facial, it ends with a tepid bath filled with mint, lime and lemongrass slices. If a detox is required, neem extract may be added.

The massage is not dynamic, so it won't irritate sore skin; rather, the gentle stroking movements work on the vital energy points to promote healing and relaxation. Similarly, cucumber cools down both facial and body skin, while lactic acid in yoghurt moisturises and restores the skin's natural pH balance. Before you know it, tender, red skin is on the road to recovery – and you're significantly less hot and bothered.

Opposite and above: Aura spa's sunburn soother at Park Hotel Chennai does the trick after an over-indulgent beach trip. Comprising a cucumber wrap, Esalen massage, cucumber facial and herbal bath, it is a balm for over-exposed skin and frazzled nerves.

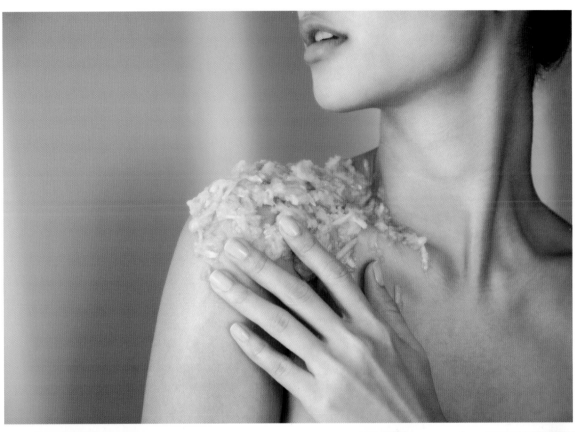

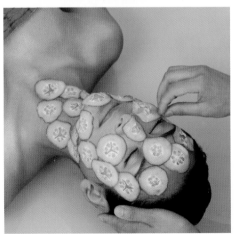

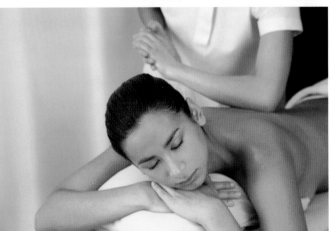

The Body Wrap

There is something immensely comforting about lying swaddled in cloth, plastic or blankets while a warming, detoxifying paste is doing its work on your body. With its roots in Indian bridal tradition, as brides always have a wrap daily for a week prior to their wedding day, the body wrap in India employs a variety of ingredients. From fruits to flowers, herbs, spices and clays, a body wrap can be deeply nurturing.

Whatever the ingredients, the idea is that the warmth of the wrap allows ingredients to penetrate subcutaneously through the pores of skin. Some wraps are prescribed for their preventative and

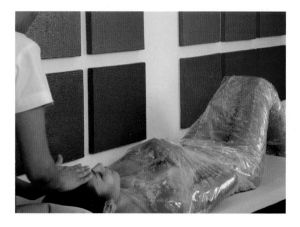

Opposite: Body wraps, traditionally using leaves for wrapping, were given in order to encourage sweating, thereby removing toxins from beneath the skin's surface. Here large shiny banana leaves have been used as in the past; today, these have largely been replaced by plastic, cloth, towels or cling wrap (as *above*).

Above: Enzyme-rich papaya is mildly exfoliating, so it removes flaking skin cells from the surface of the skin, making the body softer and smoother. At Aura spa in the Park hotel in New Delhi, crushed papaya is massaged into the skin so that it works in the subcutaneous layers too; the client is then wrapped in a plastic sheet. You'll be amazed how skin texture is significantly improved afterwards.

curative properties against colds and coughs; others are used to alleviate muscle aches, headaches and fever. Others use minerals and ingredients from the ocean such as seaweed to encourage lymphatic drainage. All aim to increase blood circulation, encourage sweating to draw out unwanted toxins, cleanse internally and on the body's surface, and leave skin soft and glowing.

In Ayurvedic tradition, the process of sudation (sweating) is considered beneficial for a number of reasons. When the body perspires, accumulated toxins are believed to "melt": they then either find their way into the alimentary tract or are expelled through the skin as sweat. It is believed that a wrap increases both osmotic pressure and temperature within the body and on the skin's surface, thereby speeding up this internal detoxification process.

In a spa, a polish or scrub may precede a wrap: As the skin has been freshly exfoliated, it is in an optimum condition to receive the properties of the wrap. We outline some innovate wrap solutions from India's top spas both here and on the following pages.

Ancient Indian Body Mask

Ananda spa, high in the mountains above the holy town of Rishikesh, utilises its beautiful pollutant-free environment with ingredients close to hand in this deeply cleansing ritual. First a combination of herbal roots with pure Himalayan spring water is applied to the body to slough off dead cells and prepare the body for the therapeutic clay application

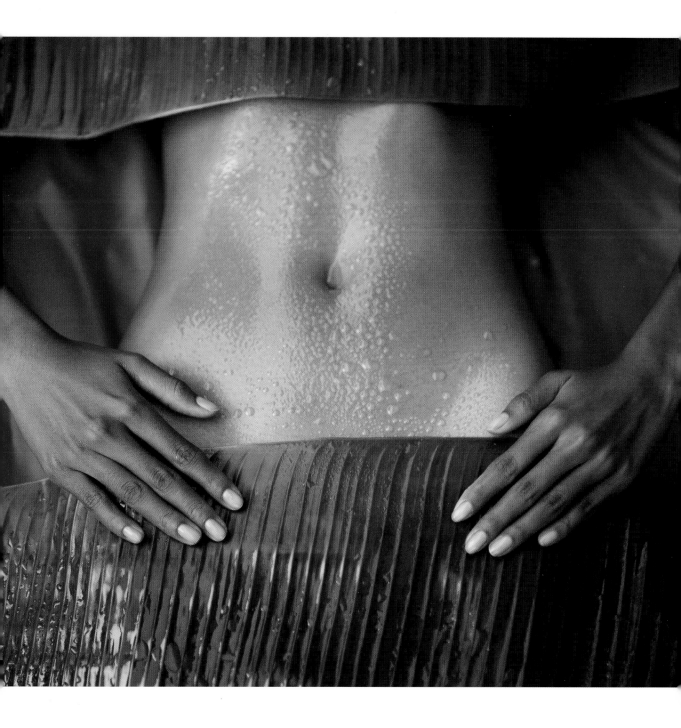

Right and opposite: Wild mint and Nilgiri honey are used in a purifying mask at Aura spa, Park New Delhi. After a sesame seed scrub, moisturising honey and antiseptic, cooling mint are mixed for this rejuvenating wrap: Be prepared for a body-blasting boost of energy after this treatment! Megha Dinesh, the spa director for Aura spas explains how it works: "Aura wraps are designed to minimise air supply to the skin so the body temperature rises, pores open, toxins are released through sweat and the properties in the contents of the wrap are absorbed."

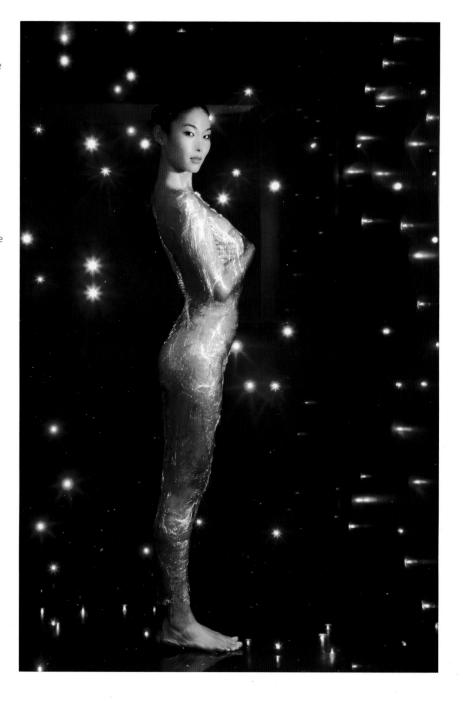

to come. This is followed by a *Multani mitti* total body mask; spiced with turmeric, sandalwood or other herbal powders, it is applied evenly over the body which is then wrapped in a sheet. While the mask works its magic, the client receives a gentle facial pressure point massage. Pure bliss.

Anna Lepanam

A paste similar to that used for Oberoi spa's Navara *kizhi* treatment is used as a wrap at Rajvilas in Jaipur. Based on a clinical therapy from Kerala formulated for muscle strain and fractures, it is here used for skin conditioning. The traditional treatment is called Navara *theppu* (*theppu* means "paste application") and ingredients include Navara rice with the addition of a *bala* root decoction. *Bala* root comes from the *Sida cordifolia* plant and is considered balancing for all three *doshas* in Ayurvedic medicine. Astringent, diuretic and tonic, it has *rasayana* (rejuvenating) properties, so is useful in topical applications. When the paste is applied to the affected area for 30–45 minutes daily for a period of 21 to 28 days, the healing ingredients penetrate deep into the skin and activate muscles after a serious bone fracture.

In the amended Rajvilas treatment, Navara rice, milk and a *bala* root decoction are combined with turmeric, fenugreek seed and sandalwood powders to make a gruel-like paste. This is applied all over the body ("rice" is *anna*; *lepanam* means "application

on to the body"), and the body is covered with warm towels. Considered excellent for firming and contouring, *anna lepanam* increases skin elasticity and flexibility of the joints and leaves skin smooth, toned and warm. Skin colour is usually warm and glowing too.

Dr Yogesh, the resident doctor, explains that if Navara *kizhi* or *anna lepanam* were part of a clinical Ayurvedic treatment, at the end the gruel would be wiped completely off the body with a coconut palm leaf strip. As Rajasthan has few coconut palms, any excess is removed with a cloth, and the treatment ends with a bath (without soap) enabling the ingredients to penetrate further. "Expect to feel a little drained," he says. "So take some time out for herbal tea and relaxation after."

Papaya Pamper

The beneficial effects of papain, the enzyme contained in papaya, have been well documented. A popular meat tenderiser, papaya is also used as a home remedy for stings and bites as it has the ability to break down protein toxins. In beauty therapy, it is popular for its ability to break down and remove cosmetic blemishes, skin secretions and dead skin cells. In keeping with their tradition of using fresh ingredients in treatments, Aura spas at Park Hotels offer a wonderful fruity papaya body wrap that is preceded by an oatmeal scrub. Ideal for sensitive skin, it isn't too harsh and leaves the body tingling and skin glowing afterwards.

171

The Body Polish

I have loved the sunlight, the sky and the green earth;
I have heard the liquid murmur of the river
through the darkness of midnight;
Autumn sunsets have come to me at the bend of the road
in the lonely waste, like a bride raising her veil to accept
her lover.
Yet my memory is still sweet with the first white jasmines
that I held in my hands when I was a child.

– Rabindranath Tagore from The First Jasmines

A good body polish is a wonderfully invigorating experience. Floral, herbal or other natural ingredients (usually of a gently abrasive nature) are combined with oil and massaged all over the body to increase circulation and metabolism and open the skin's pores to receive the healing properties contained within the polish. A polish also exfoliates the skin's surface of dead cells that build up on the outer layer; these tend to give dull skin tone, so a polish literally does as it says. Skin is always smoother, brighter and more translucent after an exfoliating polish.

A body polish is also helpful for lumpy cellulite, although it does not constitute a miracle cure. Pockets of cellulite – deposits of fat, water and other wastes – build up on hips, thighs, buttocks and upper arms and not only look unsightly, but are difficult to disperse. It is believed that these toxins and wastes become "trapped" within the cells' hardened connective tissue, so releasing them is not easy. A healthy diet, a strong lymphatic system, regular exercise and vigorous skin brushing can all help with the problem.

Using an abrasive cloth or natural bristle brush, include a daily skin brush in your beauty regime. Starting at your feet, head upwards and outwards, being sure to use a reasonable pressure. Skin brushing increases blood and lymph circulation, and helps to eliminate toxins from the body. Regular anti-cellulite polishes help too, but be aware that profound changes need to be made if the condition is severe. Try some of the options outlined below.

At Quan Spa at the JW Marriott Mumbai, the choice of body polishes reads like a geographical tour of the Indian subcontinent. Usually offered in conjunction with another treatment, namely a wrap to infuse substances into the body system, a massage to improve circulation and also allow herbal oils to do their work in the deep tissues, a steam or a Vichy shower, they are deeply nourishing. Choose from the alluring menu below:

Allepey Body Polish: Taking its inspiration from the backwaters of Kerala, this is a coconut and cardamom combo that is antioxidant and full of nutrients.

Kollegal Body Polish: The Kollegal region has been India's source of sandalwood for centuries, so antiseptic sandalwood is combined here with a mud high in mineral content mud, for an uplifting, energising experience.

Madurai Body Polish: The pretty temple town of Madurai in Tamil Nadu forms the backdrop for this polish; jasmine scented oils, along with the lighting of oil lamps and ringing of bells, anoint the body on a balancing, aromatic journey.

172

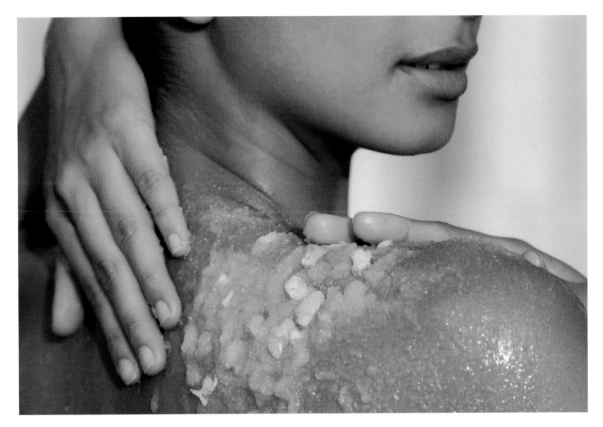

Malabar Body Polish: India's Malabar coast was the port of call for Arab traders in their sturdy *dhows*, so this polish takes its name and ingredients from the Spice Trade. Combined with a cooling lentil exfoliant to moderate the heat of the spices used, it is intense and warming.

Salt is a major ingredient in many scrubs and the spa at Ananda in the Himalayan foothills utilises natural sea salts with a variety of essential oils and herbs to remove impurities, dull surface cells and rough textured skin. Therapists there suggest having a scrub before any of their extensive menu of treatments as it prepares the body for the deep penetration of healing products that follow. Another surefire winner is the tangy *tintri* treat offered at Aura spas at Park Hotels across India: tamarind (*tintri*) is the main ingredient here. Rich in Vitamin C and a natural cleanser, tamarind juice is mixed with oats and humectant honey and milk to provide a deep moisturising polish that leaves skin radiant and glowing.

Opposite and above: Hand-picked jasmine, known as *mogra* in Hindi, is a key component of the Madurai body polish, while Ananda's jasmine salt scrub mixes jasmine essential oil with natural sea salt to enliven and balance maturing skins.

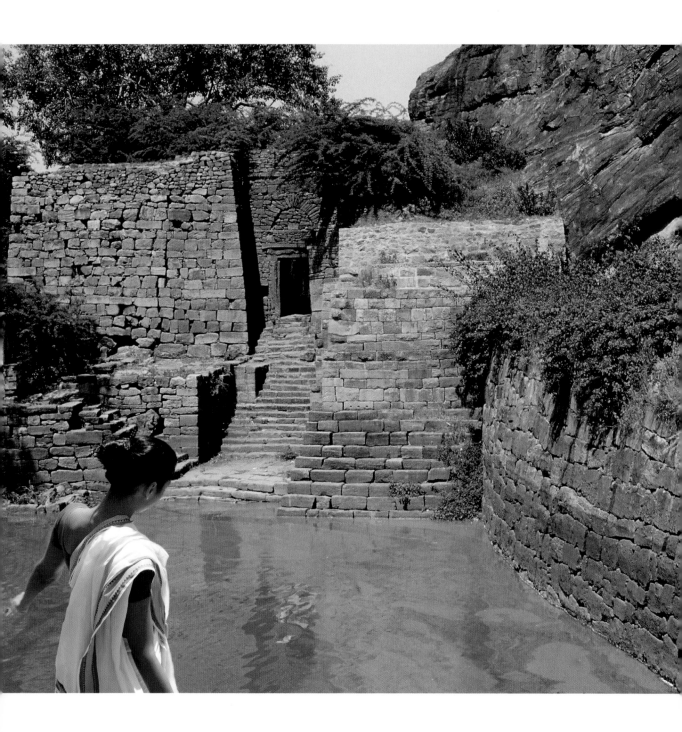

Indian-inspired Water Therapies

Bathing traditions are both widespread and deep-seated in Indian culture. For Hindus, ritual bathing is seen as a holy purification rite: Whether it is the washing of hands before a meal or a trip to a holy river, cleansing with water is imbued with significance. Pilgrimages always involve absolution by water one way or another as well. Muslims, too, use water rituals for both purification and healing, and are requested to perform ablutions before entering a mosque.

It is known that Indians prized both physical and mental cleanliness, and were bathing regularly far before most people in Western countries took up the practice. One of the most intriguing structures at the ruins of Mohenjodaro, one of the largest metropolises of the Indus River Valley civilisation, is the two-metre (six-foot) deep brick structure called the Great Bath. Waterproofed with tightly packed bricks and a layer of bitumen, it was surrounded by cloister-like rooms that are now believed to have served some religious purpose.

Whether bathing at Mohenjodaro was spiritual or physical or a combination of both is not known, but the elaborate water supply system and drain-age network indicate that the Great Bath was an important part of the city. This is backed up by

Left: Even today, morning bathing on the ghats of holy lakes, rivers or tanks is a daily ritual. Traditionally, to cleanse in holy water is to wash away sin, greed, envy and evil in order to emerge physically and metaphorically pure. Devotees submerge themselves in the water, offer up water to their ancestors and pay homage to the sun.

Above right: Situated on a north-south axis, Mohenjodaro's Great Bath has two large staircases leading down to the bath from the north and the south. It was almost certainly for ritual use.

reference to bathing in ancient Ayurvedic texts. These advocate that bathing be a daily ritual conducted to stimulate the body, remove fatigue, sweat and dirt and enhance the subtle spiritual energy or *ojas*. The Vedic texts indicate that different *doshas* require different temperatures of water.

Elsewhere in India, there are numerous tracts extant on mental and physical hygiene. A 12th-century encyclopedic text from Karnataka called *Manasollasa* gives details of scientific approaches to bathing, whilst the 17th-century handbook written primarily for royalty *Sivatatvaratnakara* provides similar details about bathing. The tongue-twisting *Kanthiravanarasarajavijaya* written by Govinda Vaidya in 1648 gives a very picturesque description

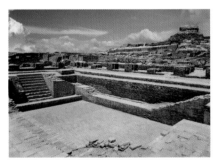

of a bathing ghat (public bath on a river-bank) and describes the importance of water supplies for the ritual act of bathing.

It is interesting to note that soap was not traditionally used in Indian bathing. Paradoxically, the combination of soap and water, although cleansing, is de-moisturising and accelerates ageing. Indians preferred to use cleansing scrubs made from grains of garam flour, wheat husks or oatmeal to exfoliate and followed this with applications of oil after drying. Because many baths were public or semi-public, it was (and is) normal to keep the *sari* or *dhoti* on whilst bathing.

In 21st-century India, a variety of therapeutic, beautifying and cleansing baths are available at spas and clinics. Oil-infused or flower-filled baths often form the fitting finale to a sequence of treatments at a spa. They take their historical cue from royal bathing practices, and leave you scented, refreshed or invigorated depending on the bath ingredients. Some bathing options are simple, and may be recreated at home, while others combine Indian traditions with hydrotherapeutic practices from overseas, such as thalassotherapy and the Vichy shower. We pick out the cream of the crop: It's interesting to see how, in one way or another, they follow ancient purification rites.

Floral Baths

Oberoi Spas offer a number of specialty baths that may be taken at the end of a spa treatment or as a stand-alone, including the visually arresting marigold bath. Each takes its cue from Indian traditions or ingredients or both (see the purifying neem bath on pages 60–61). In everyday life, garlands of marigolds are often given to welcome visitors and the blossoms are used to adorn a home altar or are placed on little leaf boats with an oil lamp at evening *aartis* (prayer rituals). Even though they do not have any religious significance as such,

their golden hues are attractive, and when used in a bath the blooms have astringent qualities. After half an hour's relaxation in this gold-and-vermilion dream water, the skin feels firm and fresh afterwards.

Another floral bath with a difference, is J W Marriott's Quan Spa's interpretation of the milk bath based on an ancient Indian recipe. Milk has naturally occurring alpha-hydroxy acids that hydrate, exfoliate and improve skin elasticity, while *ashwagandha* root, also known as Indian ginseng, is used in a number of Ayurvedic remedies. It is one of the best herbs for the mind, clearing anxiety and inducing clarity. Rose petals, of course, provide a delicate and wonderful scent. Harnessing the power of water that flows around India's busiest city, Mumbai, their rose, milk and *ashwagandha* bath can be had as a single or couple's treatment or combined in a spa package based on the five elements of fire, water, air, earth and space.

Medicinal Baths

Hydrotherapy, of course, immediately comes to mind when one considers the bath in a spa setting as people have been "taking the waters" in a variety of ways for centuries. Many venues utilise

Above and opposite: Soukya's hydrotherapy options are particularly strong, with both hot and cold water baths, jets, compresses, packs, douches and steams prescribed to clients often on a daily basis. The reflexology path (*above*) simultaneously combines the benefits of reflexology and water therapy, while the jet shower (*opposite*) hydro-massages the body to stimulate circulation and condition muscles.

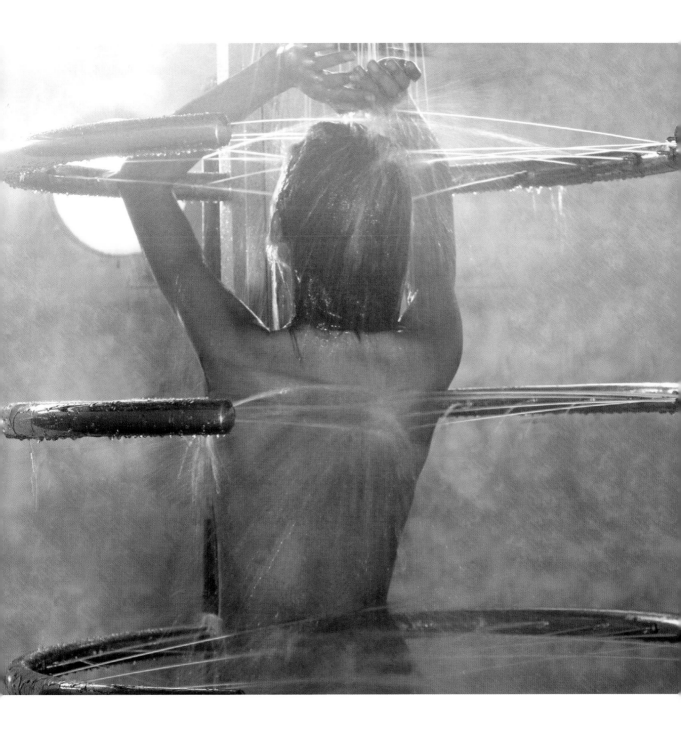

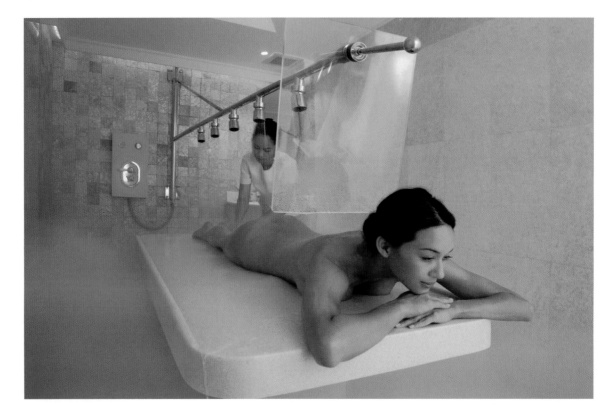

hot and cold plunge pools, Jacuzzi sprays, steam boxes and steam rooms, jets, underwater reflexology paths, and more, for a variety of ailments. One of the famous Indian inventions is the hip bath: devised by naturopath Sri Lakshman Sharma in order to concentrate water between the ribs and thighs, it helps stimulate circulation in that region, so it's good for the digestive, excretory and urinary systems. Another example is the innovative arm and foot bath: it's an important application in the case of bronchial asthma, as the reflex areas on the palms and soles are related to the lungs. It is also helpful for migraine sufferers.

In Ayurveda, medicinal baths are not overly used, though steam baths come under the category of some preparatory oleation and fomentation therapies. Described as a sudation process, medicinal steam is used to induce sweating and improve peripheral circulation to reduce high blood pressure and help in the absorption of medicinal particles present in herbal oils. The steam also augments the elimination of toxins and impurities in the excretory system and through other outlets such as sweat glands, kidneys and liver. Sometimes, a steam session will also be prescribed for skin or muscle ailments, pain and swelling.

At Kalari Kovilakom, where Ayurvedic texts are followed to the letter, steam boxes are part and parcel of the initial stages of the *panchakarma* regime. But the Palace to Ayurveda is also home to a pint-sized rosewood bath that often comes into its own at the end of a client's treatment. "After the *panchakarma* treatment, patients often break out in pimples as their toxins are released," explains Dr Jayan. "So this medicinal bath helps to restore skin conditions." Medicated warm water is also poured into this bath to soothe spinal problems, muscle ailments and skin conditions. Uterine or rectal prolapse are also helped by such baths, and people with haemorrhoids also find them healing.

One notable bath from the Himalayan region is the Bhutanese stone-heated bath or *sman-chu*. Based on the Tibetan medical system known as *So-ba Rig-pa*, it works on the same principle as hot stone massage (see pages 36–37). Using the healing power of heat from pristine mountain hot springs, the warmth from the water stimulates peripheral circulation and penetrates deeper, helping arthritic or rheumatic conditions. The Bhutanese often add herbs such as artemesia, sage and ephedra to the water, and often use a salt scrub prior to a dip.

Other spas, clinics and even hospitals use a mixture of the traditional and the modern with innovative results. At the state-of-the-art Quan spa in Mumbai, a dedicated Vichy shower room is the venue for an invigorating treatment that combines the French Vichy therapy with Indian ingredients and practices, for aromatic effect. This deep

cleansing back treatment is both invigorating and cooling, just the thing after a day's sightseeing in India's commercial capital. Fresh aloe vera is combined with the anti-bacterial and antiseptic properties of sandalwood and the power of pure water Vichy jets. Both sandalwood and aloe vera are calming for sunburnt skin, and help with heat rashes, irritated skin and general discomfort. We think you'll emerge from this one totally rejuvenated, with fresh, toned and scented skin to boot.

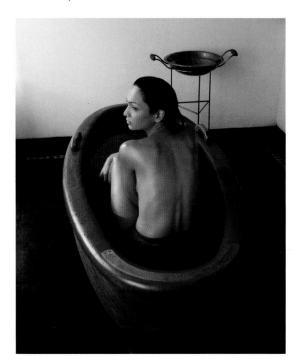

179

Opposite: Jets from the shower replicate rainfall while healing herbs are massaged into the body at the holistic spa at Mandarin Oriental Dhara Devi.

Above: Made from rosewood, this bath at Kalari Kovilakom is purely medicinal. During a prolonged detox, the skin often erupts with pustules as poisons are expelled from the body, so a soothing, medicated bath in this little tub helps surface healing.

Healing with Gems, Crystals, Metals and Minerals

"Her pendants were encrusted with diamonds and gems. On one ear she had hung the sun, on the other, the sphere of Jupiter. With two luminous orbs on either side, her face rose like the moon between the stars."

– Manjhan, 16th-century Indian poet

Many people who have made a study of gem-stones, minerals and metals maintain that they are endowed with special properties: Because they come from the ground, they are believed to have the ability to both attract and dispel negative and positive energy. As a result, they have been used in healing for centuries.

In Ayurveda, gems and precious metals are used to balance planetary influences, increase life force or *prana*, and cure certain diseases. Their preparation and prescription falls under the branch of Ayurvedic medicine known as *rasashastra* (literally "mercury medicine"). It developed relatively late in the Ayurvedic calendar (probably around the 8th century), but its practices were soon assimilated into mainstream Ayurveda. *Rasashastra* basically falls into two categories: *dehavaad* or the "treating of diseases" and *lohavaad* or the "chemical manufacture of medicines".

In today's spas and retreats, a prescription of gems, metals or minerals is rare: They are more commonly found in clinics and hospitals. However, the tradition of using such substances has found new life in a number of skincare formulations invented by entrepreneurial chemists and doctors. Tiny flecks of gold leaf or silver foil, or crushed diamonds and pearls, blended with botanical

extracts, have found their way into innovative products. Facials using such ingredients are the latest in Indian skincare: Receive the elixir of life (gold) through the skin, and detoxify; use a crushed pearl exfoliator, and see the difference in your complexion. And, for the ultimate in anti-aging, dazzle with a diamond rehydrator; you can justify the extravagance. It's doing you good.

Metals and Minerals

Less exotic, but powerful nonetheless, is the use of metals and minerals in Ayurveda. Because many metals and minerals contain certain impurities and/or toxins, they need to undergo a number of treatments before they are deemed safe to ingest. These processes are known as *shodhana* (purification) and *marana* (literally "kill"; heating and turning into ash), and may often be lengthy and compli-cated. For example, heavy metals such as mercury, gold, silver, copper, iron, lead and tin are heated and treated with such substances as cow's urine, milk, ghee and buttermilk before use. If they are to be taken in ash form, they are ground into a powder and incinerated; at other times they are added to water to create elixirs which may be drunk.

Dr Sreenarayanan of Ananda spa points out that all Ayurvedic medicines are 100 percent natural, so it is unsurprising that minerals and metals are utilised.

Right: Good as gold: Eaten, injected or absorbed through the skin, gold is the ultimate elixir of life. Ingested in Ayurveda to boost the circulation and rejuvenate sluggish organs, it may also be injected to reduce inflammation in joints of rheumatoid arthritis patients. Here, it is applied to the face as part of an absurdly luxurious four-part facial treatment by Shahnaz Husain: aptly named the 24 carat gold collection, it's an extravagant treat.

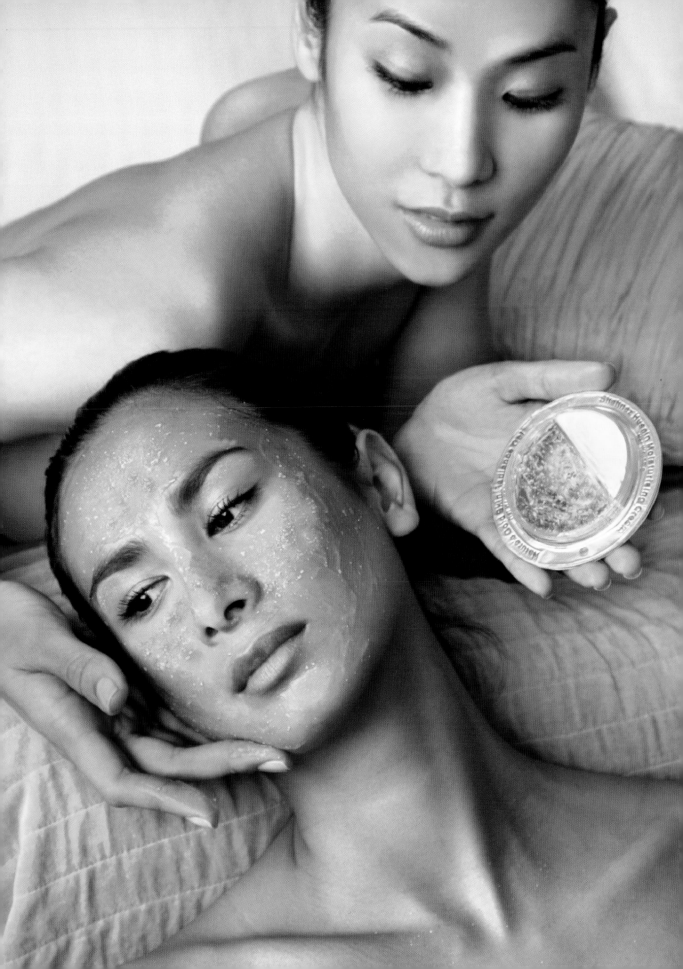

"Minerals and metals come from the earth," he points out. "And, if they are purified properly, can be very powerful." He goes on to say that in 90 percent of cases they are ingested either as a *bhasma* (ash) or as pills, but such prescriptions must be accompanied by an extremely strict diet for the medication to work. He cites mercury for chronic conditions like cancer and arthritis; silver in rejuvenation treatments; gold for vigour and vitality as well as bone problems; iron for anaemia and blood impurities; and lead for chronic skin conditions.

In the past, topical applications were quite rare, but sometimes prescribed. For example, an ointment of sulphur applied either alone or with other medications was used for skin diseases. Nowadays, applying precious metals mixed with other ingredients directly on to the skin is all the rage. Gold and silver are a case in point. According to Shahnaz Husain, whose 24 carat gold collection of facial skin products is making waves internationally as well as in India, gold has powerful anti-aging properties. "It helps reverse oxidation damage and stimulates lymphatic drainage and cell regeneration," she claims. Similarly, Aussie company Ayurda's silver leaf gel, a clear gel with glinting silver sparkles (see page 318), uses the cooling properties of silver to draw out heat from acne-prone skin. In much the same way as, centuries ago, silver was applied to cuts to heal wounds, pure silver foil helps build up skin integrity.

Gemstones

In India, jewels (often worn as uncut stones) are not only decorative, but are believed to hold certain powers. Some of these are emotional or superstitious on the part of the wearer, but others are distinctly therapeutic. Gem therapists say that the vibrational healing energies of a gem or metal may be transferred to a person if it is worn close to the body. Some people wear them for health reasons, others for luck, others for peace of mind.

According to Dr Sreenarayanan, only certain stones have healing properties and they must always be purified before use. "Gems may be soaked in running water (preferably water from sacred places such as the Ganges) and the water is drunk for health benefits," he says. "Or they may be put in the husk of rice or left out in the sun. Another way of receiving the power of stones is to simply concentrate or meditate on 'special' stones; gazing on them in a quiet meditative manner dispels negativity and calms the mind."

He goes on to note that the use of gems and precious metals is also rooted in Vedic astrological readings (see pages 90–93). The *Vedas* prescribed three methods to dispel negative planetary influences, namely the chanting of *mantras*, the wearing of gems and the taking of medicine. Today, many people choose to wear a *navaratna* or nine jewel bangle or a *rudraaksha* (string of medicinal beads) to keep harmful cosmic energies at bay.

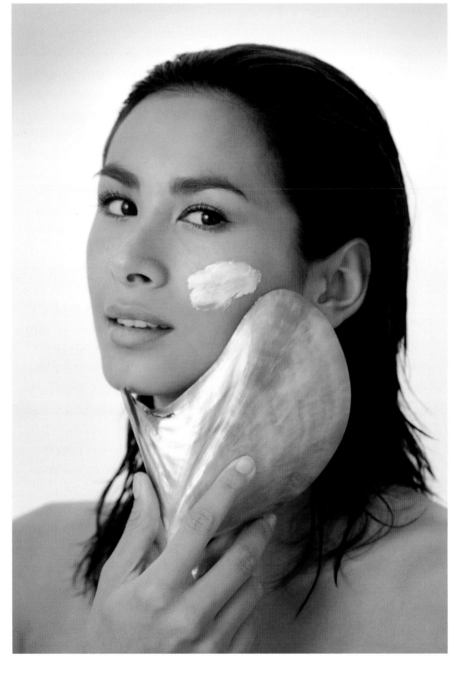

Opposite: Although not strictly gems, pearls have been used for decoration, health, good luck and cuisine for centuries in India. If the pearl is your birth stone, it will be doubly powerful. "If you wear your birth stone close to the body," asserts Dr Sreenarayanan of Ananda spa, "your energy levels open up and your immune system is strengthened."

Left: Enriched with amino acids and minerals, pearls are powerful when applied to the skin. This pearl mask from Shahnaz Husain rejuvenates facial skin at a cellular level.

183

Gems used in Ayurvedic healing

According to Dr Ramkumar of Ayurvedic consultants Punarnava, certain stones are aligned with certain planets and other celestial bodies, and may be of benefit to particular *doshas* and conditions. He shares his findings with us:

Ruby and red garnet: Aligned with the sun, these red stones are useful for *vata* and *kapha* types. They help with conditions of the heart, spleen, liver, brain, eyes and bones.

Pearl and moonstone: Although not strictly a gem, pearls are associated with the moon; they help with lung and kidney diseases, as well as problems of the mind. Crushed to a powder and dissolved in water, they help those with a calcium deficiency. Pearl and moonstone are good for *vata* and *pitta* types.

Red Coral: Associated with Mars, red coral is a *pitta* stone. It is useful for muscular, small intestine and liver diseases, and boosts the immune system.

Yellow gems: Aligned with Jupiter, yellow stones help with the liver, pancreas, nerves and glands. They are good for *vata* and *kapha* types.

Diamond and clear zircon: Good for the urinary and reproductive systems as well as kidney and bone complaints, clear stones are associated with Venus. They benefit *vata* and *kapha* types.

Cat's Eye: The stone of Ketu (see page 91), cat's eye benefits all *doshas*, and is helpful for digestive, circulatory and muscular disorders.

Blue Sapphire, amethyst and lapis: Saturn stones, blue gems are useful for strengthening bones, nerves and the digestion. They benefit *vata* and *pitta doshas*.

Green gems: All green gems, including emeralds, are associated with Mercury. They help the intellect and increase mental alertness and memory. They are also useful for the nervous and digestive systems, and are particularly beneficial for *pitta* types.

Gomedha (hessonite): The stone of Rahu (see page 91), *gomedha* is good for all *doshas*, and helps with disorders of the brain and nervous system.

Crystal Therapy

Crystal therapy is another holistic therapy that utilises the power of stones. Crystal healers believe that every living organism has an energy system based on meridian lines and *chakras*, so if appropriate crystals are placed on particular spots (ie *marma* points or *chakras*) sluggish or blocked energy is revitalised. Such therapy is also reported to be helpful with certain emotional issues. Some therapists use crystals in facials and massages too: warmed jade, turquoise and quartz used in a manner similar to hot stone massage encourage energy flow and carved, polished crystals placed on the facial *chakras* help cleanse and rebalance.

Crystal healer and beauty therapist Mirjam Rahr says that crystals are especially useful because they vibrate in the same energy fields as human beings. When working with crystals and a client, she places amethyst or rose quartz around the body on the "aura web", then places the same crystals on pressure points on the face for their soothing, healing qualities. She

184

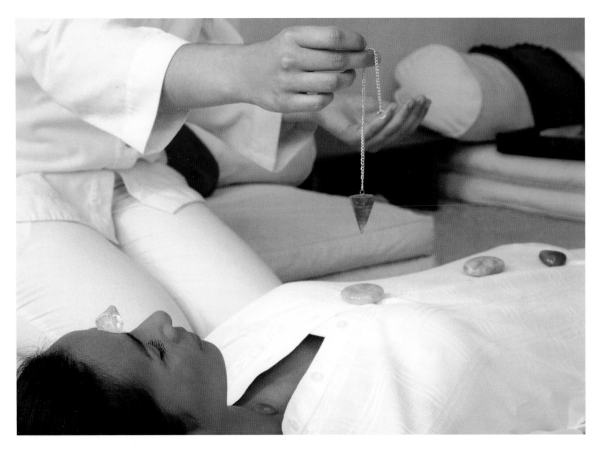

says that clear quartz is the most powerful of all crystals, so these are placed on the crown and third eye *chakras* and on the client's upturned palms, so that their energies may penetrate deep into the body. She may then use a crystal pendulum to see if there are energy blockages along the *chakras*: If the pendulum shivers, rotates or goes back and forth, that area needs attention. Then, using a combination of crystals, a *chakra* wand and Reiki (see pages 122–123), she attempts to free up energy flows and bring the body and mind back to balance.

For crystal therapy to be effective, a course of treatments is advised. "Depending on the person and their problems, this type of energetic work is most beneficial when received more than once," says Mirjam, "a course of twice a week for a few weeks can be enormously helpful."

Opposite: Green gems are Ayurvedic brain tonics, helpful for memory, consciousness and mental agility.

Above: The body's bio-magnetic field extends at least eight inches out from the surface of the skin, so when a crystal pendulum is held above another crystal positioned on a *chakra* point, it is more than likely to move. This helps give vital information to a therapist.

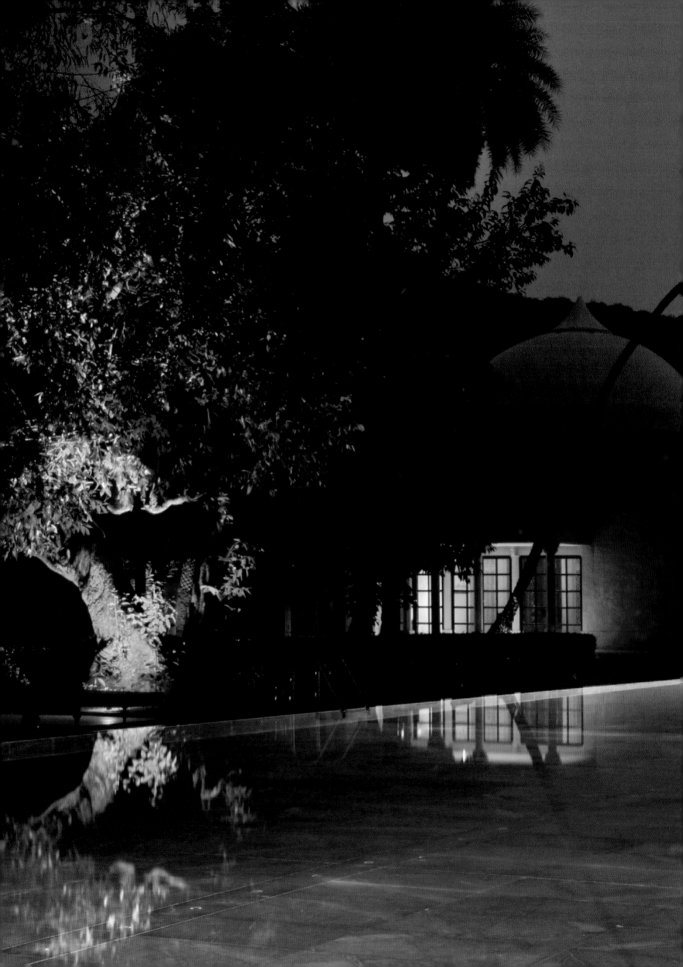

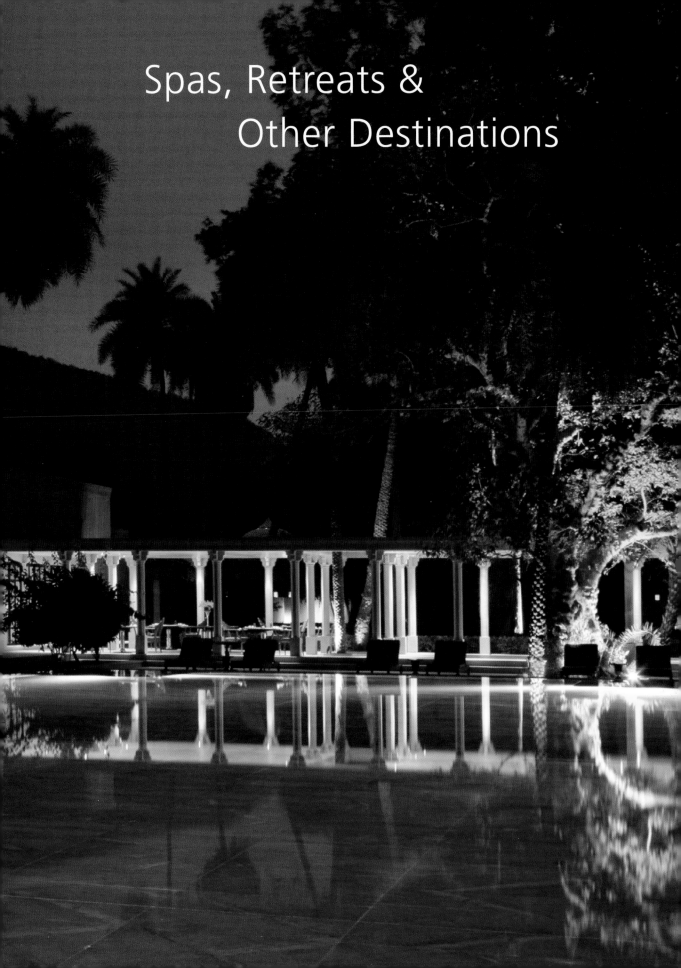

Spas, Retreats &
Other Destinations

Ananda – in the Himalayas

When Ananda in the Himalayas opened in 2000 it was something totally new to India, and more than a tad ahead of its time. Not only did it introduce the spa concept to the subcontinent, it billed itself as a "destination spa" in a country where spas were non-existent! This displayed extraordinary vision on behalf of its owners; and set the benchmark for others to follow.

Today, Ananda is well known around the globe as a holistic centre with an extremely innovative, well-run spa, exercise and wellness programme. But in reality, it is much more. There is history in the 100-acre Maharajah's estate in which it is located; there is magic and mysticism in the landscape; there is godliness in its proximity to the Mother Ganga and her pilgrimage centres of Rishikesh and Haridwar; and there is beauty and serenity in its exclusive surrounds.

A sojourn at this sybaritic spa property provides everything you could possibly desire in terms of healing. There is an enormous variety of treatments, packages and programmes and the facilities are first-rate. There is a resident nurse, Ayurvedic doctor and physiotherapist on hand, and, in addition to spa therapies, yoga, meditation, hydrotherapy, a fully equipped gymnasium, mini golf course and lap pool are offered. The spa service ethos is professional, yet caring, and the standard of therapists is among the best I have encountered anywhere. It needs to be stressed that this is not a pain-is-gain, bread-and-water retreat along the Californian model. Rather it

is a luxurious hideaway, where you can partake in as little or as much as you like of the various health, relaxation and rejuvenation programmes on offer. Food and alcohol are plentiful, yet if you are on an Ayurvedic package, tasty vegetarian Ayurvedic food is also available.

Ananda (which means "bliss and contentment" in Sanskrit) is not new to healing and devotion. The Maharajah of Garhwal, on whose estate the property is located, had a special room built on the balcony of his Viceregal Lodge for the renowned spiritual leader Ma Anandamayi. It was from here that she formulated her now well-known ashram programme propagating universal love and brotherhood. Her legacy of all-pervading love lives on at Ananda: Be it through the healing hands of the therapists, the courteous service of staff, the fresh, scented air, or simply by existing for a time in such serenity and stillness.

In addition to the extensive spa menu, there is guided hiking in the foothills of the Himalaya, visits to the *aarti* at Rishikesh (the evening ritual of song and prayer on the banks of the Mother Ganga), white-water rafting excursions to the Rajaji elephant wildlife reserve in the valley below, and more. Another option is to kick back – and chill.

Above: Inspiring mountain vistas and fresh air ensure that yoga sessions at Ananda are doubly dynamic.

Right: The Music Pavilion overlooking the annexe lawn is a peaceful spot for meditation during the early evening at Ananda.

188

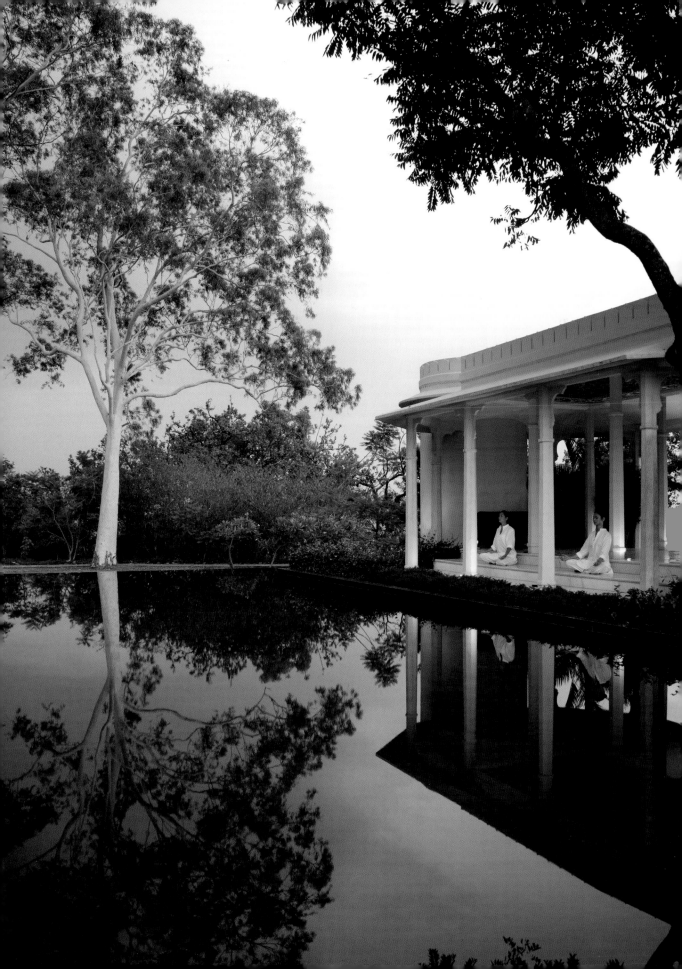

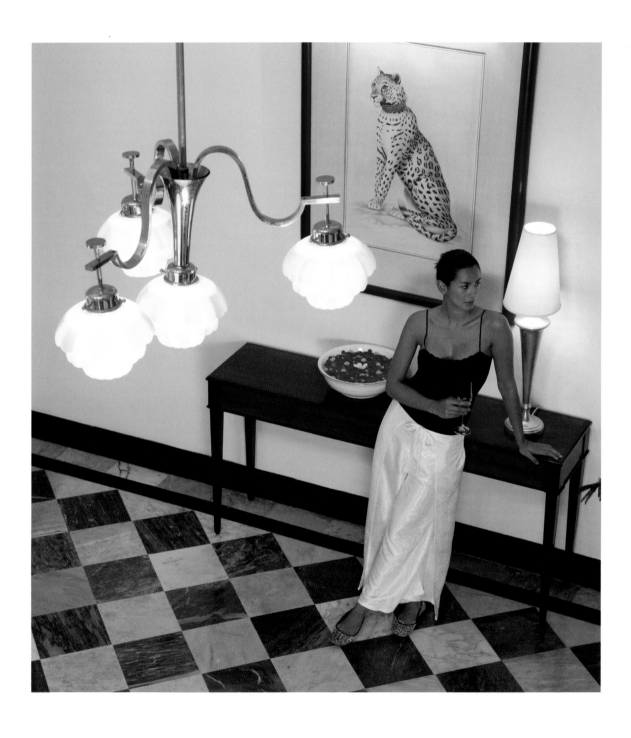

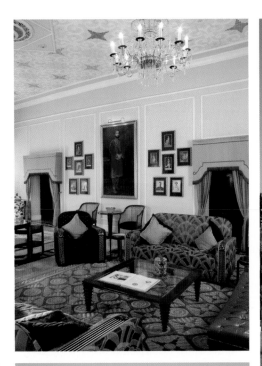

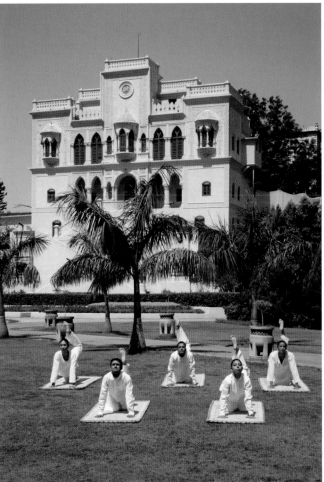

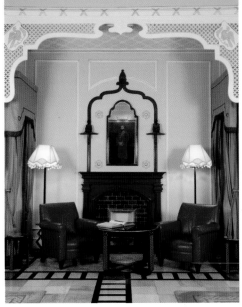

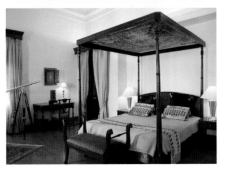

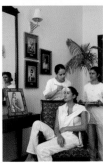

192

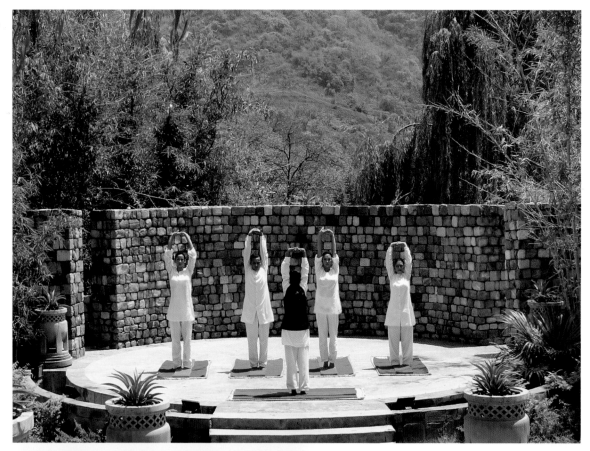

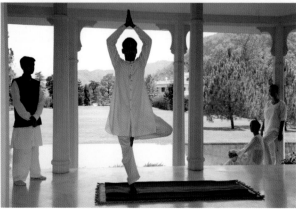

Previous pages, clockwise from left: An elegant sight in the lobby leading up to the Viceregal Suite. The Ananda reception is housed in the evocative palace annexe. The old palace, retained by the Maharajah of Tehri Garhwal, dates from 1835; the front lawn provides a peaceful spot for early morning yoga. The Viceregal Suite is the most opulent of the resort's five suites and forms a quiet setting for the Ananda facial. The bedroom is furnished with some wonderful pieces of colonial furniture including a four-poster bed, and views over the mountains are superb.

Clockwise from above: Ananda offers many and varied locations for yoga and meditation: a yoga amphitheatre carved into the hillside, a bamboo grove with resident *nandi* and the breezy, cool music pavilion. Both individual tuition and group classes are offered throughout the day.

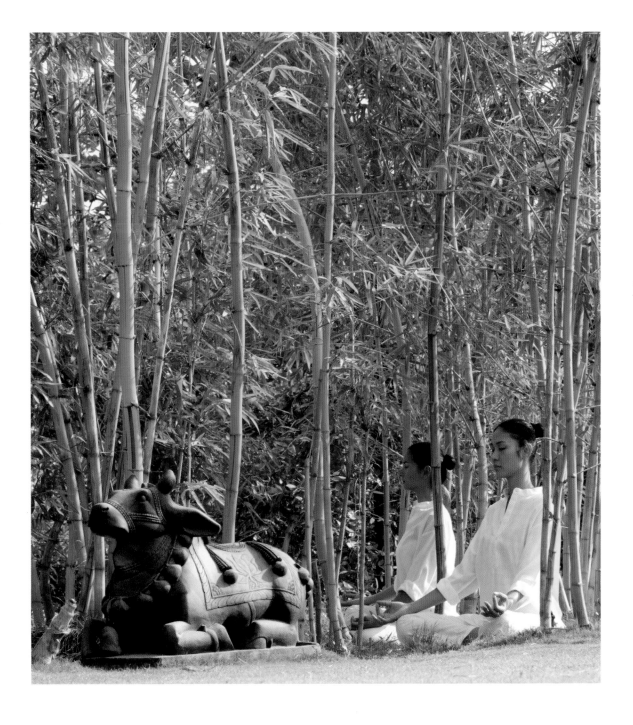

The spa itself is refreshingly modern, with a reassuring no-nonsense air of quiet professionalism. That doesn't mean to say that it isn't beautiful too. Employing a cool combination of green marble, sandstone and granite, it is characterised by signature reds and golds.

Right: A *sirodhara* session in one of the spa's tranquil treatment rooms. All rooms have their own individual showers attached, so guests are able to maintain maximum privacy.

Opposite, from top left: Holy stones: A hydrotherapy circle, complete with hot and cold water and stones from the River Ganges, is invigorating, not to mention attractive. A short stroll here combines the long-term benefits of hydrotherapy with reflexology. The slightly painful walk opens the capillaries and stimulates circulation in the legs and feet.

An exfoliating salt scrub waits for a client.

Ananda scrubs are given on a green granite "bed" specially crafted so that clients may be washed down after.

Ingredients for the Ananda signature facial artfully arranged on a tray. The facial is preceded by a back massage, and comprises a cleanse, exfoliate, tone, facial massage, clay mask and moisturise.

194

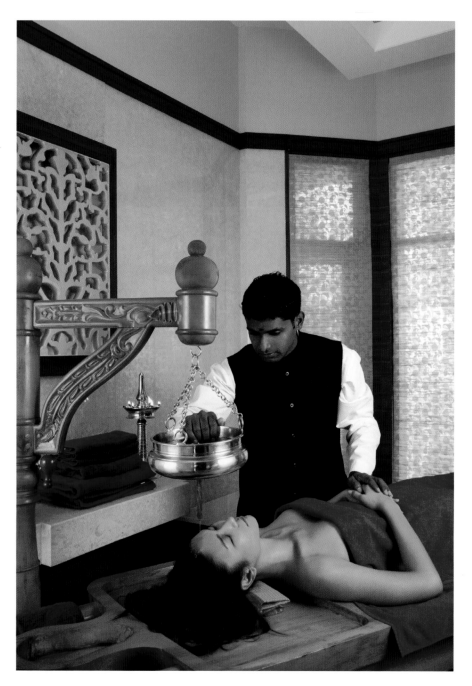

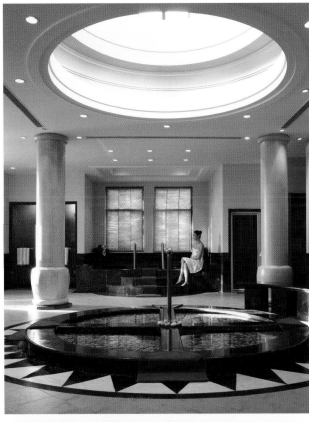

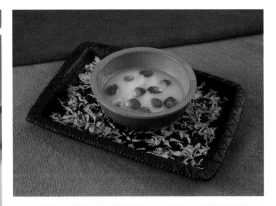

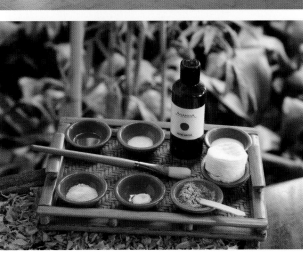

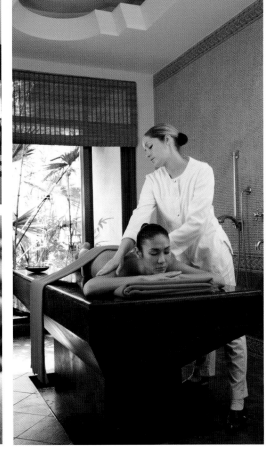

Aura Spa at Park Hotel New Delhi

This forward-looking "boutique of hotels" is India's premier brand when it comes to design and delivery. Service is slick, the hotels are über-cool in terms of decor, and the facilities top-notch. Mainly found in India's urban centres, a recent addition to their offerings is the Aura spa. With outlets in Chennai, Kolkata and New Delhi, the brand is set to grow.

A spokesperson for the group explains that the name "aura" was chosen as it implies "an individual glow, an effect or a feeling that comes from within". It also signifies a spiritual journey into the inner self, so all Aura spas are designed with calmness and tranquility in mind. They allow guests to surrender to the luxurious pampering and therapeutic treatments in an atmosphere of sequestered ease. This helps to nurture inner vitality which, in turn, is reflected by a glowing complexion, toned body and relaxed mind.

Aura spa in New Delhi is a compact space with a pastel decorative scheme that features textured walls of small mosaic tiles, embedded stones and swirling shell motifs. It has only four treatment rooms, but the addition of a beauty salon for hair and nail care and a breezy outdoor deck for yoga, meditation and more, significantly enlarges the offering.

Aura looks at the client as a whole and the menu is a varied mix of pampering and beauty treatments with something deeper, imbued with emotional or spiritual significance. Well-trained therapists guide guests to make choices that reflect their requirements: A relaxing massage, a signature

Right: An unknown artist's yogi sculpture regards a couple of clients practising yoga on the Aura terrace; cool in the early evenings, it is an ideal spot to unwind.

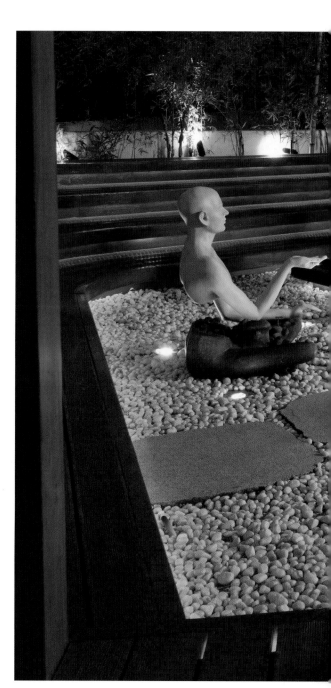

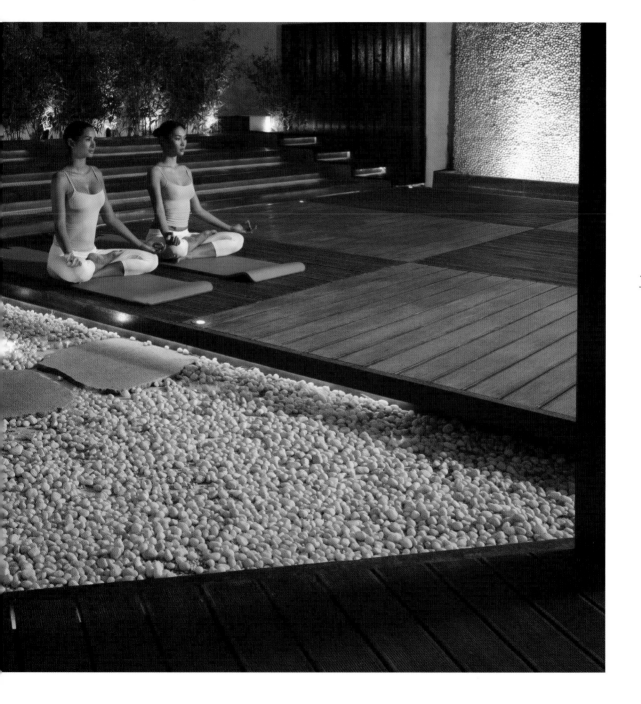

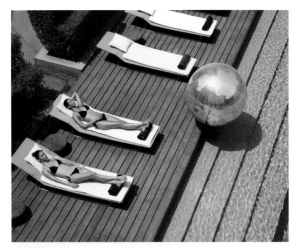

198

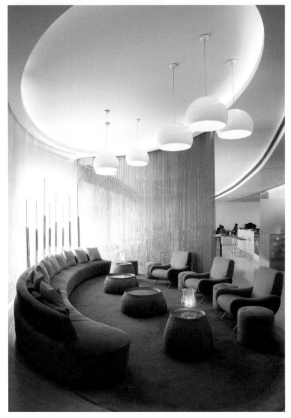

beauty treatment using a rare combination of natural herbs, flowers and spices, or a fruit-based wrap or scrub, for example. Alternatively, there are some more emotionally-releasing massages: Try the Siddha *marma* pressure point session if you want to go a little deeper (see pages 74–75), or the Esalen massage, a unique bodywork technique based on long, slow, *t'ai chi* strokes. It awakens awareness, de-stresses body and mind and helps with taut or knotted muscles.

Each Aura spa offers something that is relevant to place or context. At Chennai, each of the nine treatment rooms is decorated round one of the stunning *navaratnas* or nine-jewel tones, and the signature detoxifying Aura massge uses local *gingli* (sesame) oil with an open palm technique. New Delhi is famed for its Moghal Experience where the same massage follows a body polish composed from rice bran, rose and sandalwood. This ends with a *chamak* facial personalised to suit individual skin types.

In the same way, each hotel is distinctively designed with different decorative schemes – yet a distinctly "Park" identity. It may be difficult to define, but once you've been to a couple of the hotels, it is instantly recognisable.

Left: Designed by Conran and Partners around a *vaastu shastra* theme, the Park New Delhi uses water and fire in the design concept. The outdoor pool deck is cobalt blue, while Mist, the coffee shop restaurant (left), is cooling and quiet.

Right: A regal silver chair, cast from aluminum and bronze by Subodh Gupta, provides a throne-like seat for this floral foot soak and scrub – pure pampering!

Inset: The beauty salon is used for hair and nail treatments.

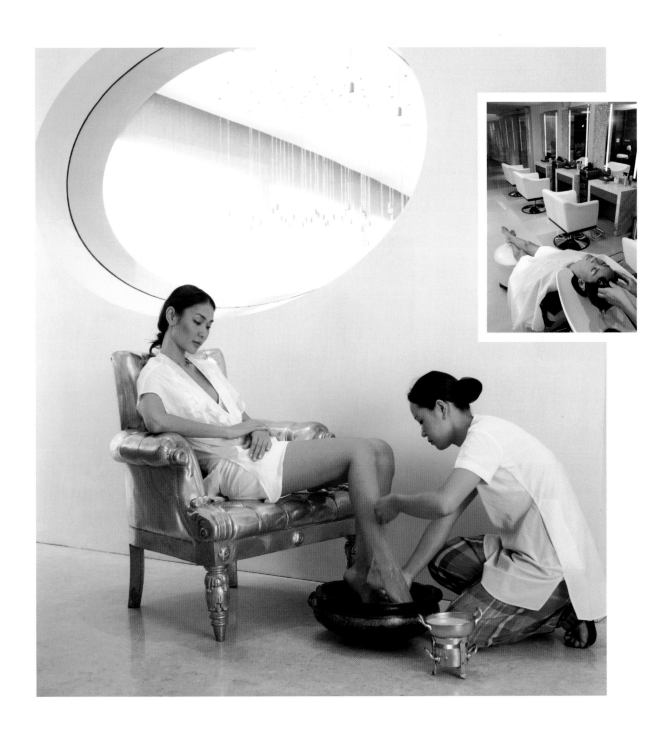

Shahnaz Husain Salons

With scores of franchised beauty salons in India and a highly successful manufacturing and retailing arm, Shahnaz Husain is one of India's best known names in the health and beauty industry. A tireless advocate of India's herbal healing remedies, Husain is well known both at home and abroad.

With over 35 years of experience in the business, Husain's is a true rags to riches story. More than three decades ago she opened a small herbal salon with little more than her savings and a crusader's zeal in the efficacy of herbal healing. Today, her Ayurvedic-based formulations are sold in Harrods, Selfridges and Bloomingdales, and she has a presence in over 400 franchised clinics, shops, schools and spas worldwide. Her strong belief in India's natural apothecary and holistic systems of healing has never wavered.

In many ways when she started out Husain was far ahead of her time. Even then, she eschewed the gold-topped, chemical-filled jar for something much more earthy – and today everybody is jumping on the bandwagon. "Everything can be found in Nature," she declares. "Be it protective, preventive or even corrective, cosmetic care should be 100 percent natural. All the answers are in our herbal heritage and ancient philosophies."

Shahnaz Herbals has researched, trialled and manufactured scores of natural remedies, and now sells over 460 products. Running the gamut from skin to hair, cosmetics to herbal supplements, they utilise many of India's famous herbals: neem, henna, wild turmeric, honey, almonds, gold, silver and pearls to name a few.

A trip to any Shahnaz Husain salon starts with a clinical assessment of skin, hair and general health; tests may even include urine or stool tests as internal purification is considered as vital as outer beauty. Hair and skin type, complexion, wellness and diet are all examined, and then advice is given as to which particular products should be used and which treatments are most efficacious. Usha Zadoo, a Shahnaz Husain beauty advisor, says that what the client does at home is also extremely important: "We try to get as full a picture as possible, before we suggest supplements, products, make-up or therapies," she explains.

Never one to shirk from a challenge, Husain is now focusing on the shift from salon to day spa, and clinic to destination spa. "The success of our herbal salon concept, both in India and abroad, bears testimony to my faith in herbal care and Ayurveda," she says. "So the next step is most definitely towards the spa." Noting that many spa therapies have their roots in India, she believes that India is well placed to become a leading global spa destination. Her first spa is soon to open outside Delhi. And, knowing this indefatigable entrepreneur, many more are sure to follow.

Above: The Shahnaz Husain name is the company's brand – and Husain, herself, is the brand ambassador.

200

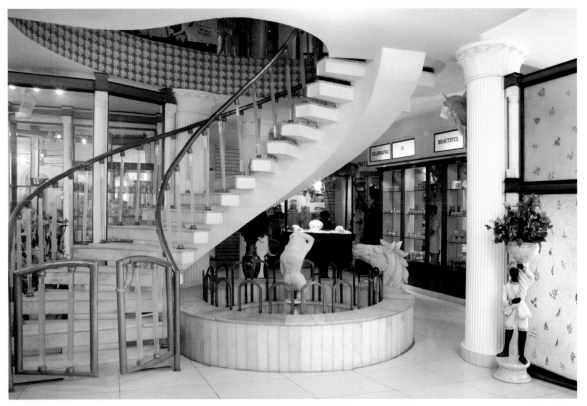

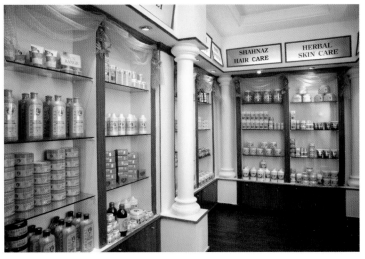

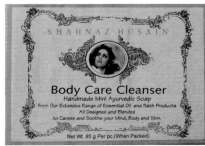

Top: Ebullient in spirit, Shahnaz Husain's salons are often extravagantly decorated.

Left and above: Building up from one basic Ayurvedic product group, Shahnaz Husain has added further ranges over the years: a neem range, a men's range, one for lightening the skin, an oxygen range – and much, much more.

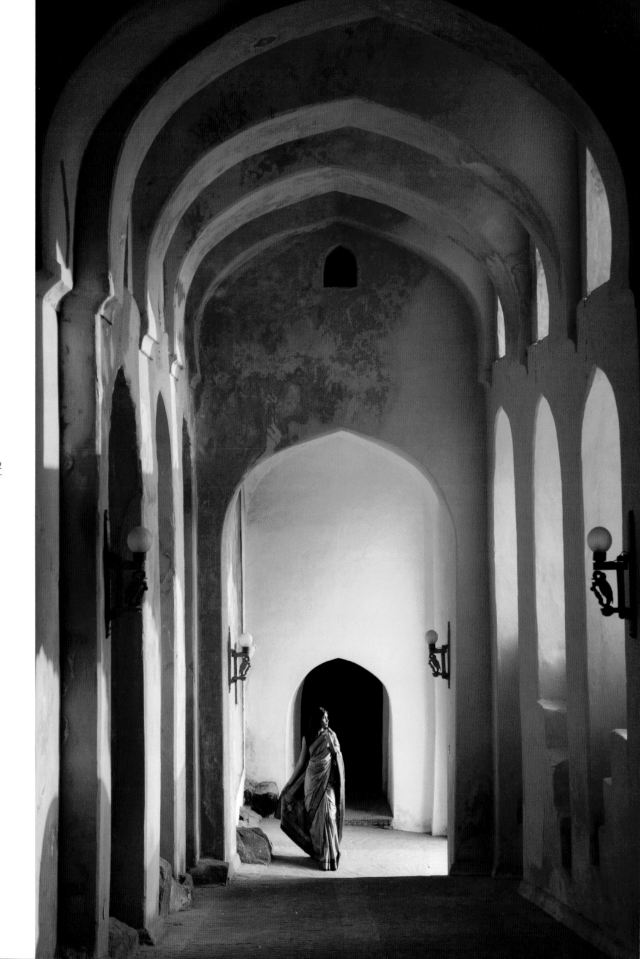

The Health Spa & Ayurvedic Centre at Neemrana Fort Palace

Opened in 1999 in association with Sansha, a herbal cosmetic firm that also runs a number of spas in luxury resorts, the health spa and Ayurvedic centre at Neemrana Fort Palace is as authentic as the hotel itself. Situated in the new wing of this magnificent heritage hotel, it offers a variety of Ayurvedic and salon-type treatments. A resident doctor supervises, and all the therapists are from Kerala.

Interestingly enough, Neemrana is situated only an hour's drive from the last resting place of the *rishi* Chyavan, a sage who is credited with formulating *chyavanprash*, one of Ayurveda's most efficacious herbal tonics. The story goes that Chyavan married a very young girl at the age of 80, and, needing to keep young, invented a *rasayana* to combat the ageing process. In Ayurvedic medicine *rasayanas* are a means to a long, healthy, disease-free life. Containing 49 herbs including *amla* or Indian gooseberry, the first historically documented formula for *chyavanprash* is found in the ancient Ayurvedic treatise the *Charaka Samhita*, where it is described as "the foremost of all *rasayanas*, especially good for alleviating cough and asthma; it nourishes the weak, the wounded, the old, and those that are of tender years as well."

Naturally, this magic elixir of youth is available at the Neemrana spa, along with an extremely

comprehensive selection of Ayurvedic treatments. All the products used, in both the Ayurvedic and Sansha ranges, are 100 percent natural, with herbs procured from India and elsewhere. In keeping with the ancient environment, treatments begin with a traditional consultation and a cleansing footbath with eucalyptus, green tea and mint and a *marma* massage on feet and legs. In addition, therapists are encouraged to start a treatment with an invocation of healing prayers and guests are given a choice of scented oils or incense.

In addition to spa treatments and Ayurvedic wellness programmes, Neemrana Fort Palace offers early morning yoga in a recently planted *mukut bagh* or "crowning garden" and other gardens, courts, nooks and crannies are perfect for sessions of quiet contemplation. Dating from the 15th century and built in stages over 500 years, the fort palace revolves around a series of such courts

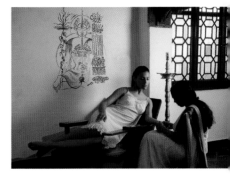

situated over nine levels. The *mukut bagh* is on the ninth level, so yoga is literally practiced in the sky with extraordinary views over the fortress below and the ancient Aravali ranges in the distance. Other diversions include a cooling blue-tiled pool, a gym, an art gallery and an amphitheatre carved from local Ghelot stone where a variety of cultural performances are held.

203

Right: In Indian salons, a manicure is usually accompanied by a hand massage that extends up the arm. In the spa at Neemrana Fort Palace, a therapist locates pressure points on the hand – for deep cleansing as well as relaxation.

Left: A serpentine cobbled alleyway leads from the fortress's first massive gate up into the palace itself where arch after Rajasthani arch reveals new sights.

For many people a visit to Neemrana is a chance to truly experience India in the raw. The sanitised environment of the isolated five-star resort is eschewed here for something entirely earthy and "real". The facilities and food are more than perfectly acceptable, but it is the warmth and willingness of the staff and the extraordinary fairy-tale fortress that fire the imagination of visitors. One guest told me that every night he discovered a different route to his room! In addition, every room houses an antique or historical artifact; every staircase or corridor opens into another secretive courtyard; and at every level, another view over the ancient Rajasthani landscape is revealed.

When the owners stumbled across Neemrana while researching a book on nearby Shekawati, it was a crumbling wreck, looted and lost, empty since 1947. Nearly half a century of neglect had reduced this once-magnificent structure to near ruin. Now, after years of loving restoration, its monumental silhouette gleams anew from the rocky plateau on which it rests – and guests from all over the world are welcomed.

Right: The exterior of the fort palace is painted in ochre tones and sports a profusion of graceful *jarokhas* (protruding balconies), cupolas, pillars and pavilions. Extremely imposing, it is far more medieval than modern. Winner in 2001 of the INTACH-SATTE award for Restoration and Tourism, Neemrana has become synonymous with the phrase "restoration for reuse". As the judges noted: "Neemrana remains the foremost example of how we can pick architectural treasures from the national dustbin and turn them around into mainstream revenue earners in tourism".

Inset: A portrait of the last Maharajah of Neemrana, resplendent in court dress, with three retainers behind.

Overleaf: Rough-hewn walls with balconies, arches and windows rise up on two sides of the beautifully lit swimming pool.

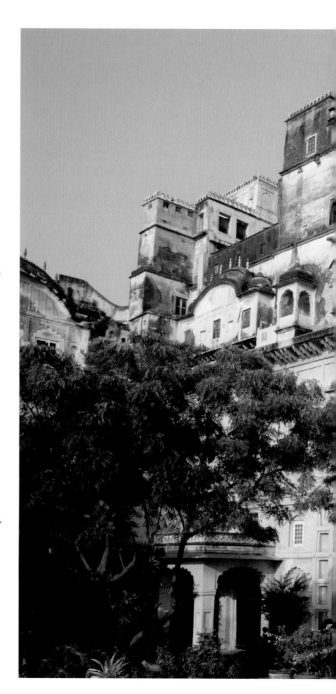

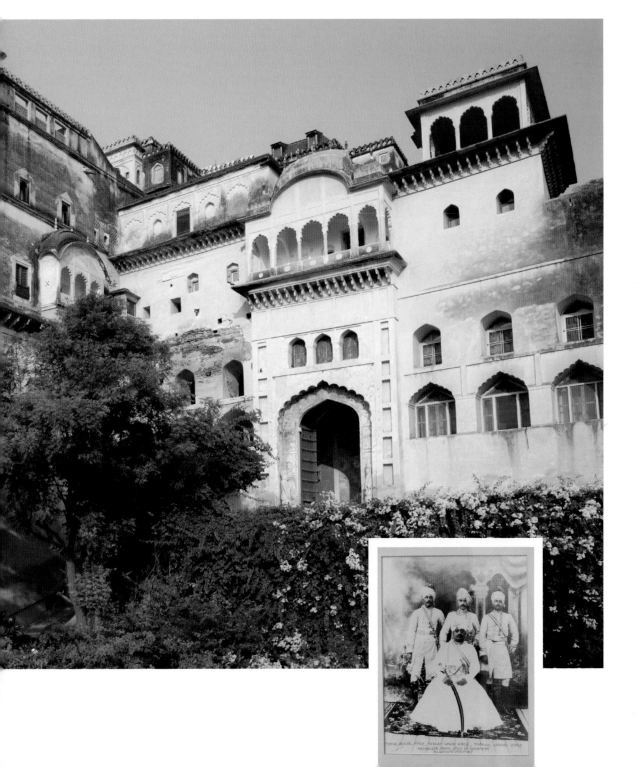

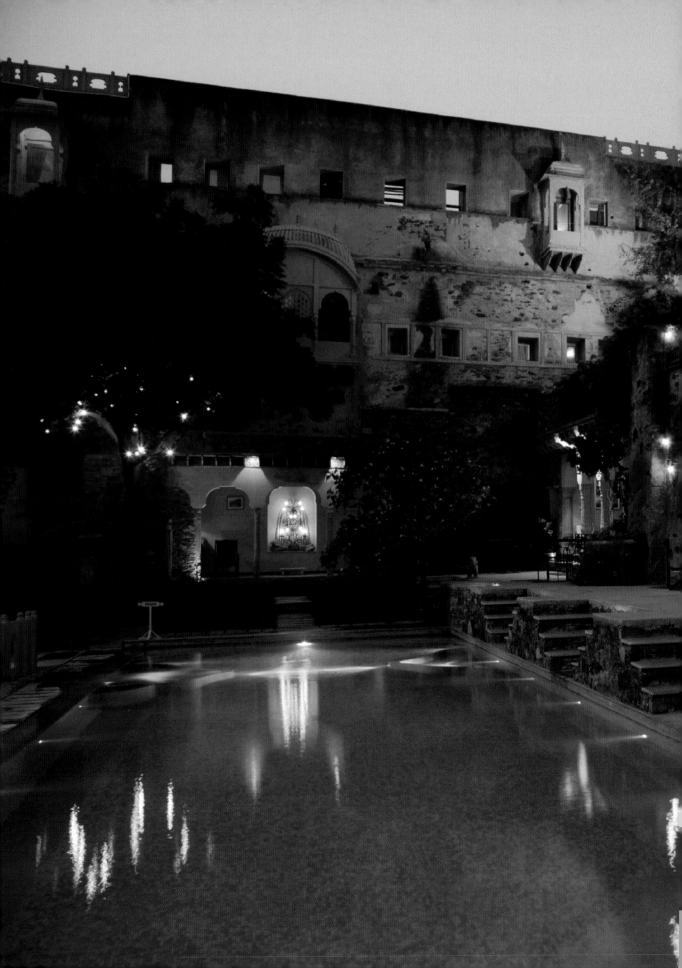

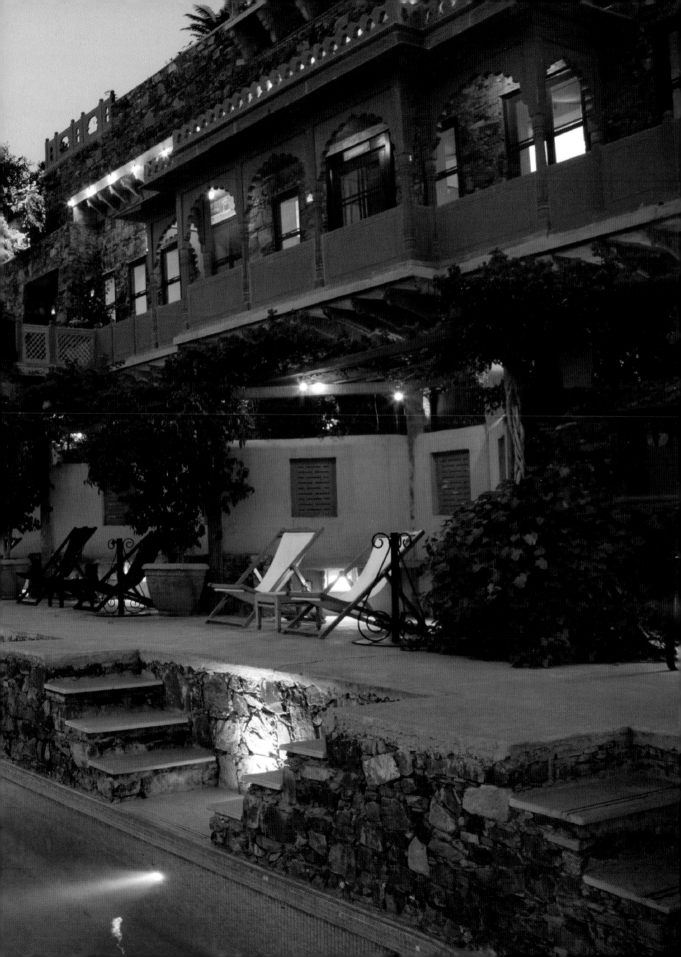

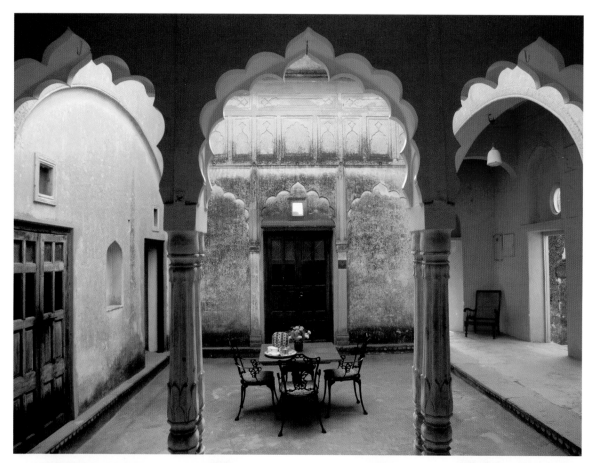

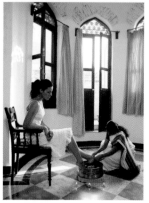
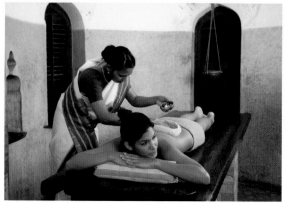
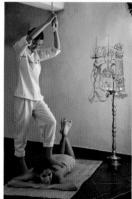

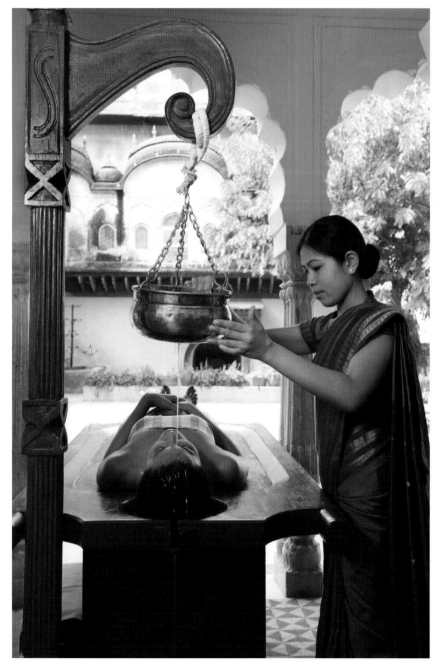

Opposite, top: Cool court: One of the many courtyards in Neemrana Fort Palace, this one is located just outside the Maharani's suite of rooms and is framed by typical scallop-edged arches and pillars.

Opposite, bottom left: At the beginning of each treatment at the spa, every client receives a cleansing footbath with a eucalyptus, green tea and mint de-stress foot soak. "It feels good up the whole leg," reported a guest. "The therapist knew where the points were and it was very relaxing."

Opposite, bottom middle: The spa is fully equipped with Ayurvedic beds, steam boxes and sitz baths to remove oil after treatments. Here a therapist ensures the client is comfortable prior to administering *kathi vasthi.*

Opposite, bottom right: A form of massage that was formulated to condition the body of *kalari* fighters, *chavitti thirummu* massage is given by a masseuse suspended from ropes on the ceiling; the masseuse uses dancing movements with the feet all over the body.

Left: The Durbar Hall features a series of pillars and arches illustrating the Rajasthani love of architectural adornment. It is a truly royal setting for the mind-expanding *sirodhara* routine.

209

210

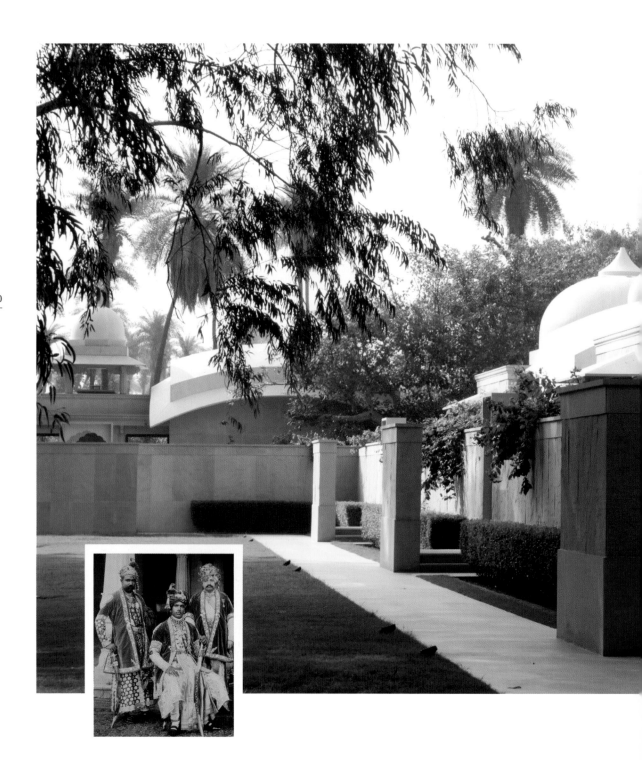

Aman Spa at Amanbagh

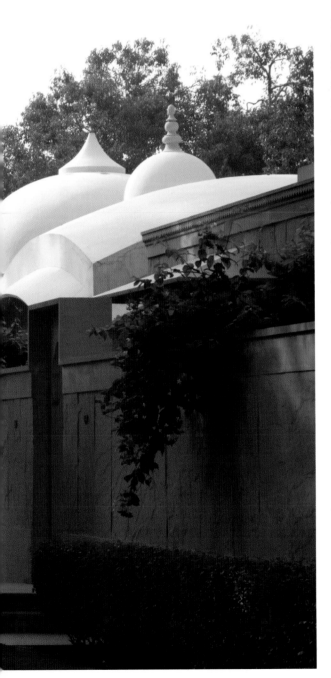

Rural India – a world that Gandhi called the "heart and soul of the country" – is where most Indians still reside. It sports an extraordinary range of environments, from snow-capped mountains and lush forests to seemingly endless plains, verdant jungles and harsh deserts, and an even greater variety of peoples, with their own distinctive cultures, religions and languages. It is, however, little visited by outsiders, with most holidaymakers and business travellers sticking to India's cities.

All the more reason then, to visit Amanbagh, where the destination should not (indeed cannot) be divorced from its location. Situated in a narrow valley on the site of the old 19th-century hunting encampment of Maharaja Jai Singh of Alwar, an area little explored and little visited, Amanbagh has fully embraced the locale in its hotel experience. Visits to villages, cultural and historical tours, exotic wildlife spotting and other excursions are as integral to the Aman experience here as is lounging by the pool and savouring the highly specialised service. The hotel has all the modern Aman amenities; its surrounds have all the exotica of a bygone age.

211

Left: Circled by an old stone wall that served as a boundary to the Maharajah's hunting camp, the property is serene and isolated, as unexpected as it is beautiful. Ancient date palms, planted by the Emperor Akbar's army who stopped at the sheltered place between long marches, and more recently-planted eucalyptus trees form the backdrop to this veritable retreat. The entire property was designed by the Paris-based American architect Ed Tuttle, with surfaces that are, for the most part, purposefully unadorned. The only decoration is some simple *jaali* screening and the flocks of parakeets and other birds that call Amanbagh their home.
Inset: Jai Singh Prabhakar Bahadur (1892–1937), the Maharaja of Alwar, flanked by two retainers. The princely state of Alwar nestles in the Aravali hills; it has always been prime hunting land.

Right: A flautist entertains guests in the central courtyard. Often you'll see a *rangoli* artwork here. Made from grains, seeds or other organic matter, the *rangoli* is a symbol of welcome for guests. At the annual Diwali festival, owners traditionally clean their houses and leave a *rangoli* at the doorstep to welcome the goddess Lakshmi. Lakshmi is the goddess of wealth, so it is hoped that good fortune and happiness will be bestowed on the home-owners after.

Opposite top: The lobby is a magnificent soaring room, fit for a queen. Two rose petal strewn fountains and a double-height space greet guests on arrival. In keeping with the traditional saying *aatithi devo bhavah* or "Guest is our God", each visitor is welcomed with marigold flowers and a symbolic string tied to the wrist.

Opposite bottom: It seems that pomegranates are always in season at Amanbagh. Spa treatments begin with refreshing pomegranate juice served in a simple silver cup and a hot towel scented with coriander and jasmine.

212

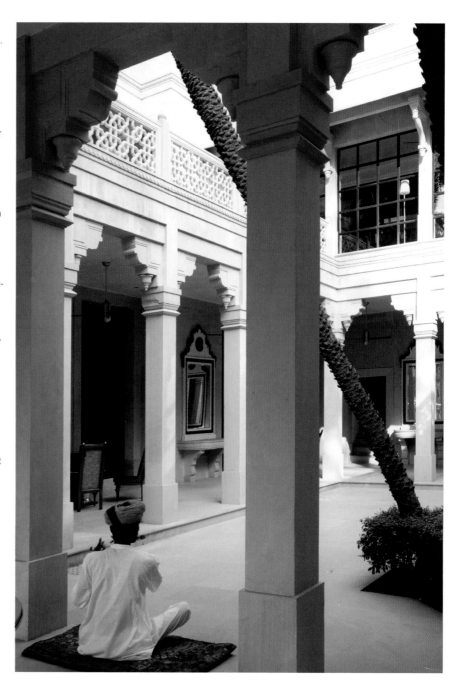

In keeping with the Aman ethos of respect for local traditions, architecture is inspired by the grandiose Moghul tradition. Domed cupolas, colonnaded courtyards and *jaali* screens in pink sandstone and marble are clustered in a garden of palm, eucalyptus and fruit trees. Outside this walled compound, life continues much as it has done for thousands of years. The hotel employs many of its staff from the surrounding villages – and of particular note is the highly dedicated team at the superlative Aman spa.

As befits such a remote property, the spa is a calm, serene space with pink marble floors and walls of teak wood and mirror geometric patterning continuing the *jaali* theme. With a spacious reception and three large treatment rooms set around a cooling pool, it aims to give complete relaxation, not just to the body, but mind and soul as well. As such, its menu includes meditation, yoga and yoga-stretching therapies, Reiki, and a couple of Ayurvedic treatments, as well as some beguiling body and face sequences.

The names of the treatments are in Hindi, and many incorporate the spirit and traditions of the former princely states that now comprise Rajasthan. The Maharana and Maharani massages are indeed fit for a king and queen; many ingredients are locally sourced and taken from Rajput rituals – saffron for skin conditioning, rose and milk for bathing, local clay with hibiscus for wraps, oatmeal powder, turmeric, sandalwood and essence of rose for traditional *ubtan* scrubs, to mention a few; and some items on the menu are offered outside the hotel grounds in the surrounding countryside. Sunrise yoga at the extraordinary deserted fortress of Bhangarh (see pages104–105) or a meditation session at the nearby Sam Sagar lake are two that immediately come to mind.

Amanbagh's site is known as *Jhil-mil* which translates as "Sparkling Waters". This is apt, as it could be argued that the whole property is one huge healing spa. There are numerous water

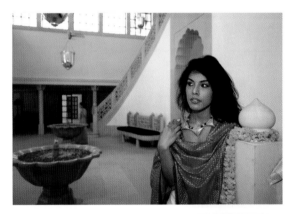

bodies within the grounds – two large swimming pools, individual plunge and villa pools, fountains and Jacuzzis – and there's a huge lake with *shikara* (Kashmiri boat) trips less than a mile away. The stunning Aravali hills form

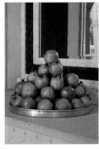

a suitably private backdrop, while the purity of the environment, the love and care of the staff who call themselves an Aman family and the tailored wellness excursions all contribute towards balancing the mind and nourishing the spirit.

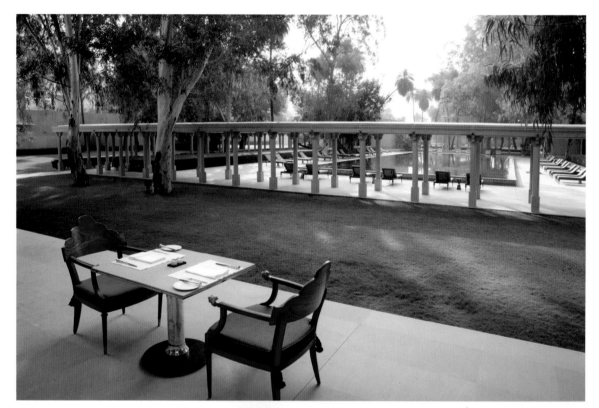

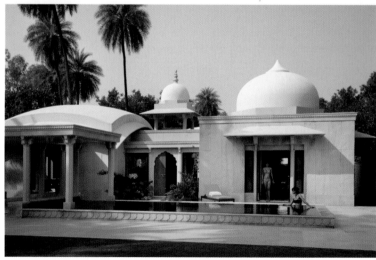

Above: Situated in a green oasis behind a large lake, there are copious water bodies within Amanbagh's walls. This view from the dining terrace shows the huge swimming pool behind an open colonnade. Behind it is a smaller spa pool, while fountains and private pools are found elsewhere.

Right: Some of the sumptuous freestanding villas have their own private pools. Each uses pink marble, green granite from Udaipur and local Rajasthani sandstone.

Opposite: The final stage of the sumptuous Royal Experience, a Rajput regime of scrub, steam, wrap and massage, performed by a therapist at the edge of the spa pool. In the background is a therapy room and a small, domed restaurant that serves healthy snacks at lunchtime.

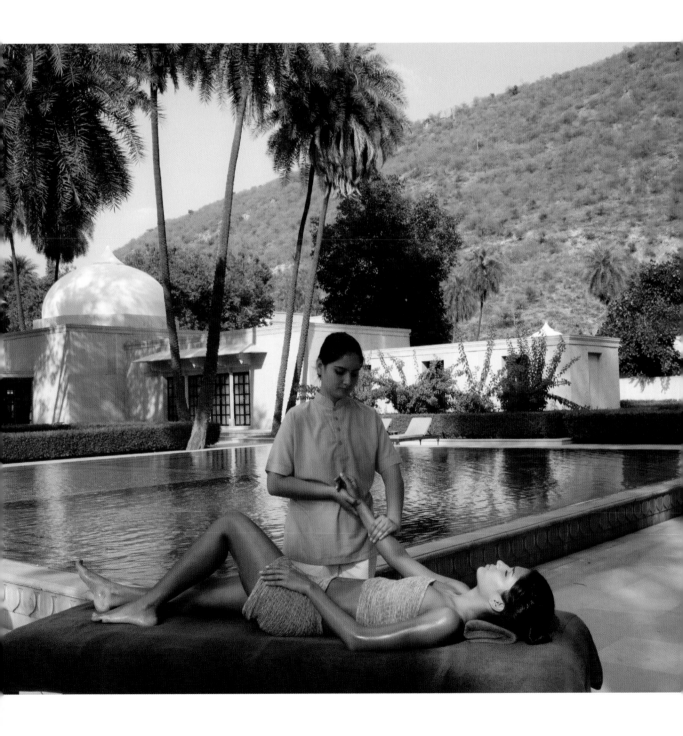

Oberoi Spa at Rajvilas

When word got out that Mr P R S Oberoi was building an enormous hotel fort on the outskirts of Jaipur, people cried, "Fort or folly?". It was the mid 1990s and rumour had it that the intention was to recreate a fanciful version of a Maharajah's court. There was to be a massive Rajasthani fort at the entrance, numerous *havelis* or mansions and tented rooms in the gardens, pools and ponds, landscaped gardens, and more. Eight hundred workers had been employed for three years to realise the vision. The budget was astronomical, the scale unimaginable.

People muttered about the cost, the design, the grandiose ambition. They worried about the 250-year-old temple at the centre of the 13-acre (32-hectare) site. Surely it wouldn't be razed to the ground? Phrases like "pride comes before a fall" were furtively whispered.

Thankfully, Mr Oberoi took no notice. Having dedicated his entire life to running hotels, he had decided the time was right to start building them. He had recently completed a painstaking and architecturally accurate restoration of a traditional fort at nearby Naila, and the success of the project had inspired him. He wanted to create a setting where visitors to Jaipur could be pampered like the personal guests of a Rajput prince, and, God willing, he would do it.

It certainly wasn't easy, but Rajvilas opened in 1997, and was an instant success. It took standards of hoteliering in the country to another level, and people flocked from within India and abroad to experience its excellent food and service, opulent décor and extraordinary architecture. Bill Clinton came not once, but twice, and the hotel won just about every award going in the hospitality industry. It became the top topic of conversation amongst the chattering classes and also led to the building of other Vilas properties and the creation and consolidation of Oberoi Group's top-tier brand.

More than a decade on, the hotel is as fresh and inspiring as when it opened. The main building is a faithful recreation of a Rajasthani fortress, the suites, rooms and villas resemble a leafy Maharajah's city, and outside the "walls" is a desert encampment of luxurious tented accommodations. The gardens, with fruit trees, shrubs and flowering plants have grown to maturity; the decorative pools and fountains continue to cool the site; its staff is as enthusiastic as ever. And the ancient Shiva temple, within a cocoon of lotus and lily ponds, still sits at the epicentre of Mr Oberoi's domain.

Opposite this is an open-sided Rajasthani pavilion or *chattri*, a cooling blue-tiled swimming pool, and a reconstructed *haveli* that houses the

Above: The grounds of Rajvilas are dotted with marble fountains and elegant water features. At the hotel forecourt, guests are greeted with cool scented towels and the sounds of trickling water from this traditional Moghul-style water feature.

Right: Traditional architectural forms from both Rajput and Moghul styles are utilised in Rajvilas. The private pool of the Royal Suite is a glittering combination of lapis blue tiles, hand-fired in Jaipur, and blush pink decoration.

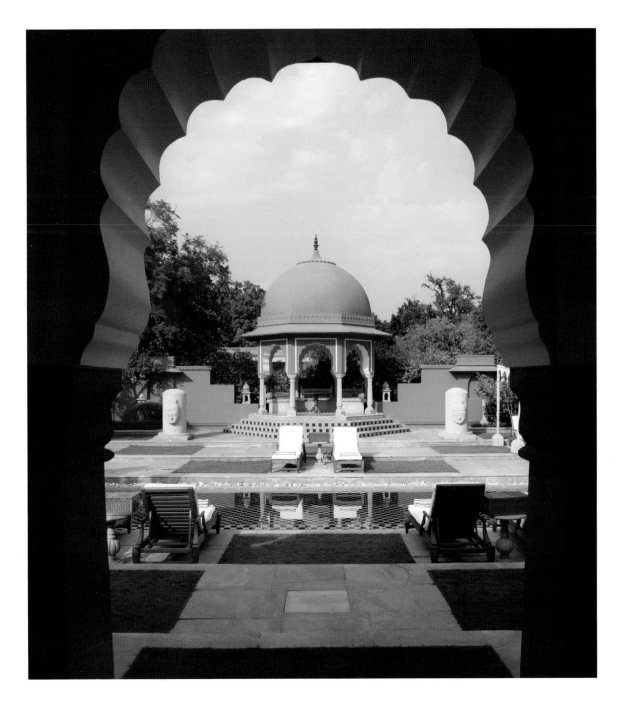

spa. Managed by Banyan Tree as are all the Oberoi Spas, it is accessed by a few stairs with the reception area at front. Within are white marble plunge pools, saunas, a central courtyard with cooling Jacuzzi in blue and white marble, opulent changing rooms, and 10 treatment rooms including four suites. In addition, there is a large gymnasium overlooking a formal herb garden that is a recreation of one at the nearby Amber palace, a beauty salon and a room for manicures and pedicures. It would be difficult to find more soothing surrounds for a pampering treatment: The interiors feature colonial-style loungers, hand-painted frescoes and warm wooden floors, while the nurturing hands of highly trained therapists ensure every visit is very special.

The recently revamped Ayurvedic treatment menu, formulated by the resident physician, offers a number of non-clinical therapies and massages including an inspiring package called the Spirit of Ayurveda (see pages 60–61), while the rest of the menu is dedicated to Western and aromatherapy treatments. True to Asian traditions, all products are 100 percent natural and are environmentally sensitive. Whether it is a soothing Ayurvedic facial, a purifying bath or a vigorous rub you require – the spa is fully geared up to guests' needs.

Right: Jaipur is famous for its blue pottery tiles. Hand-made in rich shades of lapis, turquoise and ultramarine, the craft was originally brought to India from Persia. The stylised designs of Persian pottery were revived in the mid 19th century by Maharaja Sawai Ram Singh II of Jaipur. In the water therapy areas at the spa, hand-fired versions, this time in off white, are utilised on floors and steps for a slightly rustic effect.

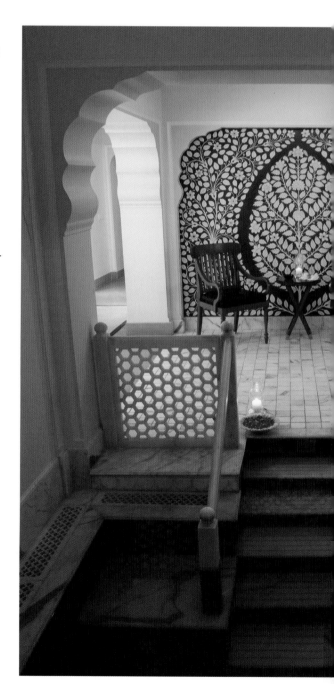

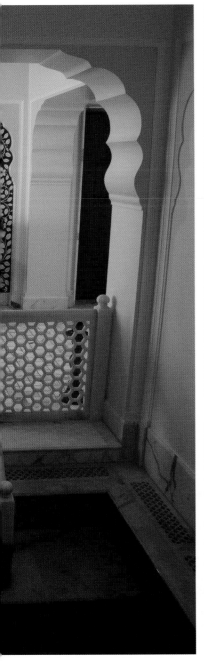

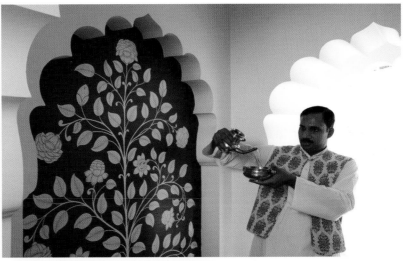

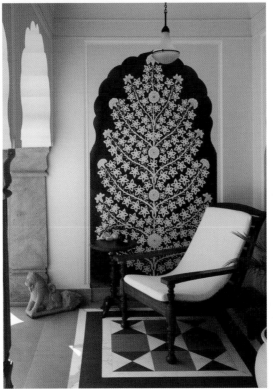

Above: Ayurvedic medicated oils are individually chosen and blended according to the guest's *dosha* by the resident Ayurvedic physician. Other oils that originate from China and Thailand are carefully selected and hand-blended for the Hawaiian, Balinese and aromatherapy styles of massage.

Left: At the entrance to the spa, a colonial-style lounger has been thoughtfully placed for a guest. All the blue-and-white wall paintings in the resort were painted by master artist Ghanshyan Nimbark and a team of painters from all over Rajasthan.

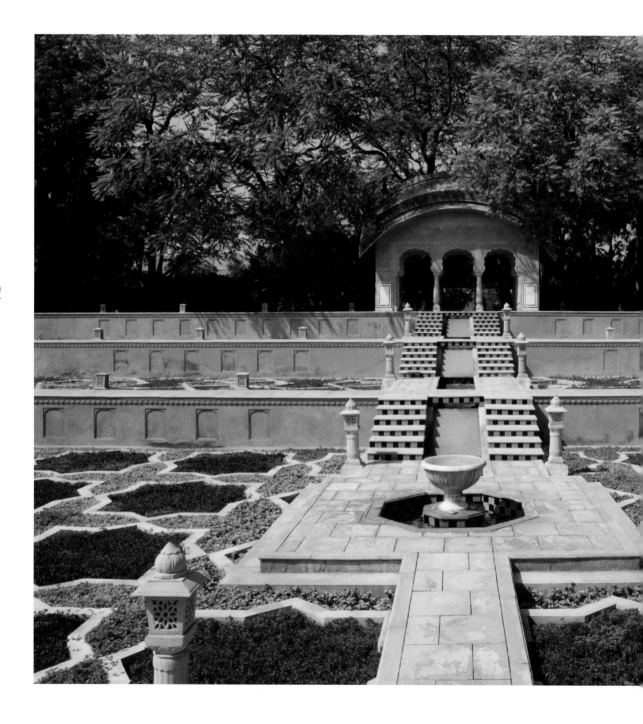

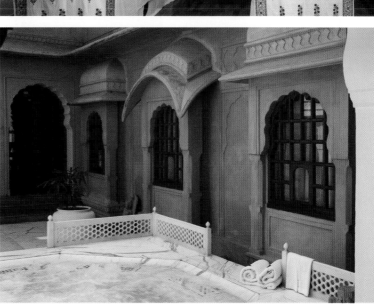

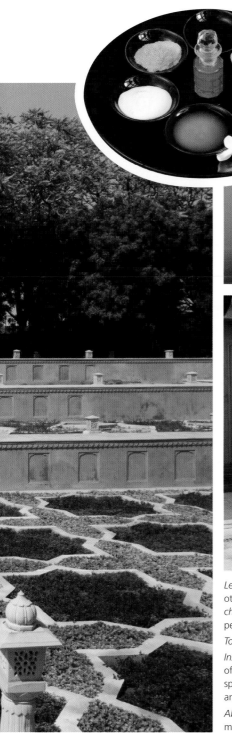

Left: The gym and some of the treatment rooms overlook this formal spa garden, whilst others have views of lotus pools or beds of fragrant jasmine. The recreated Rajasthani *chattri*, accessed by a flight of steps laid with glowing blue Jaipur pottery tiles, forms a perfect spot for quiet contemplation.

Top: A treatment room ready for a therapy.

Inset: All the Oberoi spa menus feature the signature Oberoi facial, the lotions and potions of which are pictured here. Various ingredients ranging from honey to watermelon are specially selected for each skin type. The sequence consists of a cleanse, exfoliation, mask and moisturise for healthy, glowing skin.

Above: A central courtyard, surrounded by *airaish* lime plastered walls, houses a cool marble Jacuzzi pool. Made by hand by local craftsmen, it is an artwork in itself.

Oberoi Spa at Udaivilas

Visitors to Udaivilas arriving by plane are transported by chauffeured limousine from the airport to Lake Pichola, from where they board a small boat that ferries them across the peaceful waters of the lake to the hotel's landing jetty. There can be no better way to arrive at what is surely one of India's most romantic hotels: views of Udaipur's lakeside City Palace are glorious, and the glimmering Lake Palace Hotel and Jagmandir Palace on their private islands are enduring testaments to the Mewari clan's connoisseurship of art, architecture and culture.

It is this legacy that the Oberoi Group has emulated at Udaivilas. Working to the instruction of Mr P R S Oberoi's vision of "building a palace", the past is present in every aspect of Udaivilas. Covering a staggering 32 acres (13 hectares) of undulating lakeside land, the resort comprises a collection of predominantly single-storey buildings topped with domes, chattris and pavilions, interconnected by reflecting pools, grandiose courtyards and lush gardens. All the buildings are painted a creamy white with a traditional lime-plastering technique that imbues the resort with an unabashed air of serenity.

Mewari motifs are to be found at every turn: The Mewari princes claim to be descended from no lesser figure than the sun god, so sun sculptures and artworks adorn cool stone surfaces at every turn. Intricate thekri (molten glass mosaic) work and floral and vegetal frescoes painted with natural dyes are to be found on walls, while scalloped edge arches, domes and cupolas (ghummats and ghumtis) and a variety of fountains and pools anchor Udaivilas with a strong sense of place. The main swimming pool is lined with steps of black granite and white marble to resemble a traditional stepwell, while another courtyard sports a decorative pool with a seemingly floating luminous white marble lotus.

As with every aspect of Udaivilas, at the spa nothing has been left to chance. Under the management of Banyan Tree, but with a resident Ayurvedic doctor and yoga master, it is as impeccable as a Mewari miniature painting. Reaching their pinnacle in the 17th century, Mewari painters skillfully applied natural pigments and effervescent colours to articulate human, animal, vegetative and floral forms in minute details; at this Oberoi spa each part of every treatment is perfectly and seamlessly formulated to create a wonderful and satisfying whole.

On offer are a number of non-clinical Ayurvedic options, along with a mixed menu of massages, scrubs, facials and beauty treatments. Of particular

Above: Legend has it that the Mewari dynasty was descended from Lord Rama and the Sun God, so its members are known as the *Suryavanshi* or "Children of the Sun". At Udaipur's newest palace to hospitality the sun is a recurring motif: here it is represented as a massive metal sculpture at the base of a cascading water body.

Right: The Indians are master craftsmen with stone; Udaivilas contains a profusion of domes, arches, cupolas and pavilions, all lovingly created by hand from sandstone and marble.

222

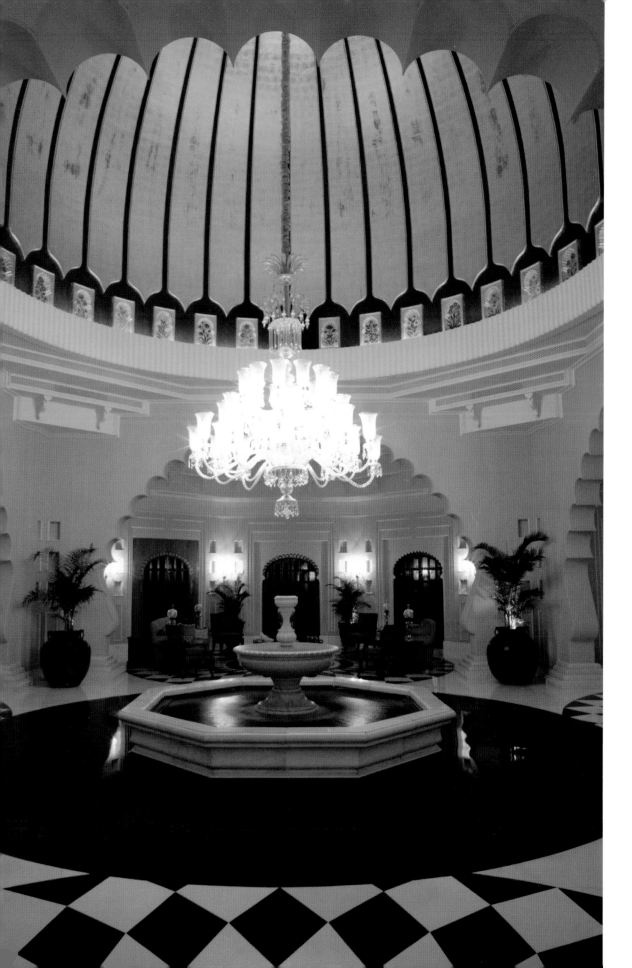

interest are the two to three hour packages, where guests are pampered in the manner of the Mewari princesses of the past. Every treatment takes place in the opulent spa premises, where therapy rooms radiate off a central, circular and domed ante-chamber, or in one or other of the adjacent spa suites. All have wonderful arched windows that frame spectacular vistas of Lake Pichola, the private spa pool and meditative gardens.

If an introduction to Ayurveda is an option, you couldn't be in better hands than those of Dr Yogesh. Trained in Kerala at some of the top Ayurvedic colleges, the physician has modulated some of the Science of Life's invigorating massages, scrubs and therapies for one-time healing. Even though they aren't clinical, the treatments do take into account the client's state of health, *dosha* and imbalances, and only take place after a consultation so that the correct oils may be prepared and used.

Alternatively, there are yoga sessions for all levels of practitioner and inspiring lakeside walks and excursions. For those who want to stay within the resort's confines, the menu of inspiring baths is the ultimate in self-indulgence. Choose from purifying neem, warm and relaxing marigold, the detox herbal soak to shed excess subcutaneous toxins, or the fragrant milk and rose petal treat. You'll be sure to come back for more.

Right: The Oberoi spa is situated in its own freestanding building with a circular interior balcony opening to a central dome with crystal chandelier. It is housed at the furthest point of the resort near Lake Pichola and has its own private spa pool. The super long water body in front may be accessed from some of the private sun decks that are attached to guest rooms.

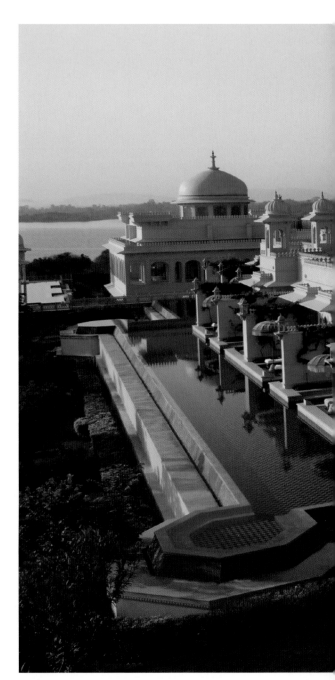

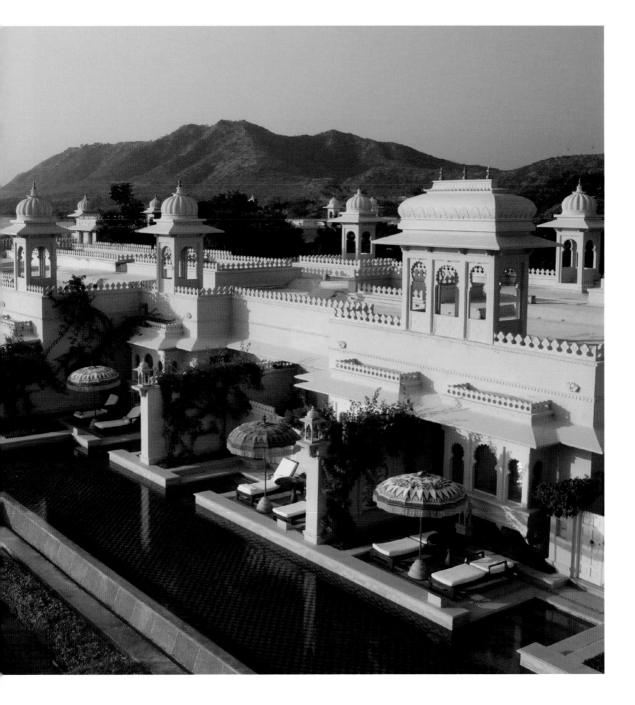

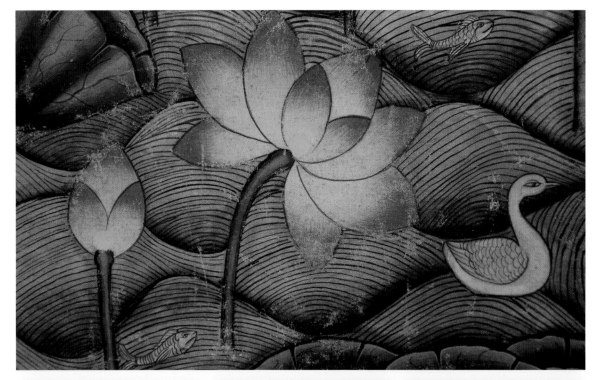

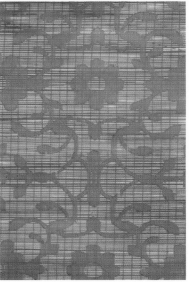

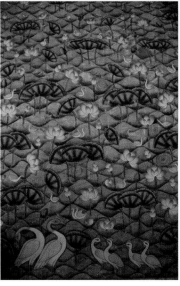

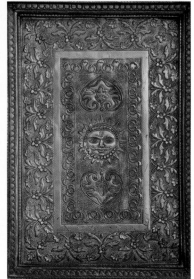

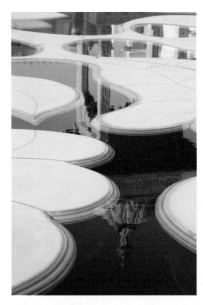
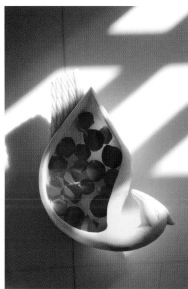
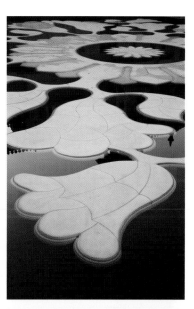

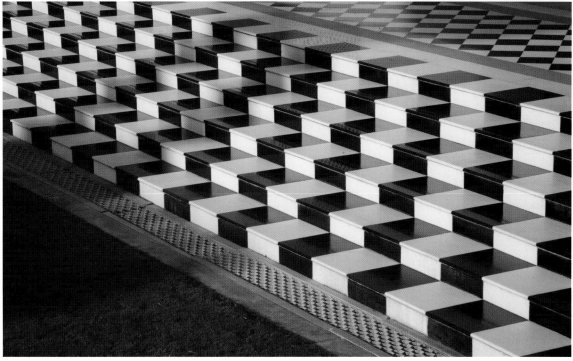

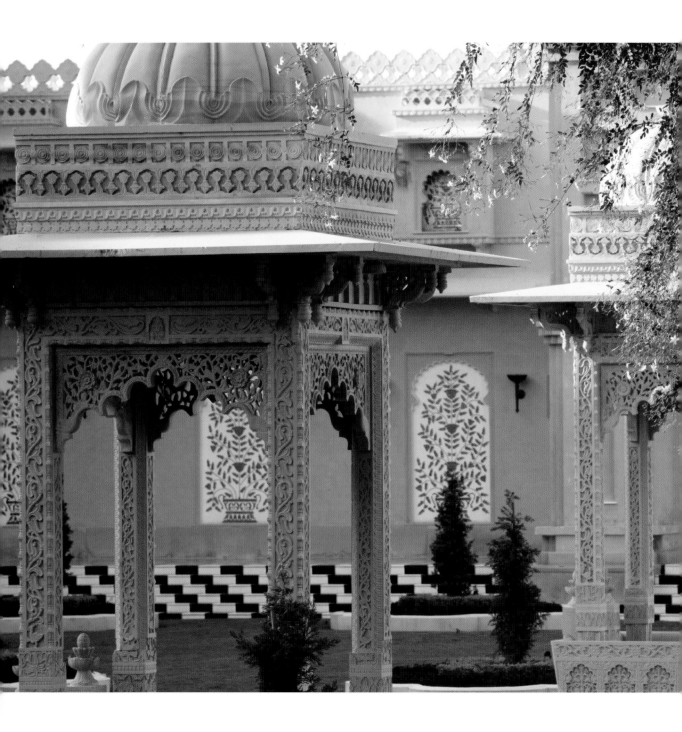

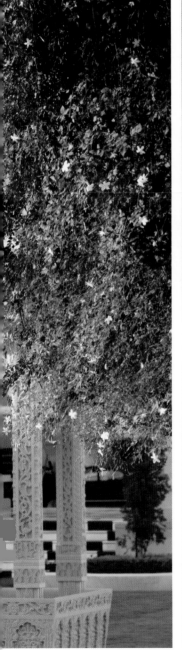

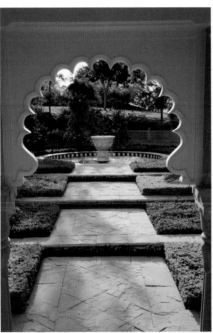

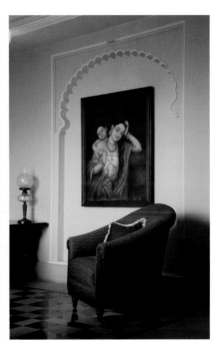

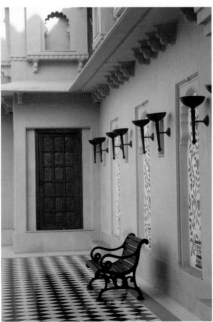

Previous pages: Every detail has been lovingly conceived at Udaivilas. As miniature painters of the Mewari School created scenes of the lives of the Maharanas of Udaipur using only a single squirrel hair as a brush, here artist Ghanshyam Mimbark and his team have created frescoes of unimaginable beauty. The same can be said for the hand-crafted brass doors and the intricate stonework throughout.

Left and above: Udaivilas treats its guests like kings and queens in a palatial environment. Whether you choose to lounge in a chair, walk in the symmetrical herb garden or wander amongst the profusion of grandiose courtyards and water cascades, you will never be short of wonderful sights to see.

Right: The resort is dotted with exquisite water features, many decorated with fresh flowers. Here a hand-crafted marble fountain sits before a decorative scalloped-edge arch motif embedded with *thekri* work.

Opposite, clockwise from top left: Some of the treatment rooms in the spa overlook the lake or meditative gardens and have claw-foot tubs for bathing with a view.

A therapist sets up the room for an Ayurvedic *sirodhara* session.

One of three treatment suites for couples: Clean and simple with a white-and-black palette, the only decoration is the Rajasthani arched windows and a colourful tapestry hanging from the wall.

All the therapy rooms have views over the expansive gardens and Lake Pichola beyond.

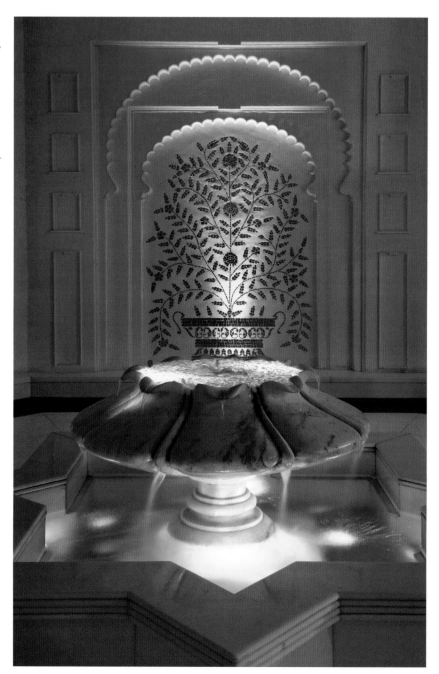

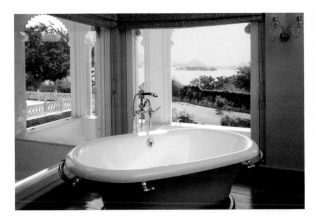

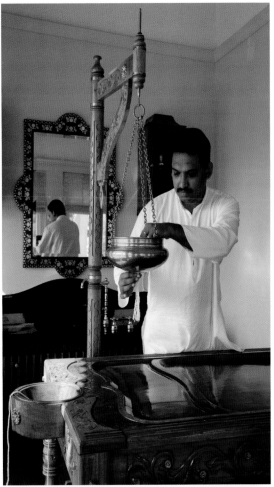

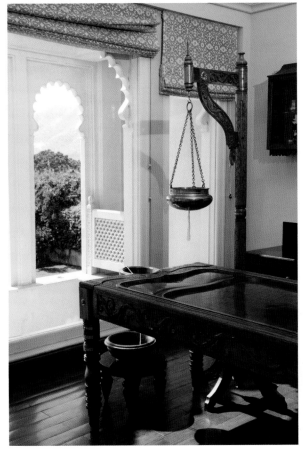

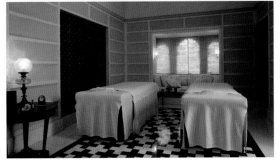

Soukya International Holistic Health Centre

On arrival at the 30-acre organic farm estate one hour's drive east of Bangalore, the first thing you notice is the green. After the dust, dirt and scanty vegetation that characterises this part of India, appears a green, water-filled vista with low-lying buildings, bright smiles and an air of organised efficiency. What a contrast! What a relief!

"Five years ago this was almost a desert scrubland," says founder Dr Isaac Mathai. "Now look at it. We are totally self-sustaining on water and food, our heating is from solar sources, we have instigated a bio gas plant, and we have 72 species of birds. Before we had none."

Certainly the environment is pleasant, green and relaxing, but that is not all that is available at Soukya. Soukya is a holistic centre that combines a number of different health systems under the one roof. Ayurveda, naturopathy, homeopathy, Western or allopathic medicine, Unani and Siddha are all offered, and are complemented by over 30 other therapies. Doctors and consultants from both modern and traditional medical systems and a large number of well-trained therapists look after the guests, while a no-smoking, no-alcohol policy and a vegetarian diet complement the system. Much of the food comes from the farm's extensive organic gardens and Soukya also makes its own 100 percent natural herbal oils and products.

If this sounds just a little too regimented, it needs to be stressed that this is a healing centre, not a holiday spot. Nonetheless, the facilities are

Below: A thatched roof (behind trees on *right*) crowns Soukya's yoga pavilion, an open-sided structure made entirely of local mud. On *left* are the therapy suites. Running through the grounds is a two-km pathway made from crazy paving with grass insets: guests are encouraged to circumambulate the route at least once a day. "When they arrive they find it difficult to walk on the uneven surface," says owner operator Dr Mathai, "but slowing down and relaxing helps them to build up to it."

Right: The special Ayurvedic treatment of *ksheera dhooma* is prescribed for patients with facial palsy and trigeminal neuralgia (the trigeminal nerve is a cranial nerve that supplies the face). Selected herbs are boiled with milk, then steamed through a papaya stalk onto the paralysed area. The steam, along with papain from the papaya, makes a fomentation on the face allowing the medicinal properties to be absorbed. The idea is to stimulate nerve endings and open up the micro-channels (*srotas* in Sanskrit) just below the skin's surface. This treatment is a good example of a traditional therapy offered in modern surrounds.

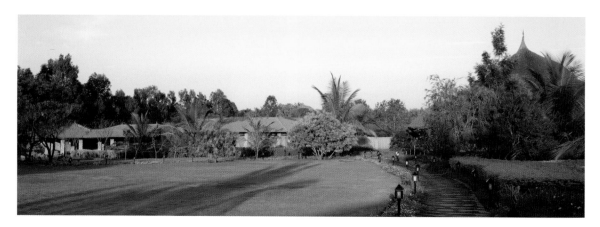

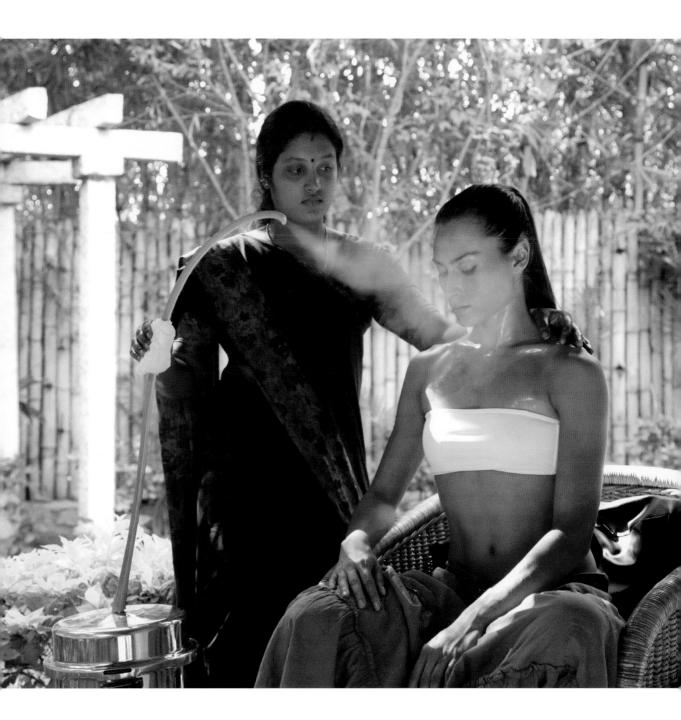

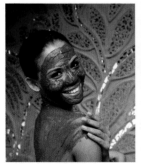

Above and right: Ayurvedic therapies at Soukya are closely monitored by skilled, caring doctors and administered by professional therapists. Above, an *ubtan* scrub used to rinse off any medicated oils from face and body; right a *greva vasthi* therapy whereby warm medicated oil is poured into a sealed area on the neck.

Opposite: Soukya has a small but well-run Ayurvedic oil and medicine production centre: Herbs and roots are stored in airtight containers, and oil production is a complicated and time-consuming affair. However, all are agreed that the benefits of freshly-made oils and powders are far more efficacious than their bought counterparts.

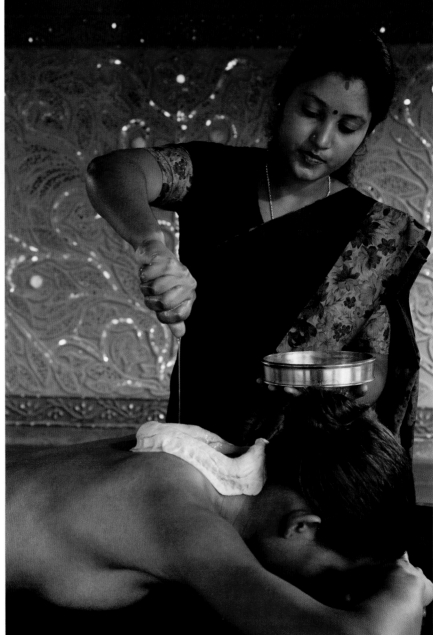

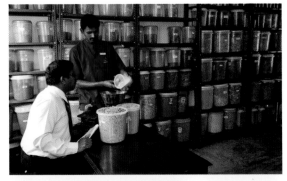

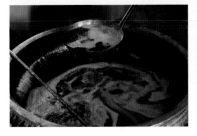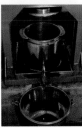

and used immediately before their efficacy has had time to fade. Some of the treatments are tried-and-tested traditionals, while others are inventions or adaptations: for example, Dr Mathai has combined Tibetan hot stone therapy with Ayurvedic *abhyangam* for a bliss-out two therapist signature massage (see page 37), and has formulated an Ayurvedic adaptation of a traditional facial to improve skin pigmentation. He also combines the Indian invention of the hydrotherapeutic hip bath (a naturopathic therapy) with an Ayurvedic decoction.

Dr Mathai explains that he tends to cater to two types of guest: The serious medical patient, who experiences a bespoke programme on site, then follows this up with medication and monitoring at home, returning for repeat visit(s) as and when necessary; and the guest that comes more for general health improvement, detoxing or weight management. "We have an integrated model with

235

modern and comfortable, with 16 spacious suites or rooms, a swimming pool and recreation area, and everyone is extremely friendly and kind. If you simply seek rejuvenation of the body or detoxification, Soukya could be for you. A timetable of exotic and interesting therapies will be prescribed, you can join in the daily yoga sessions, and who knows, you may even find that the no-stress, no-frills environment has more than just physical benefits.

The brainchild of Dr Isaac Mathai, Soukya is the first of its kind in the world. Treating each guest as an individual, it seeks to heal and comfort using, in Dr Mathai's words, "solid deep protocols from the past and traditional Indian hospitality". In the same way that physicians used to have healing herbs to hand, Soukya has enormous herb, plant and fruit gardens where ingredients are plucked, prepared

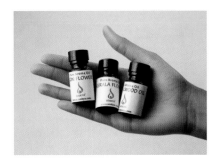

a holistic approach," explains Dr Mathai, "and we believe that healing is collective work." As such, many staff members are sourced locally, team bonding and teamwork are highly prized and doctors and therapists work closely together.

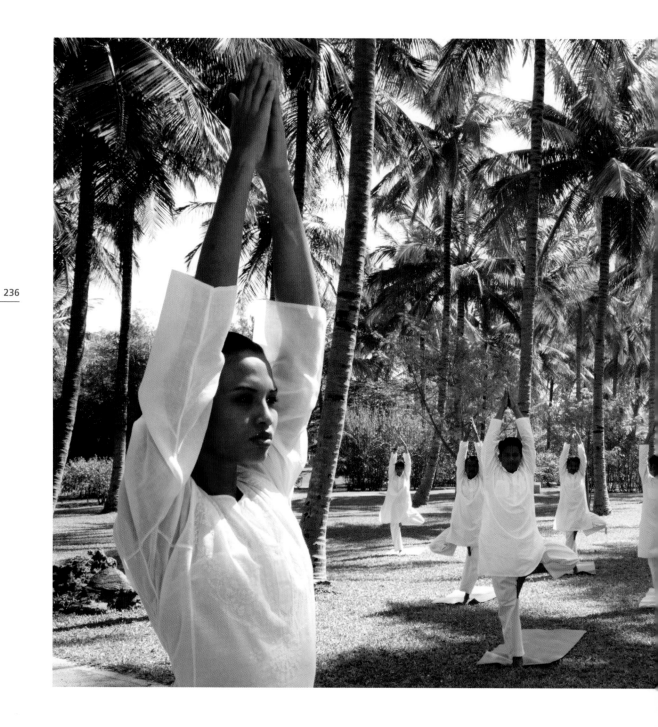

Shreyas Retreat

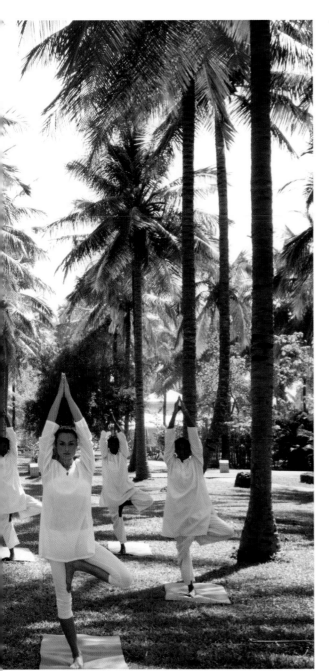

The architecture is Le Corbusier-inspired. The environment is a rural coconut plantation. The ethos is imbued with the ancient spirit of India. This may sound like a hodge-podge on paper, but in reality Shreyas Retreat is a sublime combination of the old and the new, the traditional and the modern. And surprisingly, it really works.

On the one hand, it's a luxurious resort with facilities and levels of service that easily match, or surpass, the five star. Extremely tasty meals, using mostly homegrown ingredients, are served in innovative, creatively-decorated settings. Dedicated, genuinely friendly staff cater to guests' every need. The staff number 60; guests at a maximum reach 25. On the other hand, as the owner explains, Shreyas is about "living an ashram-style life with daily yoga, meditation sessions, organic vegetarian food, no alcohol, community service and farming."

The brainchild of investment banker turned soul searcher, Pawan Malik, Shreyas is a place that helps guests to find their "inner core". Shreyas translates from Sanskrit as "excellence", so guests are encouraged to find excellence in themselves. Similarly, the resort strives for excellence; Malik's aim is for it "to be recognised as one of the finest yoga retreats in the world".

Left: A yoga session in one of the estate's coconut groves: "The wellbeing of our staff is paramount to the vision of Shreyas," explains owner Pawan Malik. "All staff are encouraged to practice yoga and meditation and to apply the principles of yoga to their particular vocation. Guests are free to join staff yoga classes and vice versa." In this particular session, attendees are photographed in *vrikshasana* or "tree pose" with hands above the head rather than in traditional *namaskar* greeeting pose. Holding the *asana* is beneficial for balance and strengthening the spine.

237

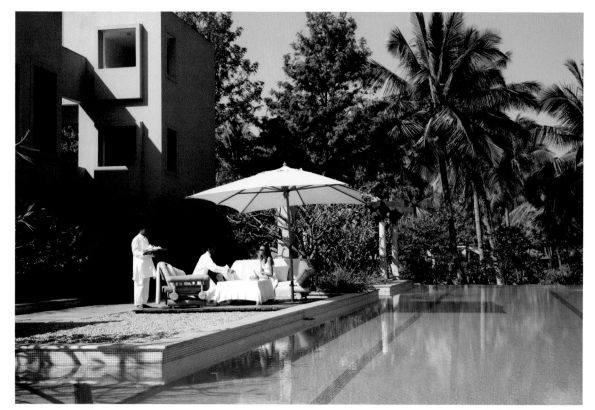

Above: Shreyas Retreat's 25 acres were landscaped by landscape designer Akshay Kaul who reinstated the original waterway that ran through the property to help harvest water in the rainy season. In keeping with the ethos of the property, boreholes provide the rest of the resort's water needs, and solar heating is used to heat water. The pool is ozonated as an added bonus.

Right: The library lounge is a vision of calm in monochromatic tones with silver accents. Malik's wife Leesha was instrumental in setting the interior design tone.

Opposite top: The airy yoga pavilion.

Opposite bottom: Many of the retreat's guest accommodations use tented canopies for a Maharajah hunting camp feel.

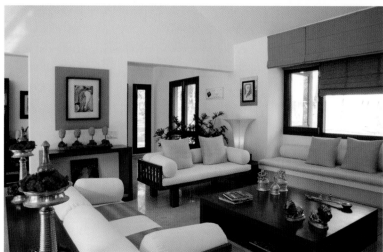

The facilities are of an extremely high quality, and both built environment and landscaping are pristine, clean and calm. Guest pavilions are well spaced one from the other, so privacy is paramount. Malik says you can choose to mingle with like-minded professionals from across the world, or choose to be alone. The contemporary interiors are comfortable, relaxed and user-friendly, not in the least Spartan. Rooms eschew TV and DVD players (leaving viewing for a large projection screen room) as well as baths for showers (saving water is a priority), but thoughtfully provide high-speed Internet access. In addition, natural landscaping with palm and fruit trees, scented shrubs and expansive lawns contribute to the overall feeling of wellbeing.

The modern architectural vibe is countered by friendly, old-fashioned hospitality and yoga practice, as well as the concept of "finding oneself". "At Shreyas, guests can learn and practice different facets of yoga," explains Malik, "for physical strength, balance and flexibility, for physiological and therapeutic benefits and, if they are interested, for pursuing a spiritual path through various types of meditation." Well-versed yoga teachers offer thrice-daily sessions and extensive vegetable gardens serve a dual purpose: they provide many of the raw materials used in the excellent vegetarian cuisine and also provide a *karma* yoga service whereby guests are encouraged to work in the gardens with no reward for themselves. A huge variety of herbs, vegetables and fruits are cultivated, and it is a wonderful place to linger.

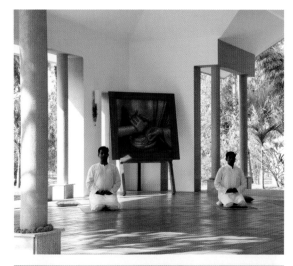

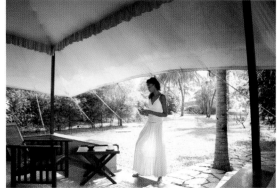

239

Alcohol is prohibited and smoking restricted to small areas around the accommodations, in keeping with the healthy lifestyle Shreyas promotes. There is also a short spa menu of massages and scrubs, a Jacuzzi and steam room, a gorgeous 25-m (82-ft) ozonated swimming pool and a small gym. How much physical, mental or spiritual exercise you engage in is left entirely up to you, but it's hoped that a stint at Shreyas will help you focus a little more inward – at least for the duration of your stay.

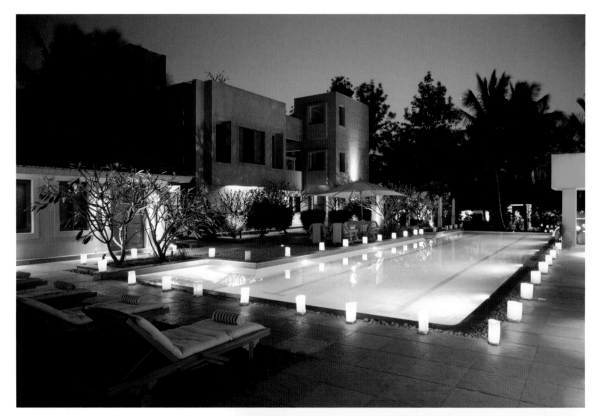

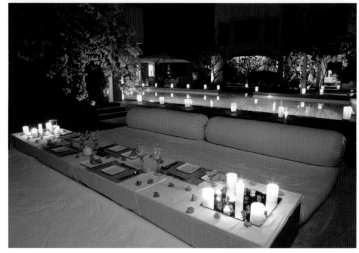

Above and right: Pawan Malik, the owner of Shreyas Retreat, left the high-stress world of high finance for a voyage of self-discovery, first setting up Inner Challenges, a life coaching company, then turning his hand to designing a retreat that is "dedicated to promoting the authentic spiritual tradition of yoga in an environment more normally associated with exclusive star hotels." As night falls, that five-star ethos comes to life in beautiful traditional candle decorations poolside and exquisitely detailed table decor. Days may be dedicated to austerity in the form of meditation, yoga and mental introspection, but dining at night time is everything – and more – that we may imagine about Indian princely extravagance.

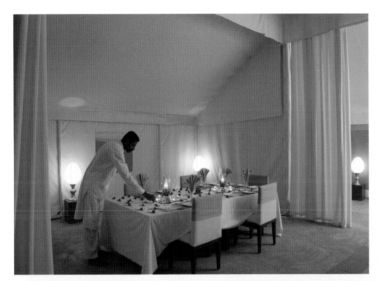

This page: Preparation for a candlelit dinner in the resort's evocative tent is meticulous. Just one of the beguiling and romantic settings for eating, other dining options include poolside, garden al fresco and in the small restaurant itself.

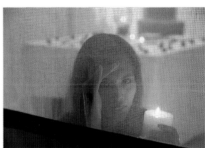

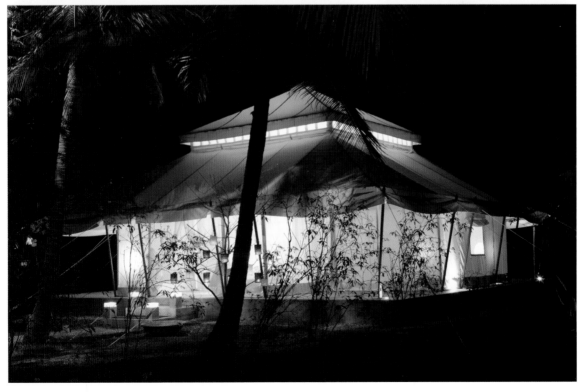

Indus Valley Ayurvedic Centre

The environment at the Indus Valley Ayurvedic Centre is fresh and breezy, set within spacious gardens with coconut trees and ornamental water bodies. Nestling beneath the famous Chamundi Hill, the landmark that overlooks Mysore, it has views over scrub countryside to the city beyond. Set up in 1996 by Dr Talavane Krishna who is an expert in *vaastu* (the Indian version of feng shui), all buildings, shade trees, fountains and streams have been positioned so as to create a harmonious whole – one that is particularly conducive to healing.

Treatments tend towards the relaxing and rejuvenating rather than the hardcore, but there are specific bespoke treatments for chronic ailments. The ethos, none-theless, is professional and nurturing. On arrival, an Ayuvedic physician listens to guests' requirements and tailors bespoke programmes for them; well-trained, willing therapists carry out instructions to the letter. However, it needs to be stressed that if you are after more than rejuvenation and a gentle detox, this is not the place for you. The IVAC version of the *panchakarma*, for example, doesn't comprise the five steps as laid down in the *Vedas*, but rather follows a gentler, less invasive programme of decoctions and massages.

There is a concise menu of therapies that includes massage, *dhara* and *vasthi* therapies, as well as some innovative beauty therapies with an Ayurvedic slant. The treatment suites and cottages are beautifully appointed with bamboo walls, slate

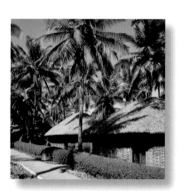

roofs and warm wood finishings (including gorgeous Ayurvedic beds designed and made on site from single pieces of African teak), and the centre also produces its own range of herbal powders, oils, pills, teas and more. There is a large yoga hall and a fabulous swimming pool for laps.

Accommodation options range in price and style, and include rooms in the main reception building as well as in garden cottages or *kutir*. These are crafted from bamboo with red oxide floors and thatch roofs, and have a private verandah. They afford the most privacy and comfort and often have views of the sparkling white domed Lalitha Palace in the distance. The centre can accommodate up to 40 or so people at full capacity, but there are plans for expansion.

The property sits on 25 acres (10 hectares) in total and one of its main plus points is its almost somnolent peace and quiet. Also of note is the fact that it was the first Ayurvedic centre in the world to be certified by the ISO (International Organisation for Standardisation), the world's largest setter of standards. "The certification is an accreditation process," explains the founder, Talavane Krishna. "It certifies that our organisation has met all the requirements for the systems and procedures as per international standards. It is a very tough certification to get." For those worried by general standards of hygiene at some Ayurvedic centres, this is extremely reassuring.

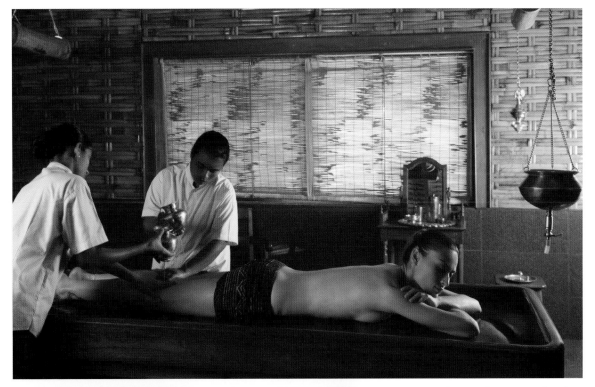

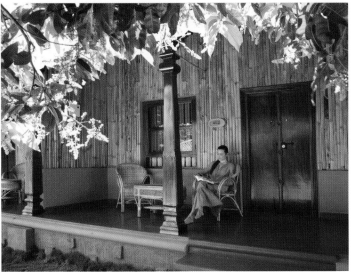

Opposite: Set in a breezy palm grove, rustic-style therapy cottages are well spaced for seclusion.

Left: Shaded by a flowering mango tree, a guest relaxes in privacy on her verandah. Privacy and hygiene are of paramount importance at IVAC. In the words of its founder, whose vision is to bring Ayurveda to "the forefront of modern medicine", the centre is designed to "take into account all three levels of human existence – physical, mental and spiritual". Judging from guests' comments and the number of repeat guests, the formula seems to be succeeding.

Above: Four oil drip procedures are offered at IVAC: *sirodhara* for the forehead, and three entire body drips – *takradhara* with buttermilk, *ksheeradhara* with medicated milk and *grithadhara* with medicated ghee. The physician decides which is most relevant to the patient's needs, then two therapists drop the liquid onto the body and give a four-hand massage to ensure it is properly absorbed into the system.

Nrityagram

Opened in 1990 by renowned dancer Protima Gauri Bedi in order to create a sanctuary for Indian classical dance, Nrityagram now focuses mainly on *odissi*, the Orissan temple dance that was revived from obscurity around the 1950s. It is also a community of like-minded spirits with choreographer, exercise and health professionals, musicians (see below) and dance teachers living side by side with students in a fairly remote location.

Set in 10 acres (4 hectares) of scenic countryside near Bangalore, the campus is an extraordinary combination of peace and meaningful activity. Even though it is a resident dance school most of the year, it runs a summer school where people can come to stay for a month both to learn dance and take part in an holistic programme of *pranayama* (breathing meditation), yoga, martial arts, body conditioning and community living.

A number of buildings, designed by Gerhard da Cunha, an architect from Goa, are scattered amongst a sylvan setting of fruit trees and vegetable gardens; many are built from locally quarried stone in hues of grey and brown, while others resemble the tribal architecture of Orissa. Bulbous terracotta-washed roundhouses with thatched roofs and white chalk geometric patterning form simple guest cottages, while dance halls (*gurukul*) are airy and open to the elements. Simple student and teachers' accommodations, a circular yoga platform with attendant Orissan-style temple, and an amphitheatre complete the built environment.

Director Lynne Fernandez explains the ethos at Nrityagram: "Our students not only learn dance and perform on various tours, they are encouraged to live as responsible community members." A working day begins at 6am with a jog and walk around the property, then students are allocated household tasks that range from cooking to cleaning, working in the gardens and more. After breakfast there are body-conditioning classes where the body is trained for the rigours of the dance. These include elements from both East and West: Pilates, yoga (see right), *pranayama*, martial arts, and more. This is followed by dance training, and after lunch and into the evening, work focuses on choreographing new dance sequences. Nrityagram has a firm reputation for taking the dance form of *odissi* to new, innovative heights, breaking with tradition in unusual and inspiring ways.

It is also an inspiring environment in which to spend some time: governed by the rhythms of nature, this is a place with no television, no mod cons, and little contact with the outside world. Translated as "dance village", Nrityagram is more ashram than university, modeled as it is on the guru-*shishya* tradition whereby students seek out teachers in the countryside. Nowadays, gurus are more likely to be found in Bombay than the boondocks, something that makes Nrityagram more than a little special. For summer school guests, the cultural ethos combines discipline with idealism, and the peaceful milieu is ideal for a rejuvenating retreat.

244

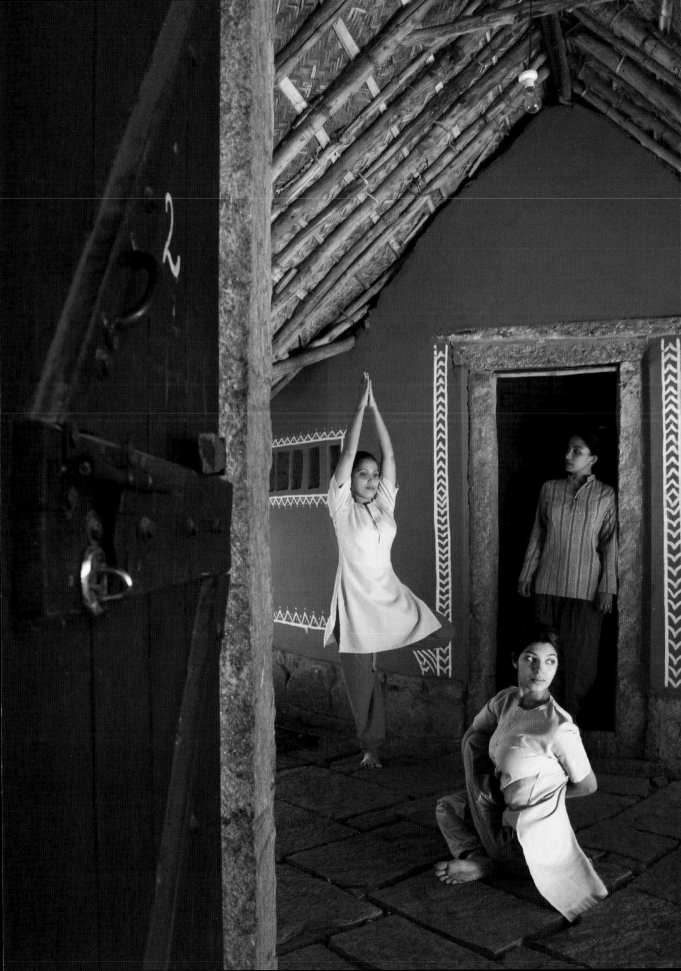

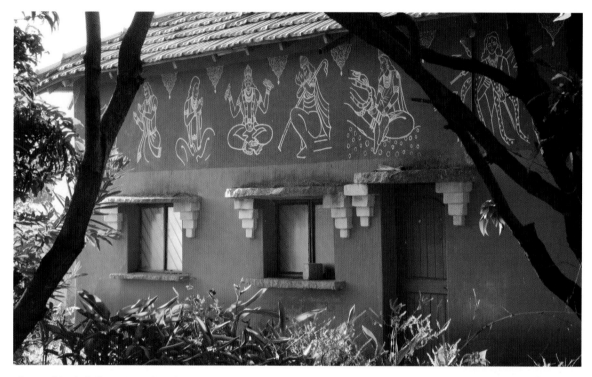

Above: White chalk illustrations adorn the terracotta washed walls of the musicians' accommodation block. *Below left:* A rustic grassy auditorium with stone stage forms the setting for an annual dance festival, as well as one-off performances. *Below right:* A puppet of the god Sri Jagannath Deva; numerous Jagannath temples in Puri, Orissa, were the original venues for the *odissi* dance.

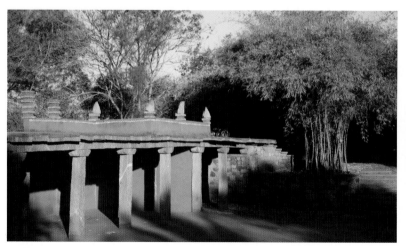

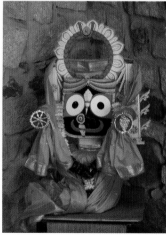

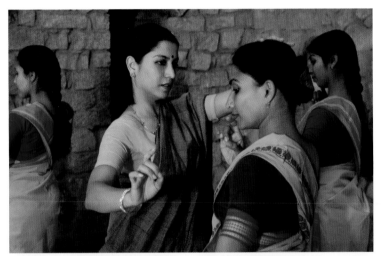

This page: The vision of Nrityagram involves living in conjunction with nature, in a manner that is not far removed from the Hindu ascetic: When the troupe is on site, they live a simple life that takes its cue from the rhythms of nature. Dedicated dance practice *(left and below)* is combined with a dawn-to-dusk regime. Organic food grown on site, composting, garbage mulching and recycling are always practiced, and any non-degradables are burnt. Those attending the summer dance programme are expected to take part in work in the extensive vegetable gardens where much of the community's food is grown.

247

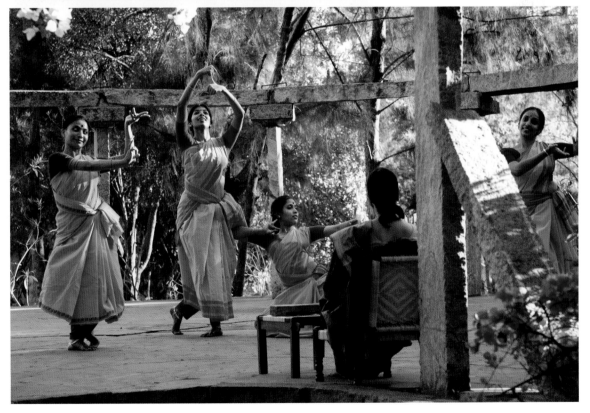

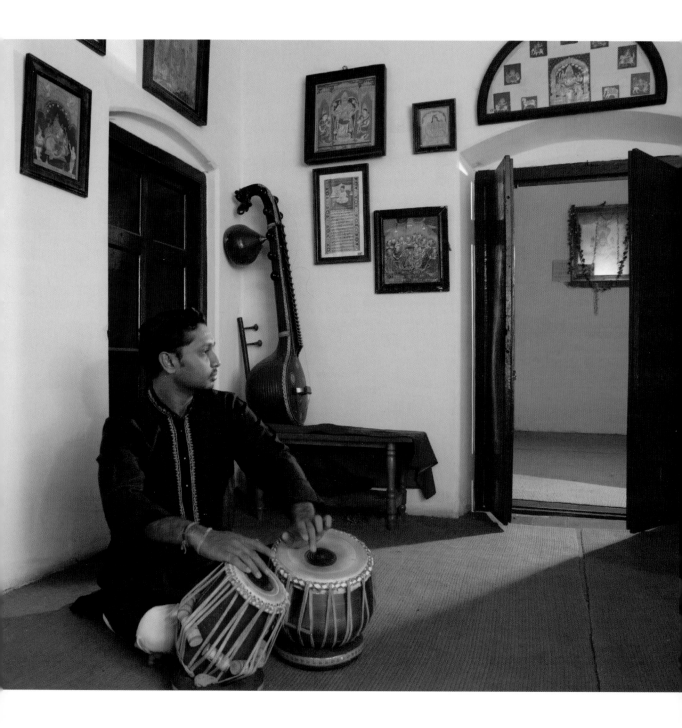

Mandala Yoga Sala

Mysore has long been associated with the rich cultural traditions of India: the Maharajahs of the princely state of Mysore, which comprises about one third of present-day Karnataka, were great patrons of the arts, and classical music, dance and traditional painting, along with more popular activities such as wrestling, flourished under their patronage. Mysore is also famous for its silk, sandalwood oil and incense production (see pages 86–89), and in recent years it has become a centre for yoga, and, to a lesser extent, meditation.

Mysore resident Sri K Pattabhi Jois, now in his 90s, is famous for refining the system of yoga known as *ashtanga vinyasa*. This is characterised by sequences of *asanas* practised in a set series that are joined by a jumping movement sometimes known as a *vinyasa*. Attention to breath, sight, rhythm and posture are paramount. He, along with his son and grandson, continues to run a yoga *sala* (school) in Mysore, while many other independent schools, of varying sizes, offer courses of tuition. Most require a month's commitment, but there are also more casual drop-in centres. Every practitioner has his or her favourite.

One of the schools we visited, and liked very much, was the Mandala Yoga Sala, housed in a 100-year old house on Dewan street in the Laxmipuram area. Dewan translates as minister, so many of the houses along this quiet, leafy road used to house high-up personnel at the Maharajah's court. As such, they are well spaced and quiet. Number 581 is no exception. Set up by Harish Bheemaiah, originally from the Coorg region, the school is praised for its excellent standard of tuition by yoga *acharya* (teacher) Mr V Sheshadri and his son. Morning and evening classes are well attended, and the centre also offers tuition and courses in other disciplines as well.

HC Paramesh is the resident Ayurvedic tutor and practitioner. His grandmother was an Ayurvedic midwife, and he learnt his trade from the Raghvendra Swamiji ashram, near Chitradurga, some 50 miles away. He offers a small service of consultation with *abhyanga* and *utsadana* massage therapy, and also gives two-week courses in basic Ayurvedic massage. His lessons are complemented by the services of a local bonesetter whose trade has been passed down to him from his father. Such small-scale health practitioners often learn their skills from other family members (see pages 304–309).

In addition, basic classical music and dance are taught, and recitals are often given in the high-ceilinged hall where the natural acoustics heighten the experience. It is little wonder that this *sala*, with its open-door policy and calm aura, has become such a success. Word of mouth ensures a steady stream of pupils, and many people return again and again. "Many of our students consider this their second home," says Harish proudly. With its little café around the back, excellent tuition and wonderful atmosphere, it's hardly surprising.

Opposite: Classical musician Bhargava warms up before a lesson. Specialising in percussion, he plays on a set of tabla drums. He especially likes a drum from south India called a *mridangam* (unseen). Its original incarnation took the same form as its present one, but was made from clay. Because of practical reasons these clay drums have ceased production. The instrument in the background is a *veenar*, the instrument that inspired the design of the more well-known sitar.

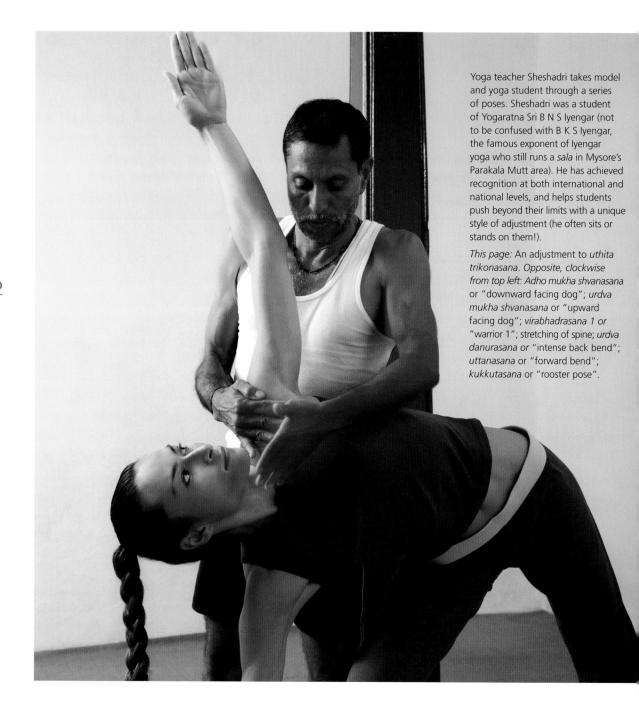

Yoga teacher Sheshadri takes model and yoga student through a series of poses. Sheshadri was a student of Yogaratna Sri B N S Iyengar (not to be confused with B K S Iyengar, the famous exponent of Iyengar yoga who still runs a *sala* in Mysore's Parakala Mutt area). He has achieved recognition at both international and national levels, and helps students push beyond their limits with a unique style of adjustment (he often sits or stands on them!).

This page: An adjustment to *uthita trikonasana*. *Opposite, clockwise from top left*: *Adho mukha shvanasana* or "downward facing dog"; *urdva mukha shvanasana* or "upward facing dog"; *virabhadrasana 1 or* "warrior 1"; stretching of spine; *urdva danurasana or* "intense back bend"; *uttanasana* or "forward bend"; *kukkutasana* or "rooster pose".

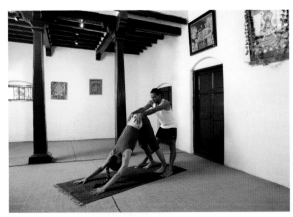
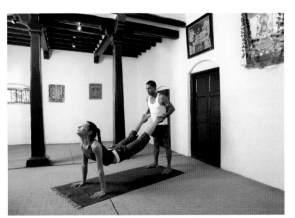

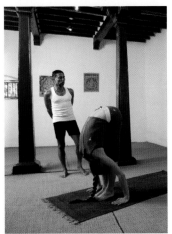
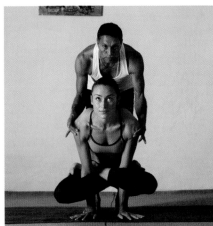
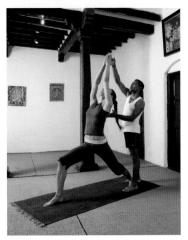

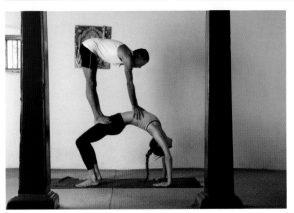
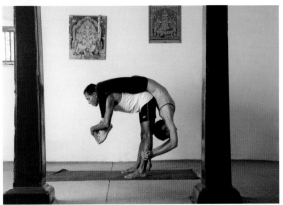

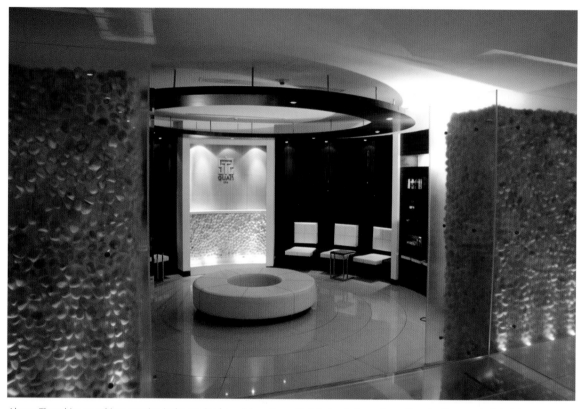

Above: The white-on-white reception is the result of a collaboration with interior designer Zoran Dzunic. Clean and clinical, it contrasts strongly with the dusky, atmospheric treatment rooms within. *Below left:* The water theme at Quan Spa is illustrated by this modern art installation in the reception area. Conceptualised and rendered by Sunil Padwal, it is a striking depiction of the importance of water on mind, body and soul. *Below right:* A simple juice bar sits adjacent to the reception desk.

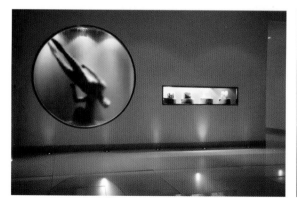

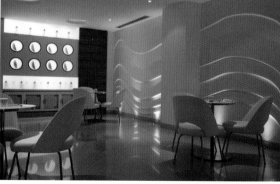

Quan Spa at JW Marriott Mumbai

Juhu, one of Mumbai's (Bombay's) northern suburbs has emerged in recent years as a hub for the city's creative cognoscenti. Most of the Bollywood set, the media crowd, the singers, models and television stars tend to congregate here, with the JW Marriott often catering to their social requirements. Parties, shows, launches and celebrations are often hosted or held at the beachfront hotel where a buzzy, busy atmosphere predominates. The hotel's modern, fashion-forward ethos is encapsulated in the open-plan lobby with its contemporary artworks as well as by its itinerary of entertainments.

Built in an international style in sandstone, the low-rise beachfront hotel is shaped like a U with decorative lily ponds, statuary and swimming pools situated centrally – and the whole facing over a sandy beach to the ocean beyond. Most of the reception areas and restaurants have the same views. Plenty of the fully functional rooms sport vistas over the sea and gardens, and at night, the grounds are illuminated by huge flaming torches set proudly on elegant pillars.

Mumbai was originally seven sleepy islands, home to Koli fishermen, and named after their Goddess Mumbadevi. Over the years the waterways between the islands have been reclaimed and now the long peninsula has expanded from the Fort and Nariman Point areas in the narrow southern tip to other pockets northwards. The design of the JW Marriott's Quan Spa uses this watery history to superb effect. The modern entranceway, with eye-catching oil paintings by Julius Macwan, leads down a flight of stairs to a thoroughly contemporary spa reception where a white circular reception desk is surrounded by a "dry riverbed" of pebbles topped by a Perspex floor. An adjacent café, with a white-on-white palette, is a relaxing spot, and an enormous and well-run gymnasium is nearby.

Off the reception area are the individual treatment rooms all with private shower/steam room – six for Western-style treatments, two for local Ayurveda, a Vichy shower room and a couple's room. The couple's room has a day bed for relaxation, a free-standing bath and a mini-bar stocked with luxe goodies for a self-indulgent treat. The atmosphere here is dusky and dim, candlelit with choice artworks in the corridors, and backlit recesses within the rooms. Each room has a different colour scheme, along with a recessed ceiling panel above the massage bed, and minimal but comfortable furnishings. Each one is identified by a *chakra* symbol on the opaque Perspex door.

The philosophy behind Quan Spa is a complete wellbeing concept within an Asian context; there are also Quan Spas at other JW Marriott hotels around the globe. In India, the spa offers a mixture of Indian elemental theory and principles from Chinese Traditional Medicine. Quan translates from the Chinese as a "source of pure water", so it offers therapeutic and pampering treatments that blend the water element with the other four elements of Earth, Fire, Space and Air. "Quan Spa's aim is for guests to leave the spa changed on a physical, mental or spiritual level in a manner that is noticeable to both the guest and to others," explains a Marriott spokesperson.

253

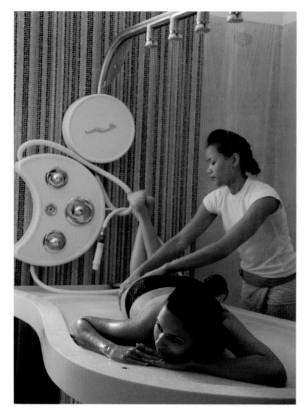

To achieve this lofty ambition, the spa has highly trained staff, quality products, superior facilities, a subtle design ethos, and an extensive treatment menu. The latter falls into four broad categories: water inspired, Ayurvedic, some Asian staples (hot stone massage, Thai massage) and European-style facials. There are also a number of themed packages, combining Ayurvedic-inspired therapies with yoga or *pranayama*, more aligned to a healing experience. Signature Ayurvedic drinks are served before and after each treatment.

The JW Marriott, Marriott's flagship property in India, is the perfect base for the modern tourist: It is close to the entertainment centre of Bandra and not too far from the airport. Many of the city's sights are close by. In Juhu itself, there is a lively beach scene with crowds of vendors and a *mela* (fair) atmosphere, a popular theatre and plenty of dining options. The added bonus is the hotel spa: After a busy day sightseeing amongst Bombay's constantly swelling population, Quan's serenity offers a very welcome respite.

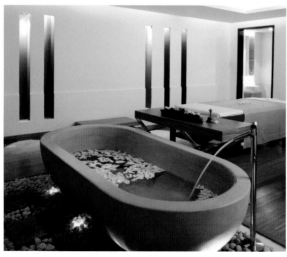

Left top: The sandalwood back treatment combines jets from the shower replicating rainfall with a healing sandalwood and cooling aloe vera full body massage.

Left bottom: As Quan Spa is in the basement and does not have any natural light, lighting techniques are extremely important here. Fiber-optics change the hues of the light in the various rooms: in the morning, it is golden and becomes cooler as dusk approaches. Deep blues and velvets are reserved for evenings. This couple's room features a handsome bath, as well as two massage beds and a wonderful couch for lounging post treatment.

Opposite: Treatment rooms are concealed behind translucent Perspex doors sporting etched on *chakra* symbols. This room is used for Ayurvedic therapies and houses a handsome jackfruit wooden massage bed.

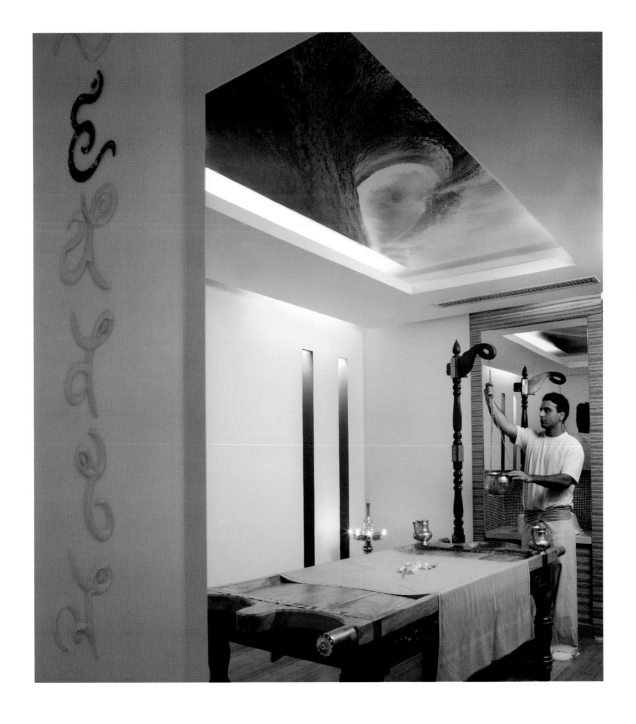

Sereno Spa at Park Hyatt Goa

Situated on a 45-acre (18-hectare) site set behind gorgeous Arrossim beach in a semi-wild area of sand dunes, the Park Hyatt Goa Resort and Spa is a good example of that rare combination – a large, multi-functional hotel that is nonetheless secluded and quiet. Constructed in Indo-Portuguese style, the resort's layout echoes that of a Goan village. Complete with "boulevards", free-standing residential blocks or *pousadas* and a serpentine swathe of pool, it sports a palette of dusky pink and terracotta. All the buildings are interconnected by bridges, walkways and paths and there is a plethora of columns, vaulted ceilings and arches in the architecture. The beautifully landscaped grounds are an added bonus.

Everything you could possibly need on holiday is on your doorstep. In addition to the huge stretch of deserted sandy beach and the longest pool in India (apparently), there is a ceramic tiled "main street" lined with a rotund Portuguese tapas bar with viewing deck equipped with binoculars and telescopes for ocean and star gazing, a library, a Western grill, a Tandoori restaurant, a wood-fired pizza and pasta restaurant, an open-plan bakery, juice bar and *dhosa* bar too. The Camp Hyatt kids' club is packed with programmes; and there are shops, a florist, a photo-developing store, a chapel and even a small cinema.

And, of course, there is the Sereno spa.

Right: Built to resemble a Portuguese mansion, the spa has trickling fountains inset with tiny mosaics, sunken ponds and arched bridges. Here, following a tradition that stretches back for millenia, a therapist sets scores of tiny oil and flower "boats" afloat on an evening journey of devotion.

256

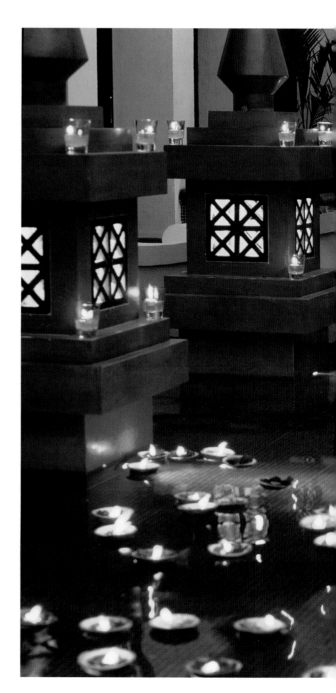

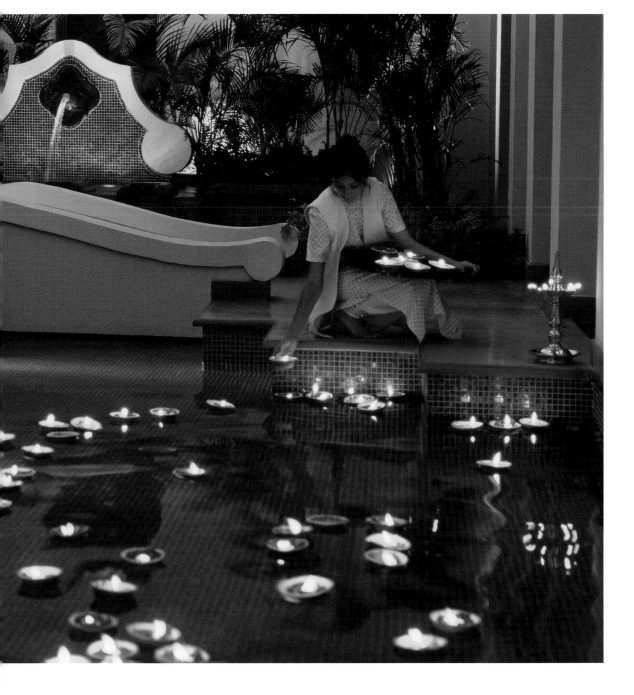

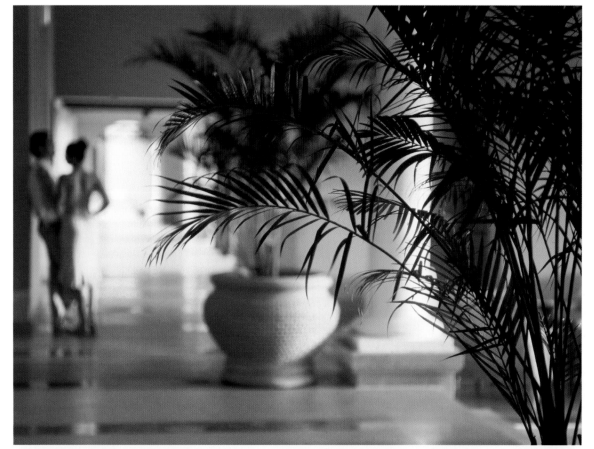

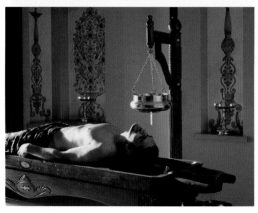

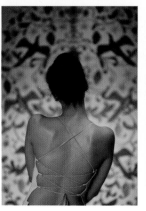

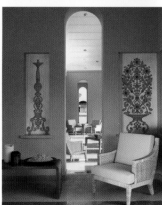

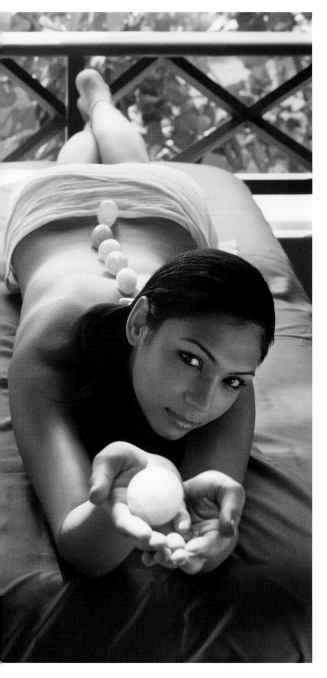

This is a cooling oasis of sweet Goan mosaic tiles, fountains and splashing water bodies, with a menu that reflects its milieu. The spa offers Indian, Western, modern and traditional therapies in nine indoor treatment rooms and several outdoor areas, as well as a menu of specials that includes an assortment of yoga, meditation and spiritual workshops. All staff members are highly trained. There's also a gymnasium and yoga room and even a beachside casuarina forest with meditation platforms dotted within it.

When three million *Conde Nast Traveller* readers were interviewed in 2006, the spa had the honour of being voted "the Number One Spa in the World" with 98.18 percent of the votes. Readers took into account the ambience, the product line, the wide range of treatments and the quality of the staff in their assessment. It was a fitting testament to the hard work of staff and hotelier, and there is no doubt that the quality control is superb.

This follows through to the standards found elsewhere in the resort. Even though there are 251 rooms and suites in total, the complex never seems crowded. This is certainly a tribute to the designer, but it is also because of the highly personalised service; guests are treated as individuals, and are helped to feel special, a rare achievement in such a huge resort.

Opposite, clockwise from top: Waiting for a therapy; big bowls of marigolds and neutral tones create a calm ambience; paintings by local artists adorn the walls; a guest gives himself up to the soothing *sirodhara* therapy.
Left: The healing vibrations of gems, stones and crystals are all used in bio-energetic therapies at Sereno spa.

259

Poomully Aramthampuran's Ayurveda Mana

One of the richest and most influential Brahmin families in north Kerala were the Poomully lords or *thampurans*. For at least 500 years their estate in Peringode near Trissur was known for its wealth and knowledge, with the present *mana* or mansion being reconstructed in 1850 by Shri Poomully Narayanan Nambudiripad. For centuries, many people, from near and far, came to the *mana* to undergo training in Ayurveda, the martial art of *kalari payattu*, yoga and other performing arts as the estate was run along guru-*shishaya* lines. Even today, the Poomully estate is famous as a seat of culture and learning.

The late *aram thampuran* or sixth Lord Poomuly Neelakantan Nambudiripad, (popularly known Arivinte Thampuran meaning "Lord of Knowledge") was the last in this great line of gurus. An expert in Vedic knowledge, his disciples were many and varied. On his death in 1997, a charitable trust was set up to continue his work, training people in Ayurveda, *kalari* treatments and *kalari payattu* amongst other disciplines. One of its projects is an Ayurvedic centre which goes under the name Poomully Aramthampuran's Ayurveda Mana.

Sitting on only a small area of the estate, the centre comprises a wonderfully preserved Sri Rama temple, a cluster of accommodation, restaurant and therapy buildings, a *kalari payattu* centre, an oil production facility and a beautiful old tank. All are

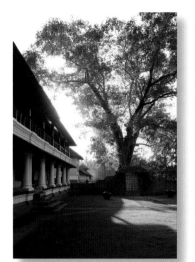

surrounded by a vast *kaavu* or forest that houses a number of ancient temples. Over the centuries, the land has been protected for ecological and water conservation reasons, and because it is considered a sacred space. Certainly, the shadowy wooded environs are wonderfully unpolluted and resonate with a strong vibe that is at once restful and healing. You can almost feel the sanctity in the air.

Poomully *mana* maintains the *kaavu* in its original state, and employs some of the estate's outhouses for its Ayurvedic centre. Twelve spacious guest rooms are housed in what used to be visiting bachelors' quarters; a handsome three-storey wood-and-stone building, it sports a long pillared verandah along its facade. Rooms have heavy, colonial furniture, the original floor tiles and wooden beams, and each has its own semi-private verandah with views out over a peaceful lawn. There are also consulting rooms, therapy suites, an open-sided restaurant, as well as a well-stocked library with priceless editions of the classical texts and a museum of historical artifacts and memorabilia including elephant ornaments.

Above and opposite top and bottom left: The *mana*'s visiting bachelors' quarters are surrounded by lawn and ancient trees. If Ayurveda Mana really takes you to its heart, or vice versa, you may get married here. Certainly, the ancient environment with its shadowy woods and spiritual atmosphere could be conducive to tyeing the knot.

Opposite, bottom right: A statue of Hanuman, beneath a sprawling banyan tree, guards the temple.

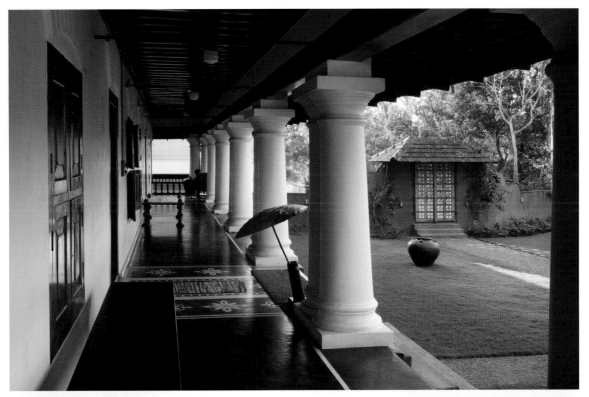

261

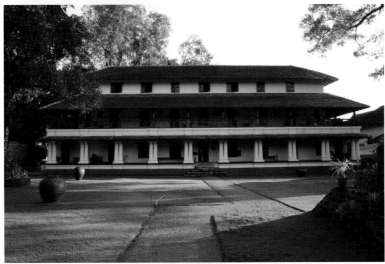

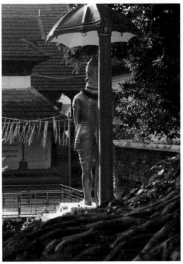

Resident doctors and visiting *ashtavaidyan* (Keralan Brahmin physicians that have mastered all eight branches of Ayurveda and are entrusted with its secrets) cater to a select group of patients. Diagnosing, prescribing and caring in what they refer to as the "Poomully way" (following ancient texts produced on site), they offer a variety of general detoxifying treatments, specialist treatments, and exclusive treatments formulated for infertility, arthritis, rheumatism and sports injuries. The latter taps into the expertise of the *kalari* masseuses with their body toning and conditioning expertise that is so important to their craft (see pages 66–67 and 130–133). Diets, formulated for different *doshas* and conditions, are strictly enforced and most medicines are prepared on site.

In addition, a visit to Ayurveda Mana can act as an authentic introduction to a cultural world that seems traditionally closed to non-Indians. Astrology and palmistry services are offered, and for those interested in the arts, workshops and training programmes in classical art forms such as *kathakali* and *mohiniaattam* dance and percussion, as well as martial arts, *panchakarma*, yoga and meditation, are available.

As the late Lord Poomuly Neelakantan Nambudiripad was reputedly an expert in taking care of elephants "the Ayurvedic way", a site-specific Day with an Elephant is another unusual option: guests spend the day with an allocated elephant, bathing it, walking it and serving it specially prepared temple-blessed food (*anoyootu*) – an experience many have found unique.

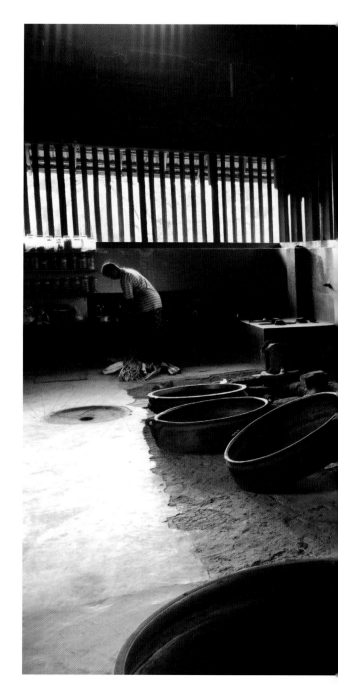

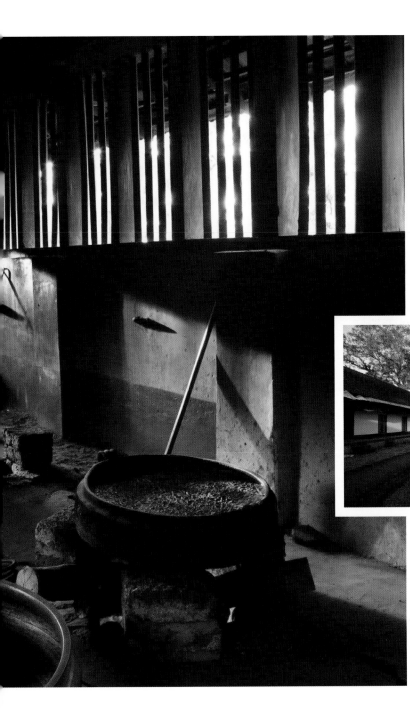

Left: Adjacent to the large tank sits an oil production centre, where ancient recipes formulated by Poomully doctors from the past are utilised for today's medicines. For more details of Ayurvedic oil production see pages 326–327.

Below: Keralan Brahmin estates were traditionally built around a temple – and Poomully *mana* is no exception. Its Sri Rama temple (below right) is a restrained example of Keralan temple architecture. The building with white walls on the left is the *kalari payattu* centre where training in the martial art is offered.

Kalari Kovilakom

Housed in a tremendously atmospheric palace estate in Kollengode in Kerala's Annamalai foothills, Kalari Kovilakom is steeped in history. Comprising a number of buildings today, it began life as a three-storey palace in 1890. The property of Dhatri, the Valiya Thampuratti or "senior-most lady" of the principality of Vengunad, it is an imposing building. So called because it is believed to have been built on the site of a ritual space for *kalari payattu*, the martial practice of the region (see pages 130–133), the *kovilakam* or palace was erected to ensure that the female members of the family would have a home of their own.

Later additions included a colonial-style guest wing, connected to the palace by an open-sided corridor, and a second palace that has since been demolished. There was also a bath house (still extant) attached to a *kulam* or water pond where the women were able to bathe, a small temple and several out-houses.

One hundred years' on, the family was scattered and time, neglect and a decline in the family fortunes resulted in the palace becoming quite dilapidated. Luckily, C G H Earth, Kerala's foremost hospitality company, negotiated a lease on the palace and renovated the existing structures over a three-year period. They added a modern Ayurvedic centre, a yoga pavilion and a *kalari* practice pit, and in keeping with the company ethos of marketing authentic experiences, decided to run the property as an Ayurvedic retreat.

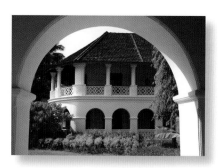

The reasoning behind this is quite straight forward. The area is remote and the large grounds are conducive to healing. The result is something unique: palatial surrounds and a guest experience more akin to an ashram than an auberge. The minimum stay is 14 days, but three or four weeks is recommended. Guests leave their shoes (and their worlds) at the door – and do not see them again until they leave. They are also asked to disrobe and wear a suit of soft cream cotton, although this isn't compulsory. What is compulsory, however, is a rigorous routine of self-discovery through Ayurveda, yoga, meditation and a Spartan diet – all timed to tune in with a dawn to dusk schedule.

Obviously, a stay at Kalari Kovilakom is not for everyone. It suits those who want to completely detox or are seeking Ayurvedic treatment for a particular ailment. It is not for dabblers or dippers; it is for serious devotees of the ancient Science of Life who do not want to go down the homestay or hospital route.

The daily routine is set in stone. Amplified temple chants at dawn act as the wakeup call, and, from this clockwork beginning, the entire day is

Above: The Vengunad rajas had a volatile relationship with the East India Company, but still built a colonial-style guest wing for visiting dignitaries. Today this houses many of the vast guest suites, some of which sport four-poster beds and ante-chambers as well as large bathrooms.

Right: The guest wing and main house are joined by this covered corridor and pavilion, a tranquil spot for yoga or meditation.

264

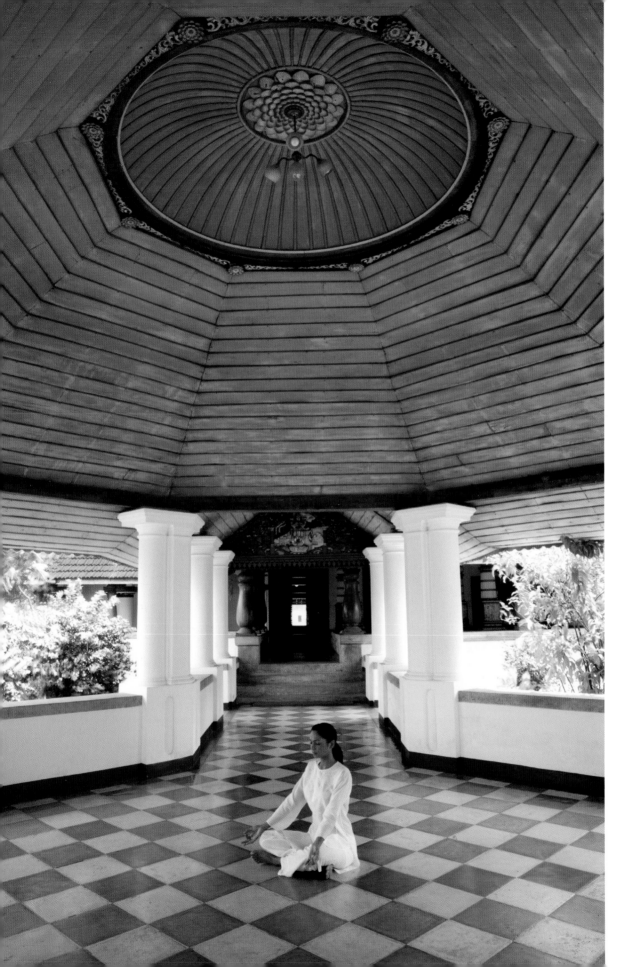

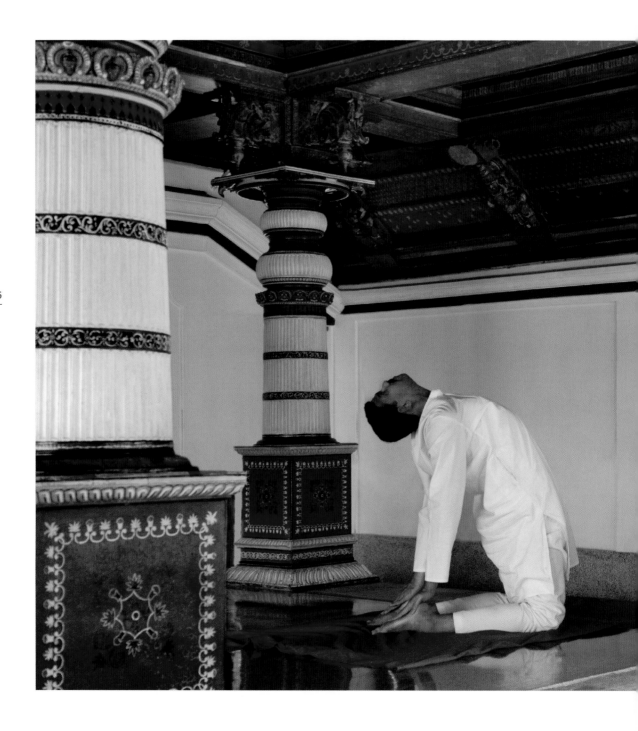

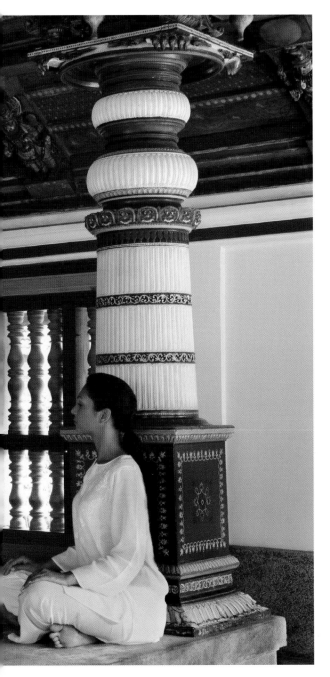

punctuated with a variety of health-related activities. Yoga is followed by breakfast, a consultation with the doctor, a treatment, then lunch, meditation, massage, relaxation, dinner before dark, then a talk or gathering of some nature before bed by eight or nine pm. Each guest is prescribed his or her own diet, medication and therapy, and members of staff are

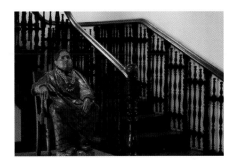

267

fully aware of all aspects of the client's programme. Flasks of medicated drinking water are individually identified and placed in each room; laundry is collected and returned; rooms are serene and tranquil with the scent of lemongrass and furniture polish.

Naturally, the Ayurvedic experience is first rate. Two male doctors and one female doctor oversee programmes that vary in content and context depending on the client's needs and wants. Each one, from diet to medication, to prescribed activity

Above: A sweeping wooden staircase leads up to the first storey of the palace. Situated at its foot in an interior hallway is a statue of Dhatri, the matrilineal head of the Kollengode clan who had the palace built in the 1880s for her family.

Left: The yoga master at Kalari Kovilakom, a devotee of the Bihar School of yoga, demonstrates the camel pose or *strasana* to a pupil in the *poomukham*, the raised dias area at the entrance to the palace in which guests were traditionally received. This posture is particularly good for stretching the back and shoulders.

(or non activity) to therapies, is individually customised and monitored throughout. Massages, herbal treatments, medicines, diet, purifying baths, yoga and meditation slowly work their magic on receptive bodies and minds. The aim is to give clients a chance to see the world afresh or "to be twice born". Anti-aging and anti-stress packages, the rigorous *panchakarma* regime (see pages 62–63), weight-loss and addiction programmes, as well as individual medical treatments for illnesses that include multiple sclerosis are all offered.

As the days progress, the healing and detoxing therapies begin to take effect, and a sense of camaraderie tends to grow amongst the group. The ambience is always hushed so as to facilitate clarity of thought and inner contemplation, but guests generally interact, share experiences and discuss health issues. However, if privacy is required, that isn't a problem, as Kalari Kovilakom has only 18 suites and a maximum capacity of 36 guests. With extensive grounds, enormous suites and bedrooms, and generous public areas, there is space to spare.

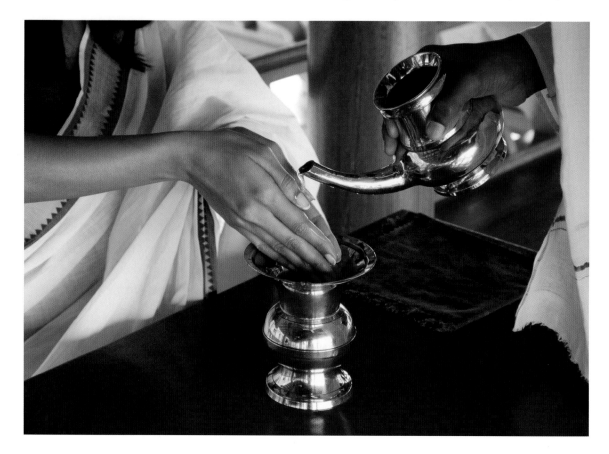

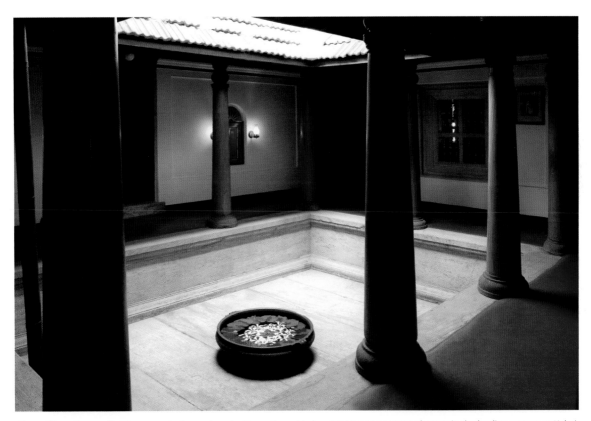

Above: The palace *nadimittam* or central quandrangle. *Opposite and below:* Diet is an important element in the healing process at Kalari Kovilakom. All food is prepared according to Ayurvedic principles: only copper, bell metal, earthenware, stone and brass vessels are used, and mainly organic ingredients are simply cooked and served in gleaming brass *katories* (cups) on a banana leaf covered *thali* tray.

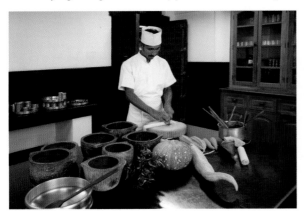

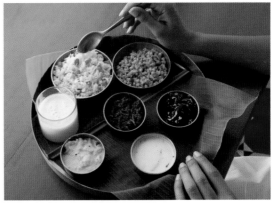

This page: A doctor discusses issues with a patient in the Ayurvedic centre.

Inset: An old herb chest made from insect-repellant wood houses roots and herbs to made clients' drinks.

Opposite top: A palace *kulam* or tank in a Keralan palace was traditionally a cool spot for bathing. Behind the tank is the modern Ayurvedic centre with 10 treatment rooms built in Keralan style with low eaves.

Opposite bottom left: Two therapists administer *pizhichil*, one of the *panchakarma* preparatory treatments. An oleation and sudation therapy, it makes the body perspire through the

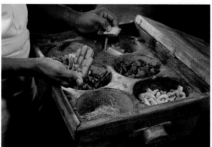

pouring of warm medicated oil from a certain height in a rhythmic manner over the entire body. "Due to osmotic pressure and the temperature of the medicated oil," explains a physician, "the herbs' properties are absorbed through skin and accumulated toxins are melted and thrown out as sweat; the remaining parts ultimately reach the alimentary tract."

Opposite bottom right: The bath house and medicines used at the centre.

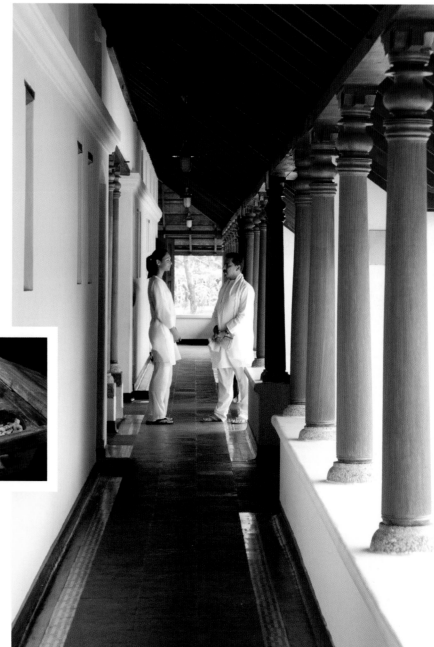

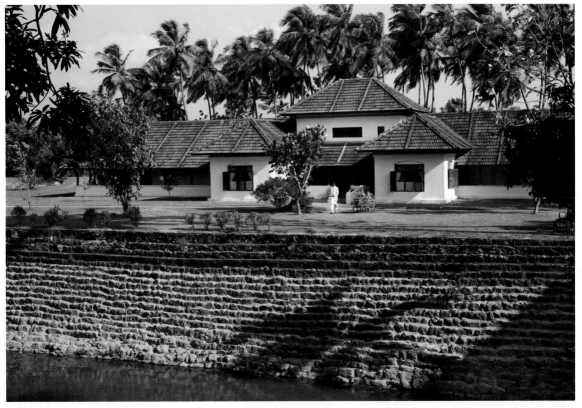

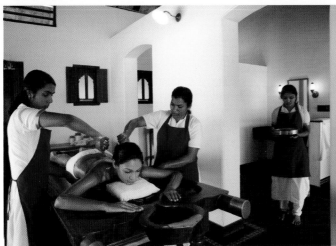

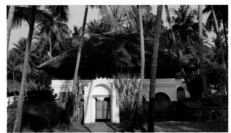

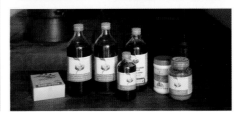

Arya Vaidya Chikitsalayam

If you are serious about treating an existing medical condition the Ayurvedic way, our advice is to skip the spas, resorts, retreats and homestays, and enrol in a full-scale Ayurvedic *chikitsalayam* ("hospital" in Sanskrit). There are quite a few reputable government and private hospitals (see listings on pages 328–335), but we have chosen to showcase the Arya Vaidya Chikitsalayam in this book because it is a leader in the field. A teaching hospital, the AVC (as it is widely known) has a well-deserved, high reputation.

It may not have the allure of a sybaritic spa, but it has the blue-chip credentials of a first-rate medical facility. Each year, thousands of Indians, and increasingly a number of Westerners, travel to its campus in Coimbatore to experience treatment sessions that may last from 10 days to up to six weeks or more. Each receives the full Ayurvedic panoply of diet, medication, therapy, yogic and spiritual techniques, and more.

The AVC is one of a number of institutions under the broad umbrella of the Arya Vaidya Pharmacy (Coimbatore) Ltd or AVP. This was originally set up in 1943 by the late Arya Vaidyan P V Rama Variar who was a humanitarian, philosopher and physician; the institute is now run by his no less able son, Sri P R Krishnakumar, who is well known for his promotion of Ayurveda on a global scale. The AVP is a massive concern: It produces both Ayurvedic medicines and over the counter products, runs a

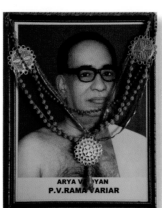

ARYA VAIDYAN
P.V. RAMA VARIAR

teaching hospital as well as many smaller Ayurvedic institutes, operates 15 pharmacies and a research centre, and provides Ayurvedic services gratis to the genuinely needy in a charitable trust. It was Sri Krishnakumar who first brought Ayurveda to the attention of the World Health Organisation.

The AVC runs like a well-oiled machine. Set in a leafy compound, it has 120 beds in wards, private rooms and cottages, an out-patients' facility that caters up to 150 people daily, a small surgical centre, a practice-based research office and an educational programme facility, all set around a central temple dedicated to Sri Dhanwanthari, the god of medicine. Its 35 licensed doctors are highly qualified – and ably assisted by a team of nurses and therapists. "We don't just look at the illness," explains Sri Krishna-kumar, an imposing man who is a philosopher as well as a doctor, "Our aim is to look a bit deeper for the benefit of the patient. All aspects are taken into consideration, the ailment, the spiritual and mental state of the patient, the astrological situation, the climate and more. Only then can we assist."

And assist people they certainly do: a priest from Badrinath with the incurable condition of multiple sclerosis literally begged me to tell the world of the benefits of Ayurveda for MS patients. He was close to ecstatic about the improvement in his health after his six-week purification regime. A couple from Singapore told me they would be bereft if

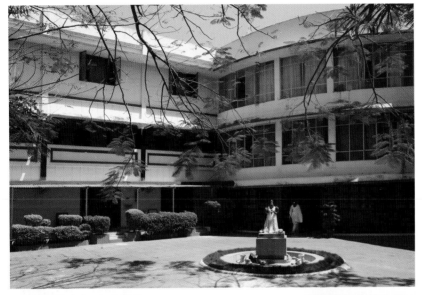

Opposite: A portrait of the late Arya Vaidyan P V Rama Variar, the founder of the AVP in 1943, hangs in the reception lobby.

Left: Set in a leafy compound, one of the accommodation blocks also contains consulting and therapy rooms.

Below left: The research centre is instrumental in the digitalisation of Sanskrit, Dravidian and Malayalam Ayurvedic texts in order to preserve their ancient knowledge. It has developed a software module so that scholars may transcribe the texts into a variety of languages.

Below and bottom right: The pharmacy works closely with doctors to ensure patients receive the correct medicine morning and evening.

Bottom left: An Ayurvedic lunch.

273

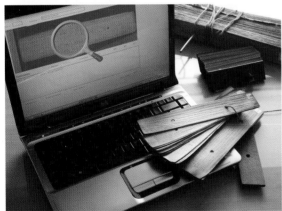

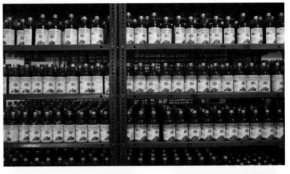

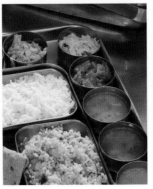

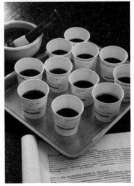

they had to miss their month-long sojourn at the AVC, as they had been coming for the past 16 years. Others, who were seeking rejuvenation or weight loss, were no less enthusiastic.

"We don't seek to cure a patient," explained one young doctor as he showed me round the facility, "We simply help the body to heal itself."

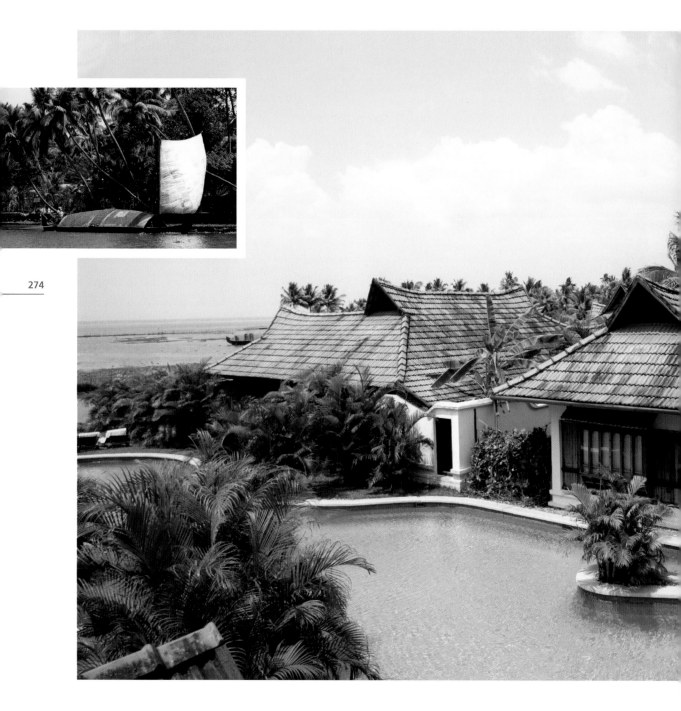

Ayurmana at Kumarakom Lake Resort

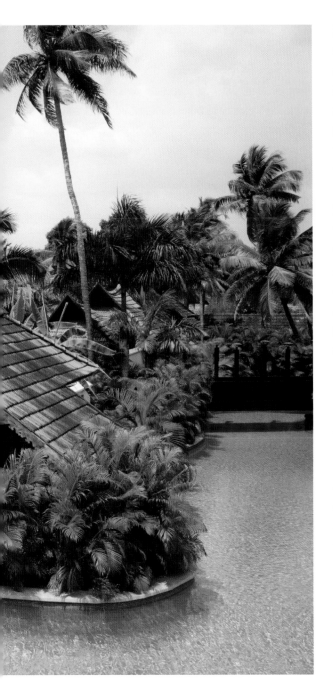

Land and water are inseparable in Kerala's back-water areas. Working irrigation channels, lakes and rivers mingle with whispering coconut groves, rice paddies and small islands to creat a patchwork topography of aquamarine and green. It's a riverine region: Fishing and farming meet where water turns to land; children paddle in dugouts to school; and the pace of life is simple, civilised and slow.

It's hardly surprising, therefore, that tourism is growing, especially as the region is also famed for its high-quality Ayurveda, plethora of birdlife, wonderful food, literate and friendly population, and ancient tradition of arts and crafts. Hotels and resorts, often eco-friendly and culturally authentic, are experiencing a boom. Kumarakom Lake Resort, set over 13 acres (5.2 hectares) of land on the eastern shore of Lake Vembanad, is no exception. It's often full.

Wholly owned by a Keralan who now lives in Bangalore, the resort sits at the heart of Kerala's green and gracious backwater country. The story goes that Paul John visited the hamlet of Kumarakom on his honeymoon and liked it so much that he wanted to return the next year. Unfortunately he was unable to reserve a room, so – to circumvent the inconvenience – he decided to build a resort! The result is Kumarakom Lake Resort: Entirely in

Left: An extremely long, serpentine pool snakes its way amongst some of the resort's accommodations. An early morning dip beneath bridges and around the houses makes for the longest lengths ever!

Inset: A traditional *kettuvallum* or Keralan rice barge made from coir and wood plies the lake's waters. Originally used for trans-porting goods, these boats have found new life as houseboats.

keeping with the natural environment, it is a maze of bridges, waterways and ancient Keralan structures interspersed amongst palm and fruit trees and flowering shrubs. The whole fronts the vast watery amphitheatre that is Vembanad Lake.

Green and leafy, with 51 villas and eight rooms, and some overwater villas in the pipeline, the resort is instantly relaxing. Public areas, such as the restaurant, bar, jetty, shop and reception area are housed in large local buildings, all sought out and bought by the hotel group in the 1990s, then dismantled and reassembled on site. Many of the accommodations are in Brahmin or *tharawad* houses that were earmarked for destruction. These have also been dismantled, the pieces – doors, windows, rafters and so on – numbered, transported and re-erected as close to their original forms as

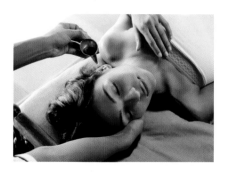

possible. Some were modified to suit their new requirements, while others were rebuilt exactly as they were.

The Ayurvedic centre is called the Ayurmana (*mana* translates as "a Brahmin family residence"), as it is housed in a freestanding 200-year-old structure that used to belong to an old family

of Ayurvedic physicians in a village near Cochin. Totally symmetrical, the four-sided building, known as a *nallekettu*, is set around a central courtyard. Every beam, wall, step and rafter is made from wood, so the entire building is imbued with a warm ambience. In addition, it carries a potent historical legacy: Generations of physicians dedicated to the oldest of medicinal sciences have practiced Ayurveda within its walls for centuries.

This Ayurvedic heritage is celebrated with a varied menu and a high caliber of staff. An experienced senior physician is accompanied by an assistant physician and 12 therapists, all of whom are well-trained, graceful and skilled. A range of therapies is offered: Long-term guests may undertake weight reduction or rejuvenation programmes, treatments for stress, tension, depression, anxiety and sleeplessness, or even the *panchakarma* regime; single visits may be accommodated with a selection of massages, skin and hair care beauty treatments. More particular therapies are aimed at individual ailments; examples include anti-arthritic and anti-neuropathic treatments.

For guests who prefer to eschew the medicinal for the recreational, Kumarakom Lake Resort offers plenty of other diversions. There is a lakeside pool with Jacuzzi, a 250-m (273-yard) meandering pool, a well-stocked shop, trips on traditional houseboats, rowing and angling, and wonderful performances of Keralan dance drama. There is also the option of lying in a lakeside hammock with the gentle breeze and birdsong for company – and chilling.

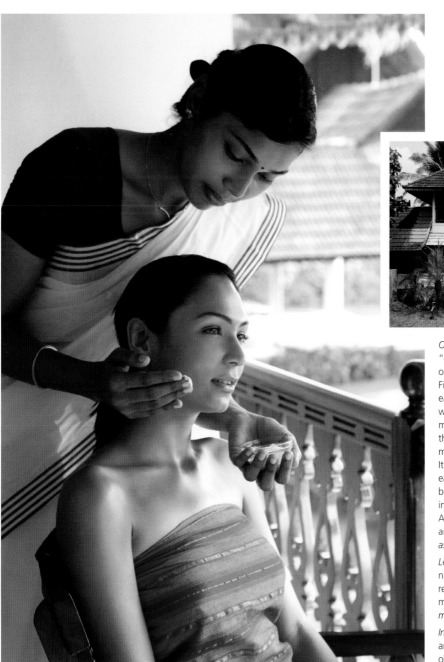

Opposite: Karna poorana (literally "ear filling" therapy) is used on and in the ear for cleansing. First of all, steam is given to the ear area which is then massaged with herbal oil; after, lukewarm medicated oil is poured into the ear, kept in place for five minutes, then drained out. It is believed to cleanse the ears, improve hearing and is beneficial for a range of ear infections and hearing disorders. At Ayurmana, the two oils used are *vachalashunadi thailam* and *asanamanjisthadi thailam*.

Left: A number of 100 percent natural facials are offered at the resort. Here a therapist applies moisturiser at the end of the *mukhalepam* (see page 143).

Inset: The resort is comprised of ancient Keralan structures with old roof tiles and ample balconies.

Right: The *siro vasthi* therapy whereby oil is poured over the skull of a client; it is recommended that the head be shaved prior to this treatment. Believed to regulate brain function and relieve stress, the therapy is surprisingly relaxing.

Opposite, clockwise from top: Ayurmana, the Ayurvedic centre, was believed to have been bestowed with the grace of the Kodungalloor goddesses and Narasimhamoorthy – so is as close to a sacred structure (barring a temple) as you are likely to get. Therapy rooms run down both sides, while behind the central courtyard lies the prayer room (now a therapy suite). According to tradition, the court is filled with pebbles and has a *tulsi* or holy basil plant at its centre.

The prayer room, with intricate carving and heavy wooden doors, today acts as a therapy room. The sheen from the all-wood interior is echoed by the sturdy Ayurvedic bed and steam box.

The senior physician takes a patient's pulse in his office.

At dusk, the lamp in front of Ayurmana is lit by some of the centre's therapists. The lighting of fire symbolises blessings to the gods, so a daily invocation of lamp-lighting is practiced. These types of multi-tiered stone lamps or *kall villakku* are either three-, five- or seven-tiered.

Overleaf: Examples of some of the exquisite craftsmanship at the resort: carving, brasswork, painting and more.

278

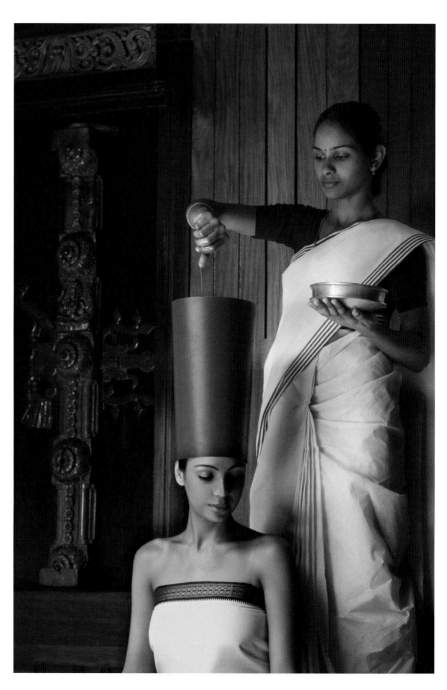

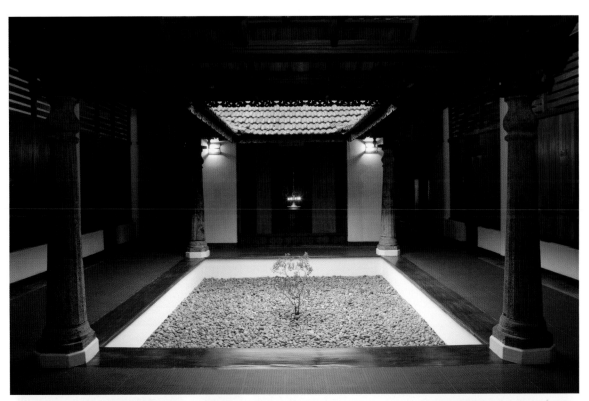

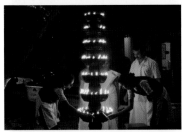

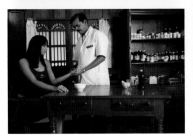

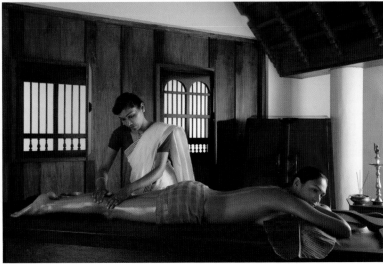

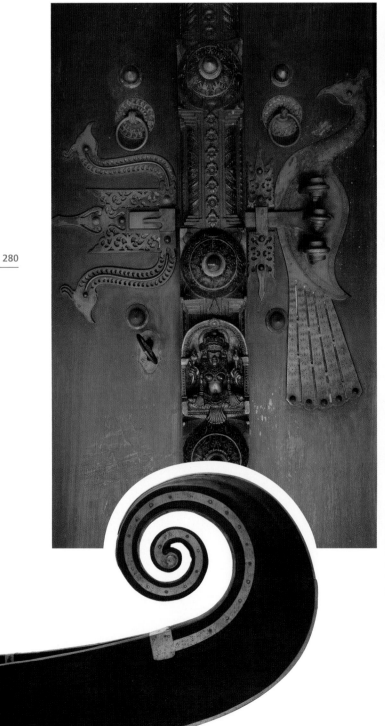

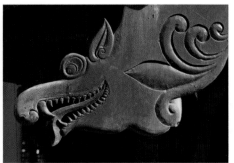

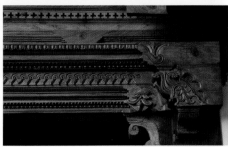

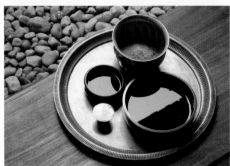

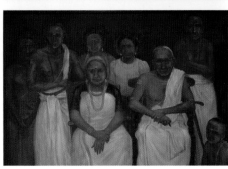

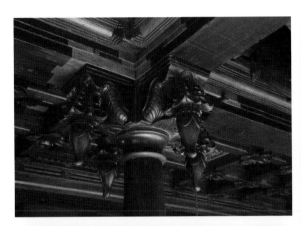

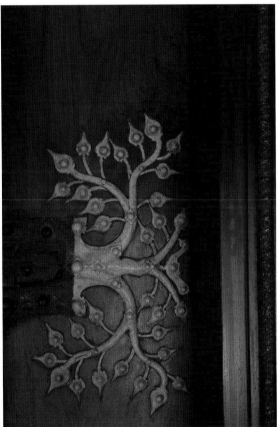

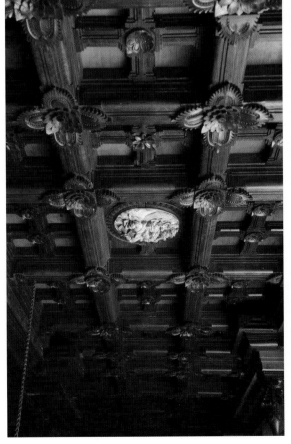

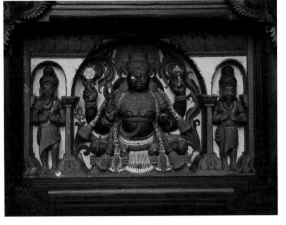

Ayurvedic Penthouse at Oriental Hotel, Bangkok

The spa at the Oriental, Bangkok has long been famed for its therapeutic, beauty and relaxation treatments, an added bonus for guests at this iconic property. Situated a short boat ride across the river from the 120-year-old historic hotel itself, it has been pampering guests and residents for a decade or so.

The recent opening of the Ayurvedic Penthouse on the top floor of the building adds a welcome new dimension to its already substantial holistic offering. Four bright, breezy treatment suites with river views, antique Indian furniture, beautiful brass vessels and Rajasthani wall hangings are not only wonderfully serene, but are filled with extremely high quality Ayurvedic equipment. Treatments are no less than should be expected from a hotel that prides itself on high levels of service.

Whether you are looking for a life-changing long-term plan for wellbeing or a relaxing and exotic pamper, the Ayurvedic Penthouse delivers. There is a careful selection of traditional and authentic Keralan treatments designed to create a healing effect on the body and soul, as well as full and comprehensive yoga sessions that include *asanas* (postures), *pranayama* (breathing exercises), *dhyana* (meditation) and *yoga nidra* (yogic relaxation).

Even though the Ayurvedic menu is short in size, it is long on sophistication. Highly trained therapists offer a variety of massages including a synchronised *abhyangam* that employs harmonious strokes, rhythm, speed and pressure, as well as a traditional *uzhichil*. This is the invigorating, deep massage that *kalari* practitioners give and receive in order to keep the body in condition and the *pranic* channels free from blockages. In addition, there are some heat therapies and a wonderful facial. Clients may also try some of the customised Ayurvedic programmes formulated to treat individual constitution and health needs. Choose from Ayurvedic Rejuvenation, Stress Relief, Body Toning and Yogic Health in three-day to three-week courses.

Below: The Author's Lounge at the hotel has hosted such luminaries as Somerset Maugham, Graham Greene and Joseph Conrad.
Opposite: The entrance to the spa, housed in a colonial-style building, features soothing water and landscaping that includes window boxes and pots with tropical flora.

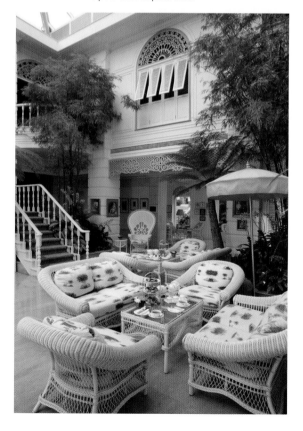

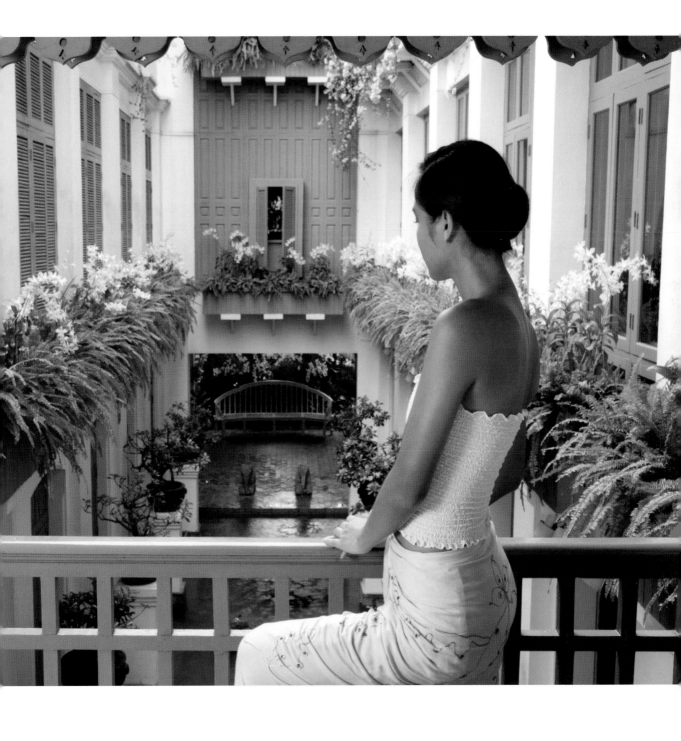

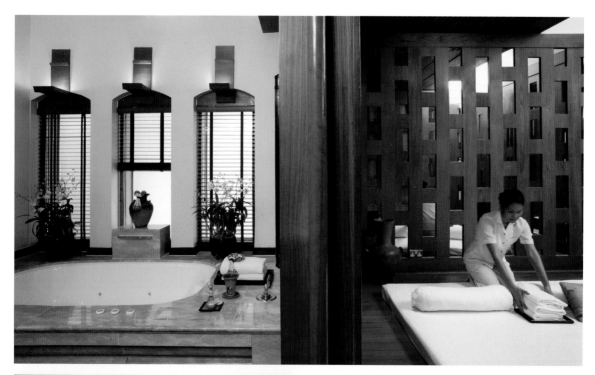

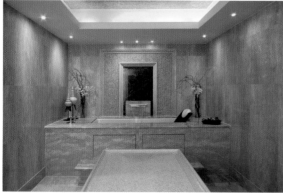

Above: Teak panelling, marble bathrooms, high-quality products and well-trained therapists make for a winning formula at the Ayurvedic Penthouse in Bangkok.

Left: One of the suite bathrooms featuring marble, cool stone and mirrors. Most treatments end with a scrub of ground beans and a shower or bath in such a bathroom.

Opposite, from top: An authentic Indian atmosphere is achieved through the use of equipment and artefacts for the most part sourced in the subcontinent. Of particular note are the massage beds made from single pieces of wood (no nasty joints) and cool copper tubs (bacteria-free and healing).

A brass tray containing a scented water shaker, as well as the exfoliating ingredients for an *ubtan* scrub and a bowl of healing medicated oil lying on a bed of jasmine flowers.

Oil and cotton "candles" create a sensual, relaxing atmosphere as a client waits for a *sirodhara* treatment.

A sweeping staircase made from teakwood leads from the second-floor spa up to the top floor Ayurvedic Penthouse.

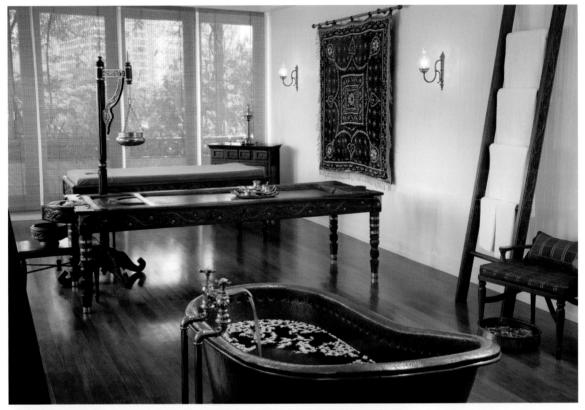

285

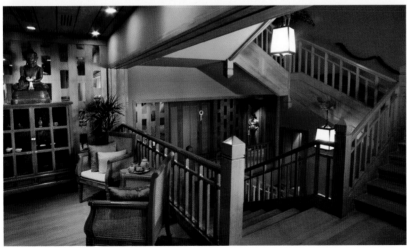

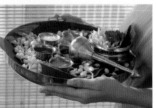

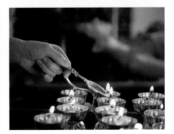

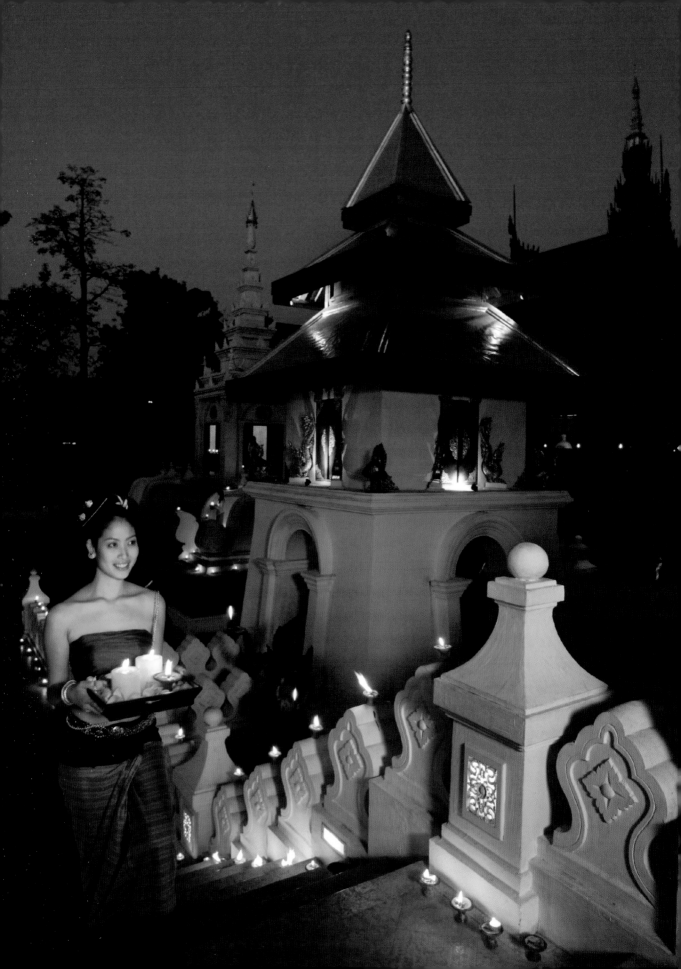

Dheva Spa and Holistic Centre
at Mandarin Oriental Dhara Dhevi

At first glance, a resort that honours Lanna or northern Thai culture may seem out of place in a book on Indian spas, but close analysis of the Mandarin Oriental Dhara Devi reveals that this is not the case. Many Lanna healing traditions are rooted in Ayurveda; much of the resort's art and architecture is Burmese inspired; and the resort has the most comprehensive and well-run Ayurvedic centre to be found anywhere outside India.

The scale of the property beggars belief. Set in 60 acres (25 hectares) of paddy fields in Chiang Mai's Sankamphaeng district, it took thousands of designers, architects, artisans, builders, and craftspeople more than five years to turn a dream into reality. The owner, a Thai businessman who moved to Chiang Mai in 1999, wanted to celebrate the Greater Lanna region; his young dedicated team produced the goods – a fortified wall on the perimeter and an interior containing moats, lakes, lawns, temples, a network of roads and a cluster of extraordinary buildings. It resembles a kingdom rather than a five-star resort.

A resort it is, nonetheless . . . and one with wonderful service and a plethora of amenities. In addition, it more than pays homage to the history, culture, art and architecture of its milieu. From its elaborate entrance gate to its breathtaking buildings with soaring roofs and spires, striking stuccowork and huge collection of artworks, it is truly inspiring.

The Dheva Spa takes its cue from the ancient palace at Mandalay in Burma. A series of teakwood pavilions cluster round a central tower that features a seven-tiered roof symbolising the ancient ideas of cosmology. At the Mandalay palace (1857), the king's throne in the Great Audience Hall was placed directly below a similar tower, but it was clad entirely in gold plate. As at the Dheva Spa, it was surrounded by teakwood structures, elaborately carved with mythological creatures, floral designs and astrological symbols. A team of 150 woodcarvers at the spa took more than three years to replicate many of these intricate carvings, and the overall atmosphere beneath the vertically stacked roofs and towers is one of almost celestial beauty.

The interiors are no less impressive. Asian antiques and artworks punctuate the public spaces, while the 25 treatment rooms and suites are a tranquil combination of Thai silks, polished teakwood and cool marble floors. In the adjacent Holistic Centre, there are also a number of private villas with their own exclusive treatment room attached.

Opposite: A therapist walks up the steps to the Holistic Centre reception carrying a tray of aromatic candles. The spa, in ornate Burmese style, may be seen in the background.

Above: The grandiose entrance stairway leading to the main lobby of the Mandarin Oriental Dhara Devi is illuminated so as to give a fairy-tale atmosphere. The series of spires etched against the night sky showcase Burmese-style architecture beautifully.

The ultimate in pampering indulgence, their luxurious complex was built according to the principles of *vaastu* (the Indian equivalent of *feng shui*). In addition, there is a health and fitness centre, accessed through tunnels inspired by the nearby 500-year-old cave monastery of Wat Umong, as well as a comprehensive meditation and yoga *sala* (open-sided pavilion).

The Mandarin Oriental cites the spa as the resort's "spiritual centre". Its aim is to help guests on their own individual paths to wellbeing, by offering what is probably the most varied menu on the planet. Treatments and services are a blend of Northern Thai, Burmese, Indian and Chinese ancient therapeutic traditions with modern Western know-how and techniques. All are a combination of wellness, relaxation and beauty. Asian-inspired treats are derived from Ayurveda, Thai and Traditional Chinese Medicine (TCM), while Western therapies include hydrotherapy, lymphatic drainage and aromatherapy, amongst others.

The Holistic Centre is dedicated to the art of Ayurveda under the supervision of an Ayurvedic doctor and a team of therapists. Treatments are bespoke according to the client's *dosha* and present state of health which is assessed using the latest in diagnostic technology. Depending on the doctor/ client discussion, recommendations may include a personalised health plan with diet, exercise, rest, relaxation and lifestyle pointers, or some therapies. The latter range in variation from therapies with herbs and spices to aromatherapy, therapeutic massage techniques, colour therapy, meditation, music and more.

Not all treatments are Asian in origin, the hydrotherapy options being a case in point. There is a Lebanese *rhassoul*, derived from an ancient Arabic cleansing ritual, where the guest lies in a steam room wrapped in mineral-rich river mud to draw out toxins, a Turkish *hamman* and an innovative ice fountain, not to mention the French Vichy shower and a special mosaic pool dedicated entirely to the unusual art of *watsu*.

The extraordinary variety of treatments on offer is complemented by the very high levels of service, and a long term view. A spokesperson sums up: "Our aim is to provide extensive holistic treatments aimed at long-term rebalance, as well as some wonderfully indulgent spa experiences that boost the self-esteem and make our guests feel, and look, years younger."

Above: The resort's swimming pool, with a central lounging platform, is surrounded by villas and rooms.

Right: A guest does some gentle stretching after a yoga session on a balcony of the Holistic Centre, overlooking the multi-tiered tile and wood roofs of the spa.

288

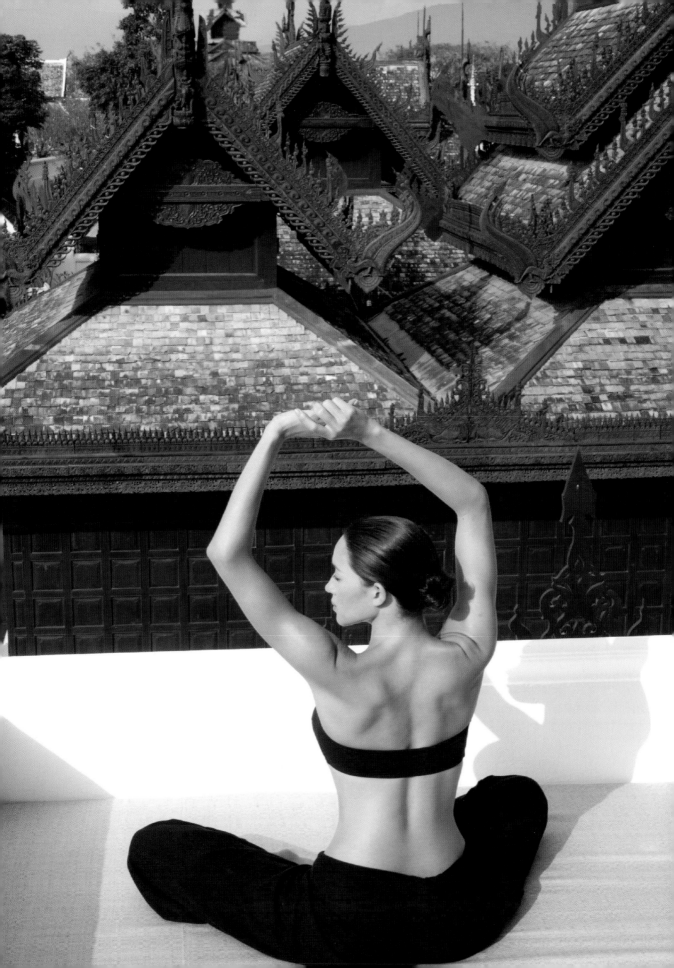

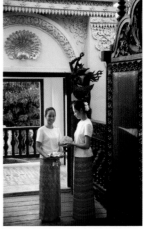

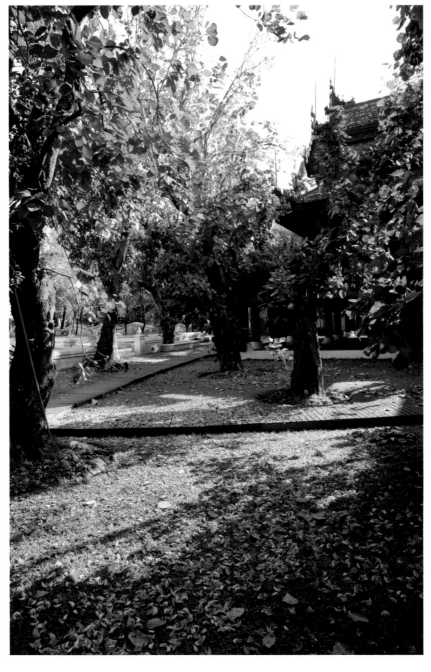

Left: Behind the spa stretches an extensive lawn where thousands of mature trees which were up-rooted and transferred to the site provide cool shade. Here a series of *Erithryna* or coral trees shower the grass with scarlet petals.

Above: Two spa therapists, dressed in traditional Lanna sarongs, stand at the entrance to the spa. Floral motifs are hand carved into the impressive door, while arched stuccowork sits atop a golden peacock.

Opposite top: The expansive site includes a reconstructed Buddhist prayer hall that resembles the *viharn* or assembly hall at Wat Lai Hin in Lampang.

Opposite bottom left: The Royal Villa, the most exclusive of the accommodations, comprises a series of Lanna-style pavilions set around a lotus pool.

Opposite bottom right: Yoga on the lawn at the resort's heart.

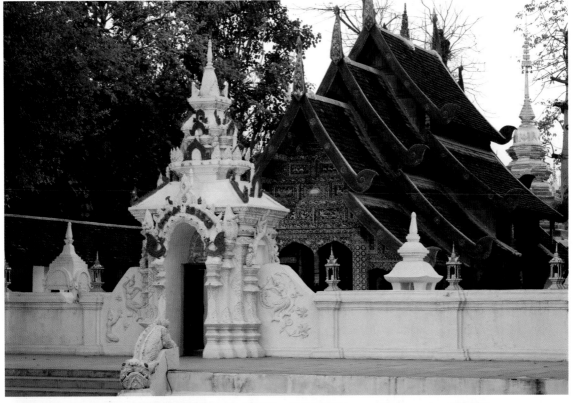

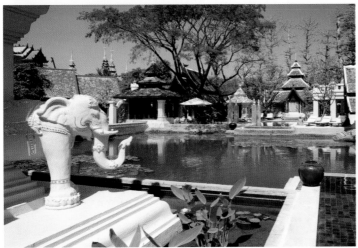

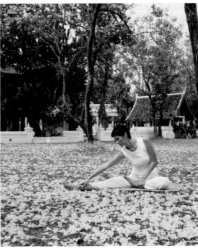

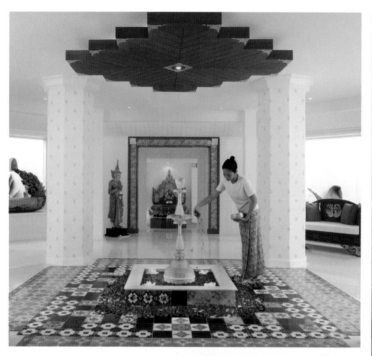

Above: The lower level of the spa is meticulously decorated with Burmese artifacts and art works. At its centre is a cooling fountain set within a mosaic tiled square.

Right: An attractive bath in one of the spa suites is used for chromotherapy as well as for relaxing with the Jacuzzi jets turned on.

Far right: For ultimate indulgence, a separate building decorated with glass mosaic tiles and soft lighting is reserved for *watsu*, a type of healing water *shiatsu*.

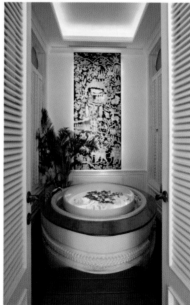

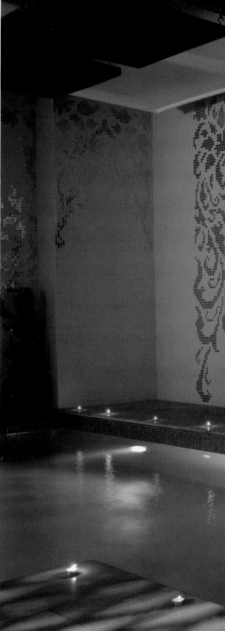

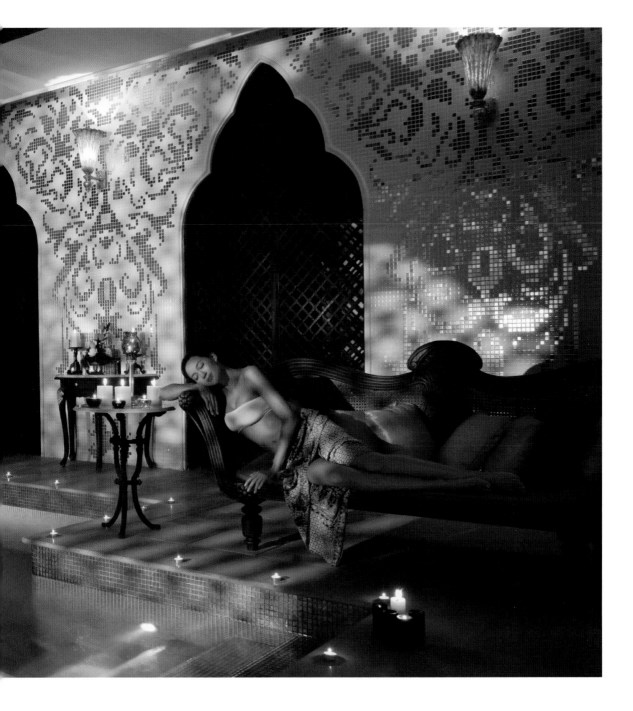

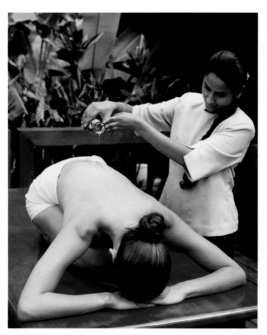

294

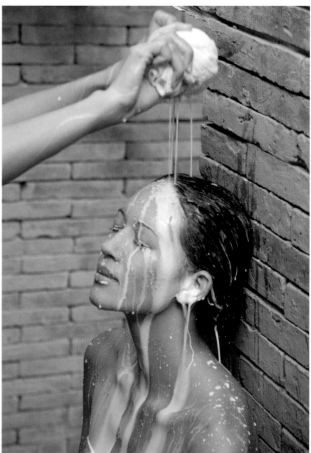

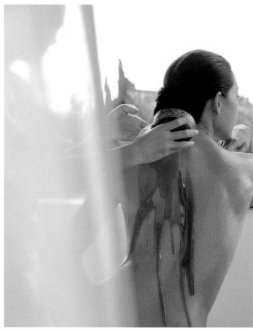

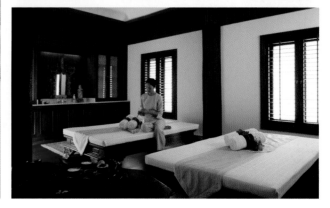

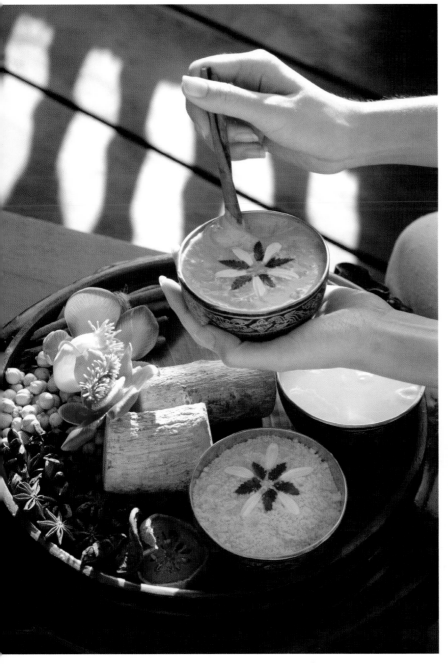

All the therapies at the Dheva Spa and Holistic Centre are designed with total wellness in mind. Many form part of extended rituals or long-term rebalancing plans.

Opposite top left: Offered to soothe the central nervous system and balance the *doshas*, warm oil is poured on to the spinal cord and then gently massaged in.

Opposite top right: Milk is used as part of a facial treatment for its emollient and nourishing properties.

Opposite bottom left: Honey is highly prized in Thailand for its regenerative and healing abilities. In the north of the country it is produced under royal patronage.

Opposite bottom right: Treatment rooms are calm and quiet in the spa. Traditional Thai teakwood beds are used for both massage and facials.

Left: A tray containing ingredients for a northern Thai scrub.

Below: Annointing oil on the feet before the start of a foot massage.

295

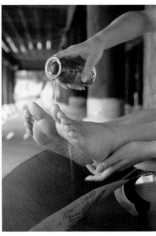

Spa Village at Pangkor Laut Resort

If a Robinson Crusoe-esque island, but one with super luxury and oodles of pampering, is your ideal getaway option, the Spa Village at Pangkor Laut Resort could be your dream holiday destination. An inspired retreat, it is globally renowned for its world-class therapies, caring and cultured staff and nature-rich environment.

The resort is situated on its own private 122-hectare (300 acre) island, 80 percent of which has been left as it was found. With no television, no cars and only a handful of guests for company, it is a place of deep peace. Divided into three sections

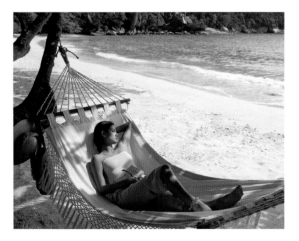

– the original resort around Royal Bay, the ultra-sumptuous Private Estates, and the Spa Village – it is favoured by both European and Asian visitors. And because it is some distance from airports, cities and transport hubs, its isolation ensures its exclusivity.

With the shrouded rain forest as a backdrop and the glittering ocean in front, the Spa Village comprises a number of breezy pavilions, baths, pools and fountains, as well as an Ayurvedic centre,

some Malay-style nap gazebos (airy Zen dens for lounging), a *jamu* bar, reflexology path and 50-metre (164-foot) infinity edge pool. Accommodations consist of 22 overwater villas (see right), all with private verandahs and restful interiors that rely on simple comfort and attention to detail rather than opulence. Hand-spun cottons, fruity toiletries, incense cones, citronella insect repellent and bowls of pot-pourri, along with views of sea and sky, ensure that nature is integral to the package.

Ayurvedic, Chinese and Malay doctors, along with a team of highly experienced therapists, are on hand and the menu is a heady mix of the local and the global. Signature rituals are based on the two medical systems that have influenced peninsular Malaysia's herbal healing traditions for centuries: Ayurveda and Traditional Chinese Medicine. There are also Thai, Balinese and indigenous Malay herbal therapies, along with yoga and meditation and *tai chi* and *qi gong* sessions. A unique addition is the special Bath House ritual that precedes all treatments: During this innovative hour-long journey, Chinese foot pounding and a Shanghai scrub are combined with Japanese hot *onsen* waters and Malay herb-and-water fountain therapeutics. It fully opens the body and stills the mind in preparation for the individual therapies that follow.

Above, left: On the opposite side of the island from the Spa Village is dramatic Emerald Bay, a horseshoe shaped cove accessed by jungle trails. Soft white sand, hammocks and the gentle lapping of the waves are the order of the day here.

Opposite: Saltwater meets pool water at the gorgeous infinity edge pool at Pangkor Laut Spa Village. Stilted accommodations are Malay-inspired and entirely made from local wood.

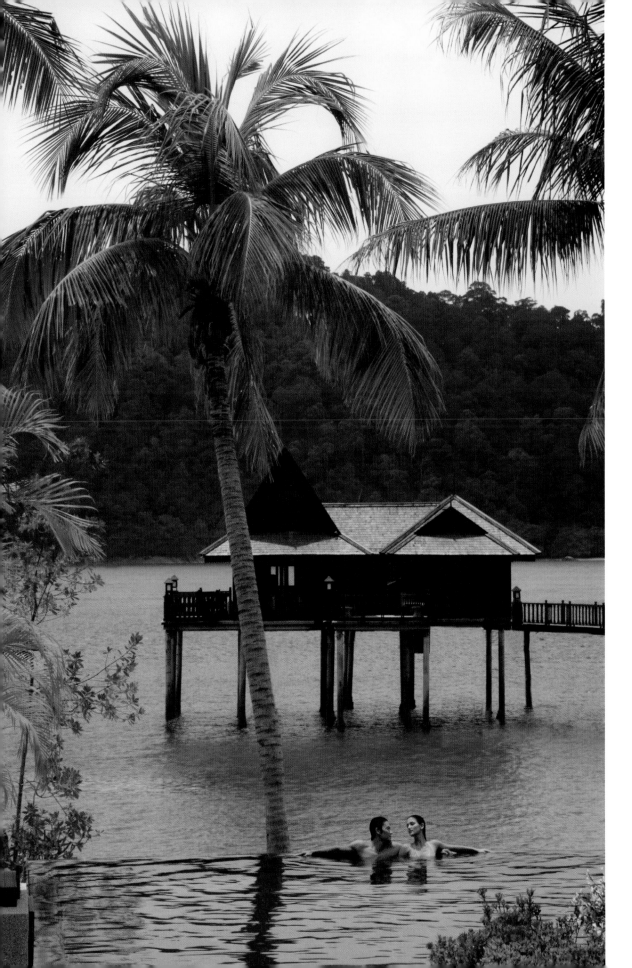

The Ayurvedic Hut, surrounded by a circular herb garden, is the Keralan doctor's "office" and it is here that guests head to if they are interested in experiencing any of the Science of Life's detoxifying therapies. All treatments are prescribed after the usual doctor/patient consultation where pulse and blood pressure diagnosis is combined with discussion. Even though the menu is not extensive, many authentic therapies, such as bone-deep, restorative *abhyanga* massage, soothing *sirodhara*, Navara *kizhi* and *pizhichil* are offered.

To complement the therapies, there is a simple spa cuisine menu where herbal teas and tonics are paired with non-fussy, fresh dishes such as rice porridge and vegetarian steamed dumplings. All the food is full of goodness, low in salt, fat and cholesterol, but rich in flavour.

Whether you want to dabble with a number of different treatments or go for a full two- or three-week programme of healing therapies is entirely up to you. There is no pressure either way. Alternatively, you may want to dedicate yourself solely to the yoga sessions. But one thing is for sure: the natural environment, the tranquil atmosphere and the healing hands of the therapists will ensure your stay is restful, calming and rejuvenating.

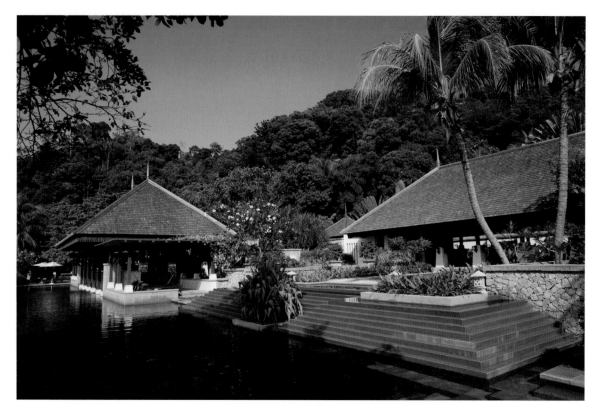

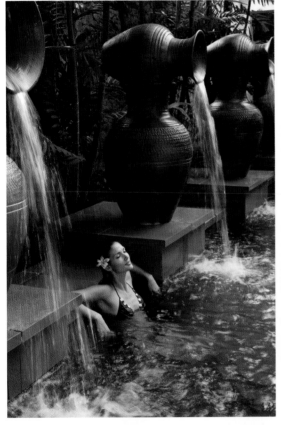

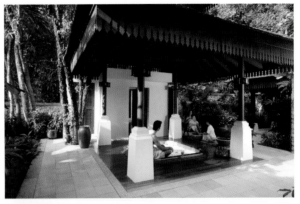

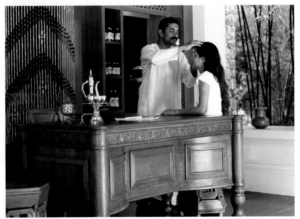

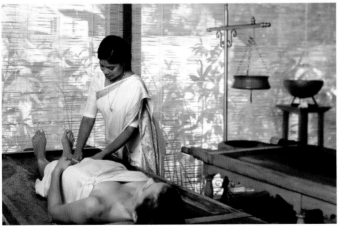

Opposite: Airy, open-sided pavilions with a jungle backdrop surround the tranquil pool.

Above left: The sunken, waist-deep Malay Bath is situated in a walled garden: water gushes from a series of terracotta pots lining one side, while each corner has a platform housing simmering essential oils that waft exotic fragrances over the water.

Above top: Some of the therapy pavilions have private Jacuzzis on the verandah; behind a customer receives a pedicure in jungle surrounds.

Above: An Ayurvedic consultation involves both physical and mental examinations, as well as a deep discussion of lifestyle and stress patterns.

Left: A therapist administers massage in one of the sequestered Ayurvedic treatment pavilions.

Prana Spa at the Villas

Discovering the wonders of Rajasthan in Bali may seem a bit like an oxymoron, but once you enter Prana Spa at the Villas complex in downtown Seminyak, you'll immediately get the picture. As with an Indian *haveli* or nobleman's house, the spa is entirely designed around a central court. There are Islamic arches and open-sided corridors, swirling motifs etched in gold on the walls, elaborate columns and cool tiled floors; the colour palette is an exotic, rich mix redolent of the saris, turbans and regalia of Rajput royalty; even the Jacuzzis and steam rooms have minute Indian mosaics reminiscent of a Moghul palace garden.

Therapies follow the Indian theme with a plethora of Ayurvedic offerings, as well as yoga, Balinese and Javanese traditional therapies and a host of water-inspired treats. Taking their cue from the spa's name, treatments, rituals and packagess are designed to revitalise *prana* or life force in the body, mind and spirit. With such beguiling names as Prana Rebalance, Sun & Moon and Simple Bliss, the two- to four-hour packages are well worth an afternoon or two.

Hydrotherapy is well represented with a Turkish *hamman*, steam and sauna, rain shower as well as complimentary hot and cold plunge pools. In addition, foot baths with fragrant tropical blooms and salt scrubs are often offered as a prelude to a longer treatment. The Indian *chai* or tea bath is spicy and warm, and, as befits its beach location, seaweed, kelp and marine products find their way

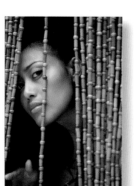

into much of the menu. Clay and minerals are also liberally used as all-over detoxifiers, and wherever you are, you'll smell the fragrant aroma of a host of natural herbs, spices and flowers permeating throughout the entire space.

The spa is spacious by any standards with 1,300 square metres (14,000 square feet) of space containing 24 massage rooms (single and double), hot and cold plunge pools, four rain shower massage rooms, two saunas and three steam rooms, as well as separate areas for reflexology and beauty treatments. The central courtyard planted with potted palms and colourful bougainvillea is the place to relax with a cup of herbal tea after treatments.

As is to be expected in an Indian-inspired environment, yoga is often integrated into spa packages, and Pilates is another menu staple. Fusing traditions from both East and West is not frowned upon: Indeed, many of the packages combine Ayurveda with Balinese massage, for example, or Western facial ingredients with such Indian therapies as *sirodhara*. The lofty aim of "fulfilling guests' dreams with exotic pampering" is furthered by the huge range of options on offer.

Above and opposite: Prana spa at the Villas is a riot of colour with royal reds and golds predominating. A theatrical space that takes its design inspiration from Moghul and Rajput decorative details, it allows guests to subliminally receive a dose of India – in Bali. Indian inspiration in the decor is accompanied by such practices as yoga and Ayurveda at Prana Spa. Bespoke yoga sessions may be arranged by request.

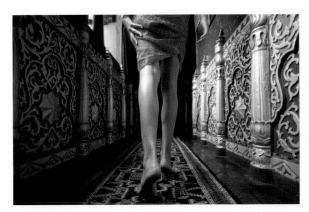

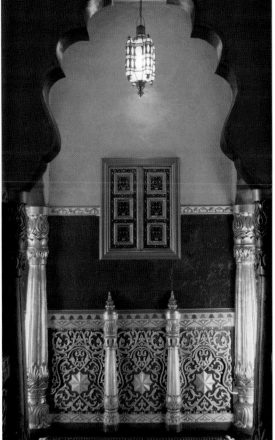

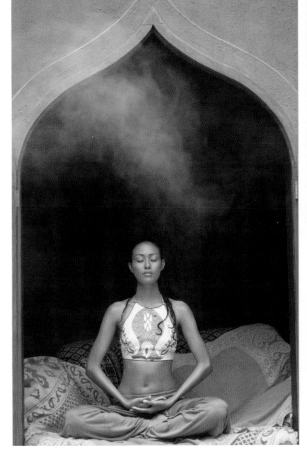

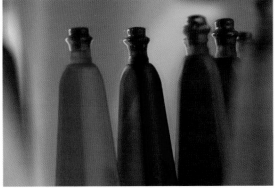

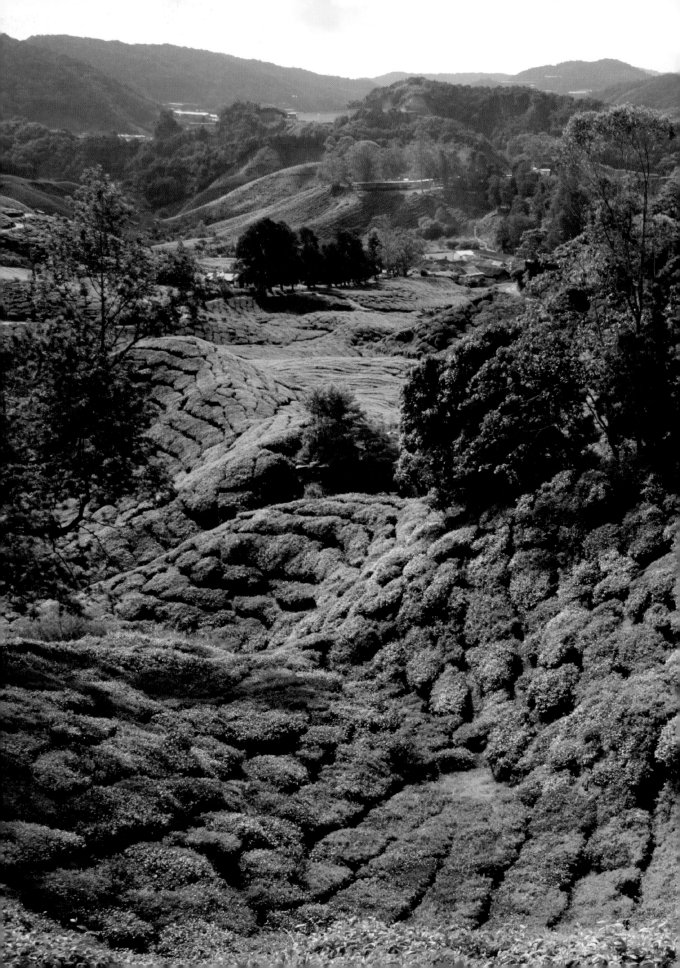

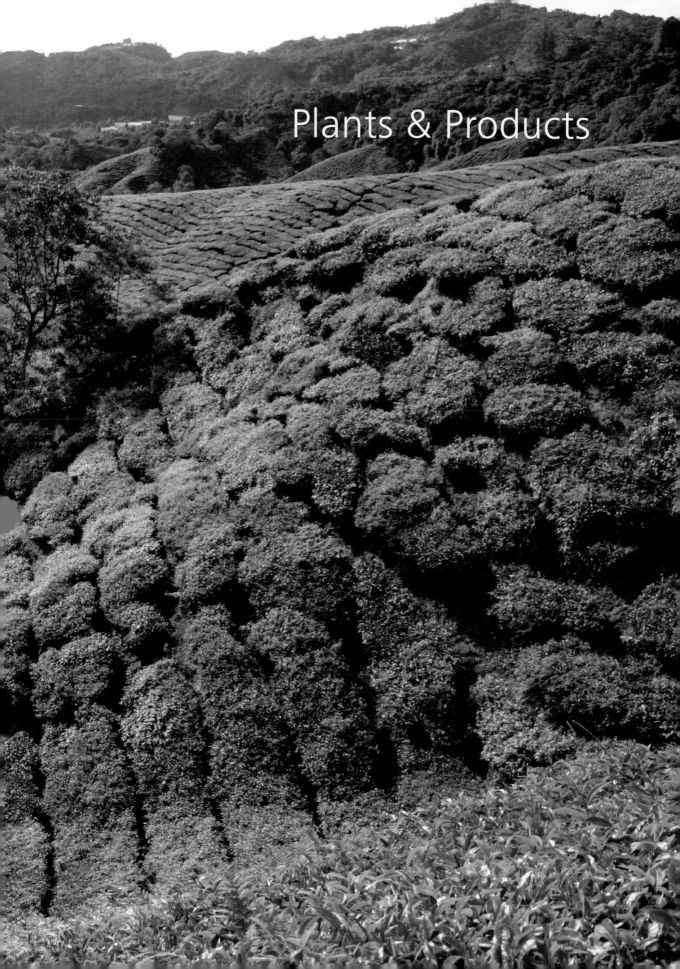

Plants & Products

The Barefoot Doctor

"Akal devayun ni aveh;
akal to heeyaon upajeh."
"Creativity cannot be given to you by an outsider;
it can only be unearthed from the heart."

– old Indian verse

India's creative health and welfare systems are predominantly plant-based (although minerals have a role) and it is estimated that most households rely upon locally available plant material for their pharmacopeia. According to the World Health Organisation (WHO), between 35,000 and 70,000 plants have been used for medicinal purposes globally at one time or another, and in India today at least 10,000 are regularly used. In line with this trend, the sale of herbal medicines and natural products is increasing all the time both within India and around the world.

Across the breadth of the country, people receive medical help from both qualified and non-qualified practitioners. As we have noted previously, there are four traditional systems practiced in India – Ayurveda, Siddha, Unani and ancient Tibetan medicine – all of which are based on humoural pathology. Since Independence in the 1940s, each has built up a solid base of medical colleges imparting education in five-and-a-half year programmes. They have been joined by a fifth: the study of Naturopathy. Currently, only graduates of such recognised medical schools are legally entitled to practice medicine in India, and it is believed that there are around 600,000 such licensed practitioners.

Be that as it may, there are, in addition, literally hundreds of thousands (some say over a million) non-qualified healers servicing the health needs of India's huge population. Often, they comprise families that have practiced their individual skills for centuries – and are well known in the community. Some such practitioners may have some rudimentary education as well, but economic and other factors may have resulted in their medical training being cut short. Others are completely unqualified on paper, indeed they may even be illiterate, but they are the recipients of a wealth of oral healing knowledge that has been handed down through many generations.

As such, they are hugely skilled – and a vital part of any Indian community.

There are numerous examples of such traditional healers, all of whom fall into a category that can loosely be termed the "barefoot doctor".

Clockwise from top: Many unqualified Unani herbalists are recipients of herbal preparations from family members. This young pharmacist follows in the tradition of his grandfather and father (on right). Some of his prescriptions include herbal powders for kidney stones and diabetes, and he was proud of a particularly noxious black paste that is taken internally for digestive problems.

Hakim Sayed Riazuddin, a Unani doctor who learnt his trade from his father, in his Mysore clinic. He makes his own medicines or *mufaras*, often in the form of tasty jams and jellies, from recipes that have been in the family for decades.

Dravidian culture is the source of Siddha's medical arts (originally, a *siddhar* was a devotee of the god Shiva; a *siddhi* is one who has achieved extraordinary power). Here, Dr S B Nithyanandam stands in the temple grounds of his local Shiva temple. Even though he learnt his trade from his father, he also trained at a Siddha medical college.

Charts and photographs in the consulting room of bonesetter Mohammed Khasim; he is the son of Abdul Gafar, a renowned bone specialist who treated the Maharajah of Mysore's family.

304

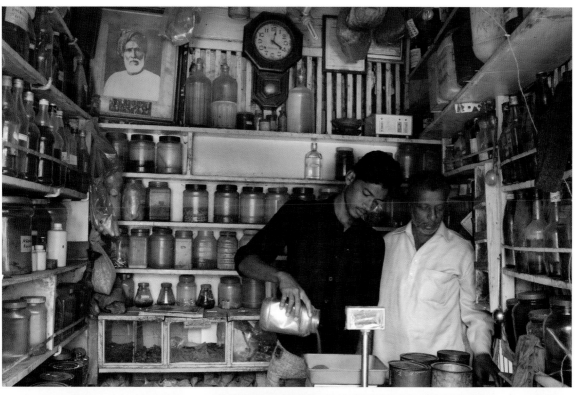

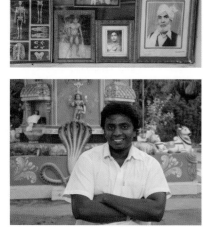

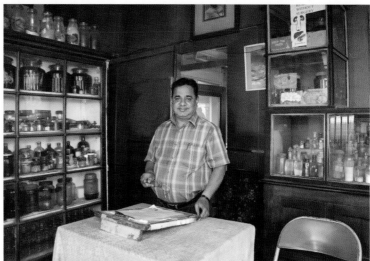

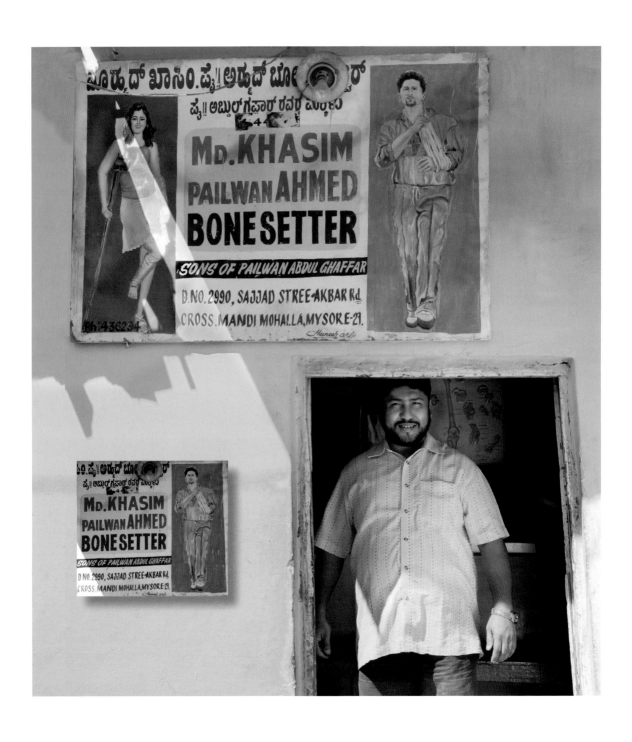

The village midwife: Each village has at least one traditional birth attendant known as a *dai*. These women are skilled in delivering not only healthy babies, but have knowledge of breach births, stillborn foetuses and babies with umbilical cords around their necks. Often coming from a family of midwives, they are skilled in ante-natal and post-natal care as well.

The bonesetter: The traditional bonesetter or orthopaedic healer is another example. In the countryside, such a person may look after the needs of the population of 20 villages or so, walking from one destination to the next to treat sprains, fractures, joint problems or muscle pain. A group involved in strengthening traditional systems of medicine called Lok Swasthya Parampara Samvardhan Samithi (LSPSS) in Coimbatore estimates that there are over 60,000 bonesetters serving rural populations and, in cities, established practitioners

Left: Having learnt his trade from his father, Mohammed Khasim set up a small practice that is always packed with patients. He uses a herbal paste on breaks and fractures, then binds them with a splint; another paste and manipulation is the favoured route for muscle and joint problems. One of his favoured plants is *Cissus quandragularis*; its ovoid reddish black fruit contains calcium and Vitamin C, so, when it is crushed and applied on fractured bones, it helps set breaks and controls inflammation.

Above: Even though there are 2,100 Ayurvedic hospitals, 196 medical colleges and a dozen major pharmaceutical companies in India, the roadside pharmacy overflowing with dusty medicine bottles, dried roots, powders and oils is a common sight. This self-taught Ayurvedic doctor and oil producer came from a family that has practised Ayurveda since 1850; his clients come to him on recommendations from previous supplicants.

may see up to 30 or 40 patients a day. It is estimated that over 50 percent of people with broken bones are treated by bonesetters in any given year.

The poison healer (*visha vaidya*): Snakebite is a common occurrence in rural India and traditional *visha* healers have specialist knowledge. They can differentiate between different snakebites, and they know which antidote works for which type of snake. Their remedies are almost always herbal and prescriptions include purgation, antidotes and topical application of specific plants. The *visha vaidya* is often called on in the case of rabid dog bites too.

Less clear cut, but no less important, are people like oil producers, small-scale herbal medicine manufacturers, wandering monks with herbal knowledge, community elders who have specialist knowledge of herbal home remedies and nutrition, martial art masseuses, and *kannu vaidyas* or eye physicians who treat eye complaints even to the extent of giving cataract operations. Following tradition, many of these care-givers have a relationship with their "patients" and don't practise specifically for monetary gain. Rather, in a similar manner to the taking of the Hippocratic oath, they place value on a code of ethics that includes service to others, the transference of skills, prayers for guidance and holistic health care for all. In some cases, practitioners accept a *kanikkae* (a kind of offering or gratuity) for services rendered.

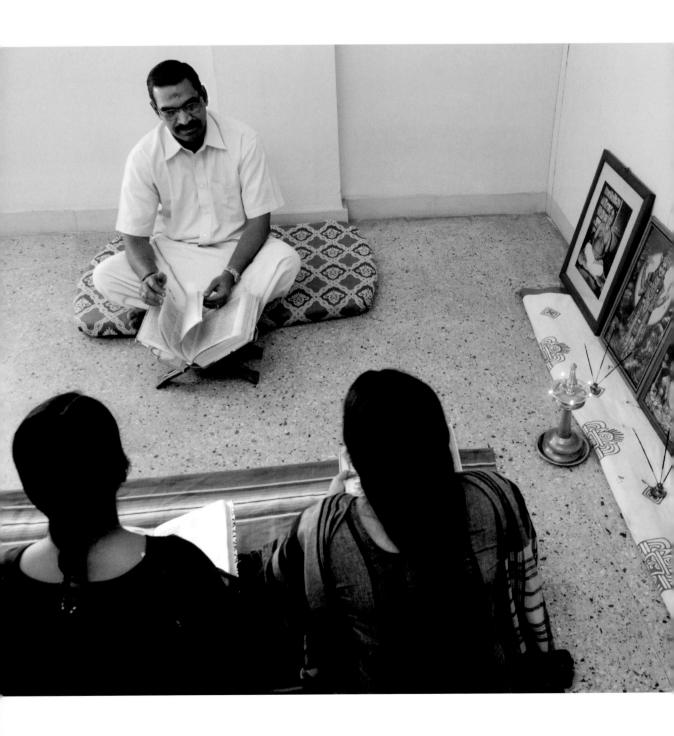

Even though most of these people do not have legal status (or only have semi-legal status) as medical practitioners, they are considered legitimate healers in their own right. Indeed, such organisations as the LSSPS are keen to tap into their specialist knowledge, some of which is invariably being lost with the passing of time. For a start, none of it is written down: Most barefoot doctors receive their healing knowledge orally via person-to-person transmission either in the form of the guru-*shishya* tradition, or commonly from father to son or mother to daughter. Secondly, with rapid industrialisation and loss of rural land, vital herbs, plants and trees are being cut down in the name of "development". Thirdly, as India develops, a worrying trend has been noticed: Such

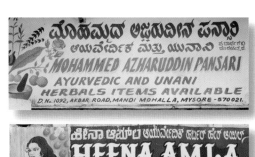
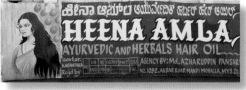

people are usually over 40 years old, and are not handing down their skills to the next generation.

In both the codified systems of medicine where knowledge is catalogued and non-codified systems where it is orally transmitted, India's local environment is its greatest asset. Most medical

Left: The belief behind the guru-*shishaya* method of transferring knowledge is a cyclical one. Knowledge from God is transmitted to a guru, who, in turn, passes it on to his disciples. The aim is for the disciple to become better than the original guru, a scholar in all subjects, so that his knowledge may be passed on for the benefit of all humanity.

Above: Examples of some of India's colourful painted billboards advertising herbals for health and beauty.

remedies are derived from plant life with all parts of a plant – roots, leaves, stems, stamens, pistils, flowers, fruits – being utilised. The government-run All India Coordinated Project on Ethnobiology estimates that about 7,500 wild plants are used for medicinal purpose by rural and tribal peoples, with most of their resources coming from forests, markets, gardens and kitchens. Steps are being taken to try to preserve local knowledge and environments – but many warn that there is a gradual erosion of both.

In recent years, some developed countries have shown a renewed interest in plant-based medicines; a distrust of chemicals with their side effects has led many people to desire more "natural" solutions to health problems. India is one of the countries they are turning to, not least because of its ancient documented herbal health systems. Yoga retreats, sojourns at Ayurvedic homestays, and visits to spas and clinics are definitely on the increase. But there is also much to learn from undocumented remedies too. Unfortunately, precisely because there is no systematic inventory of its wisdoms, much of the knowledge is fast disappearing.

On the following pages we showcase some of India's most important medicinal herbs and plants, along with their applications and history. Following that is a listing of reputable natural products.

Healing Plants

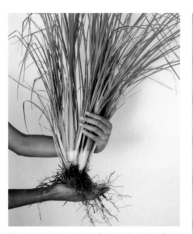

Chrysopogon zizanoides: Native to India, *vetiver* is a Tamil name. Vetiver root has cooling and calming properties, so is effective in treating burns, while oil of vetiver is a key ingredient in perfumes.

310

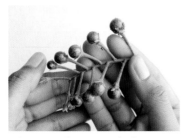

Solanum xanthocarpum: Also known as poisonberry, this spiny diffuse herb grows wild in India. The juice of the berries is given for sore throats, and roots and seeds are administered for coughs.

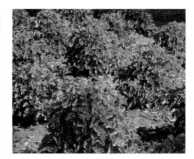

Coleus zeylanicus: Known as *ambu* in Sanskrit, this plant has anti-bacterial, deodorant and cooling properties, and is used in urinary infections. Its leaves are used to reduce body temperature or fever.

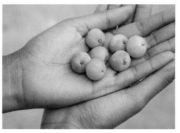

Emblica officionalis: The Indian gooseberry or *amla* (*amlika*) is a very important Ayurvedic fruit, used in the treatment of liver conditions, jaundice, anaemia and diabetes. It is an immune system booster.

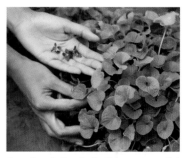

Centella asiatica: Brahmi leaves are useful in abdominal disorders, while the oil is good for the reduction of scarring. It is also used in the treatment of leprosy, epilepsy, cardiac debility and more.

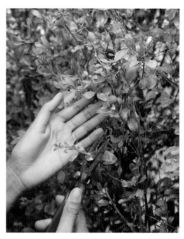

Lawsonia inermis: Henna or *mehndi* has been used as a dye on skin, fingernails, hair, leather, silk and wool since the Bronze Ages. It is also an anti-fungal and the essential oil is a good scalp stimulator.

Adhatoda vasica: Also known as the Malabar nut tree, the *vasaka* shrub has leaves that are rich in Vitamin C and carotene. It is used as a tea for bronchial and asthmatic troubles and is helpful with skin infections.

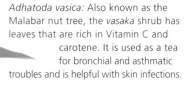

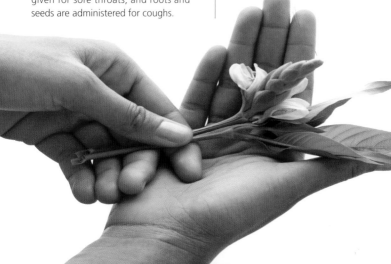

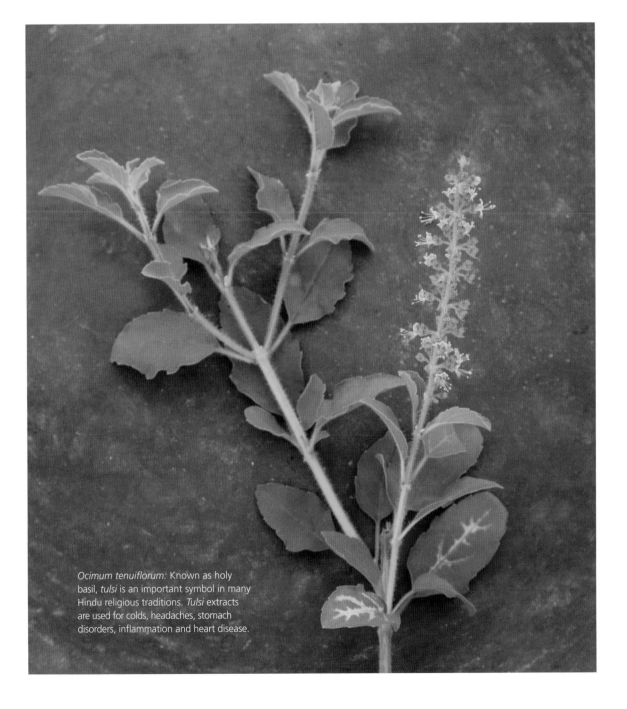

Ocimum tenuiflorum: Known as holy basil, *tulsi* is an important symbol in many Hindu religious traditions. *Tulsi* extracts are used for colds, headaches, stomach disorders, inflammation and heart disease.

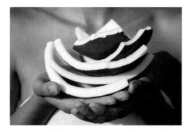

Cocos nucifera: Known as "the tree that provides all the necessities of life", the term coconut refers to the nut, which is widely used in Ayurveda as it is *vata* pacifying, cooling and strengthening. It is used externally for its oil and internally as food.

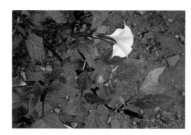

Datura stramonium L.: The thorn apple or *shivpriya* grows as a wasteland weed. Hindu physicians regard it as intoxicating, emetic, digestive and heating. The dried leaves, flowering tops and seeds are used to treat asthma and bronchitis.

312

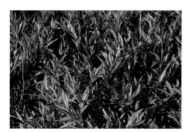

Eupatorium tripinervi: Called *ayyappana,* the leaves of this ground-covering shrub are used for digestive disorders, piles (as it has haemostatic properties), nervine disorders and asthma. It is also used to bring down fevers as it is antipyretic.

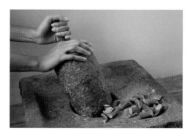

Glycyrrhiza glabra: Liquorice is used in herbal medicine as a liver detoxifier and endocrine system booster. It is also useful for a variety of bronchial problems and in India liquorice sticks were (and still are) commonly used as teeth-cleaners.

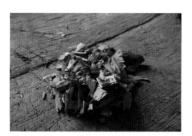

Caesalpinia sappan: The bark from this "tropical redwood" tree is noted for its blood purifying and cooling properties so it is often an ingredient in tonics; it also has anti-bacterial and coagulant properties, so is useful for wounds.

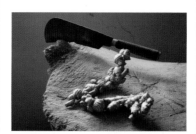

Zingiber officinale: Ginger is used widely in both Ayurvedic and Unani medicine. Charak said "every good quality is found in ginger". It enhances the digestion, clears the micro-circulatory channels and helps with joint pain and motion sickness.

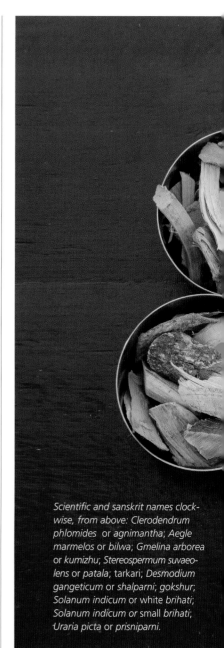

Scientific and sanskrit names clockwise, from above: Clerodendrum phlomides or *agnimantha; Aegle marmelos* or *bilwa; Gmelina arborea* or *kumizhu; Stereospermum suvaeolens* or *patala;* tarkari; *Desmodium gangeticum* or *shalparni; gokshur; Solanum indicum* or white *brihati; Solanum indicum* or small *brihati; Uraria picta* or *prisniparni.*

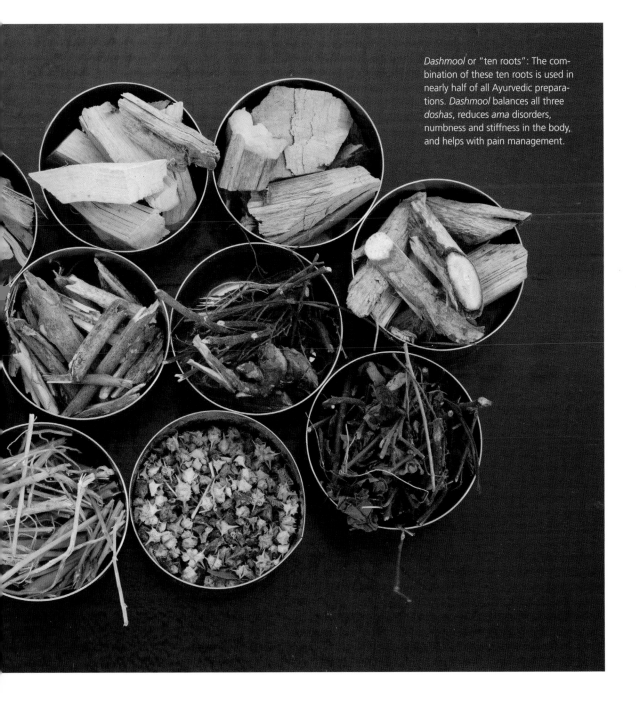

Dashmool or "ten roots": The combination of these ten roots is used in nearly half of all Ayurvedic preparations. *Dashmool* balances all three *doshas*, reduces *ama* disorders, numbness and stiffness in the body, and helps with pain management.

313

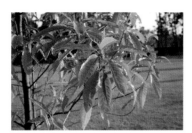

Elaeocarpus spharicus: This small tree supplies the ridged fruits that are dried and used as medicinal "beads" in *rudraaksh* or garlands worn to stave off evil or illness. The fruits are used for hypertension, mental diseases, epilepsy and arthritis.

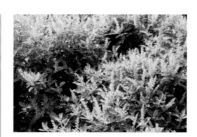

Ocimum basilicum: Also known as sweet basil and originally native to India, basil is well known as a culinary herb. However, its seeds are used medicinally in India for constipation and the leaves are used for indigestion and skin diseases.

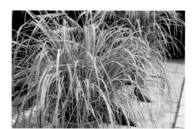

Cymbopogon citrates: A medicinal plant, lemongrass is used in Ayurvedic herbal teas for *pitta* types, while the essential oil is a useful insect repellant. It is also widely used in perfumes and cosmetics, and is a useful stress-reliever and cleanser.

314

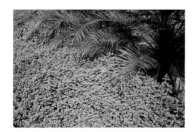

Mentha arvensis: Called *paparaminta* in Hindi, mint is indigenous to India and is widely distilled for its antiseptic and antispasmodic oil. Helpful for headaches, rheumatism and neuralgia, mint is also used in teas to prevent vomiting.

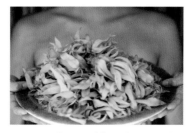

Cananga odorata: Oil from the greenish-yellow flowers of cananga (also known as ylang ylang) is relaxing and tension relieving. It is also recommended as an anti-depressant. It has an erotic, sweet smell, so is widely used in perfumery.

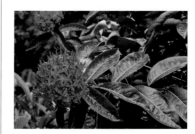

Ixora sp: A poultice of the leaves and stems is good for sprains, eczema and boils. A flower decoction helps with hypertension, amenorrhea and irregular menstruation, while a decoction of the leaves is useful for wounds and skin ulcers.

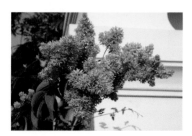

Calicopteris floribunda: Known as *pullani* or *ukshi*, this woody climber is used in Ayurvedic remedies for malaria, dysentery and snakebite. Its essential oil is reported to to be useful for depression as it has grounding properties.

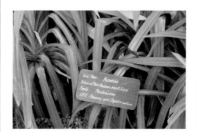

Pandanus amaryllifolius: The long leaves of the pandan or screwpine are used as a flavouring in food, but are also known medicinally for aiding digestion. The leaves are also thought to contain an anti-viral protein that is useful for influenza.

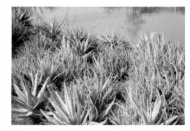

Aloe barbedensis: Highly prized for the liquid contained in its thick, fleshy blades, aloe vera is revered for its cooling properties. It is used externally for skin rashes, sunburn, itchiness, scarring and psoriasis, as it is antibiotic and antiseptic in nature.

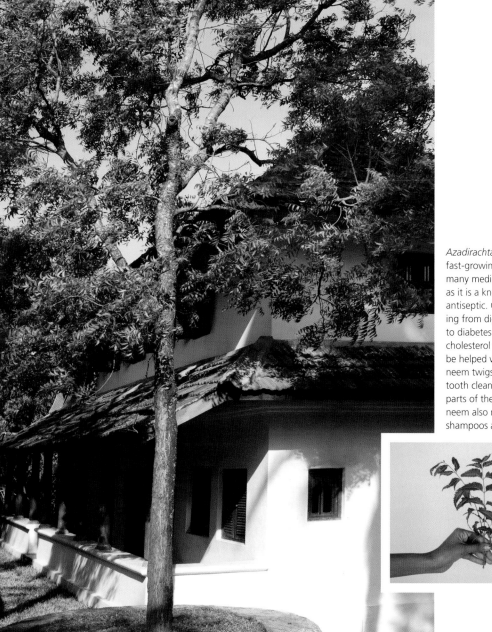

315

Azadirachta indica: The fast-growing neem tree has many medicinal properties, as it is a known purifier and antiseptic. Conditions ranging from digestive disorders to diabetes and from high cholesterol to cancer may be helped with neem, while neem twigs are a traditional tooth cleaner in India. All parts of the tree are used; neem also makes soaps, shampoos and creams.

316

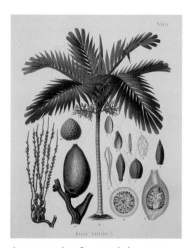

Areca catechu: Commonly known as betel, the areca nut may comprise part of the Indian recreational digestive known as *paan*. The nut has stimulant and astringent properties and is used to sweeten the breath and strengthen the gums.

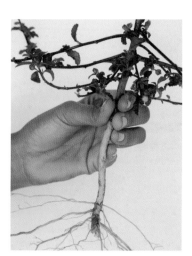

Sida cordifolia: The *bala* plant is part of the magical trio of herbs associated with women in Indian herbology. *Bala* oil is good for all disorders produced by the derangement of *vata*, and it is a proven root effective for neuralgia.

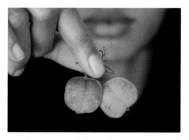

Cardiospermum halicacabume: A ground cover creeper, the balloon vine grows wild in India and is a useful hair care ingredient. Antiseptic liquid from the fruit (*indravallari* in Sanskrit) is added to hair after washing to act as a traditional conditioner.

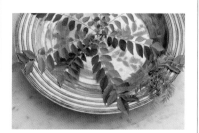

Murraya koenigi: Found in many Indian backyards, the curry leaf plant is a staple in Indian cuisine. However, its leaves also aid the digestion as they are mildly laxative, and the powdered root and bark are used for relief from kidney pain.

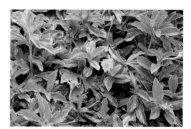

Eclipta alba: Bhrigaraja is an annual herb that is commonly used in the treatment of skin diseases and as an anti-inflammatory. It is also reported to be effective for blackening and strengthening the hair and is cooling on the head.

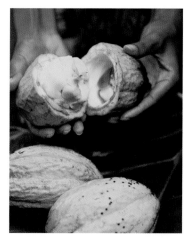

Theobroma cacao: Used to make cocoa and chocolate, cacao beans also form the basis for cocoa butter, an all-natural vegetable fat. It is used in a variety of beauty preparations, and is used for sunburn, as a skin softener and to reduce scar tissue.

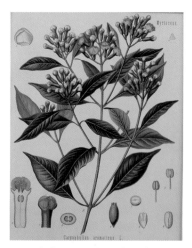

Caryophyllus aromaticus: Cloves have both culinary and medicinal uses. It is a stimulant and an antiseptic, so is used in a variety of Ayurvedic medicines: it helps gastric irritability, aids the digestion and enhances circulation and metabolism.

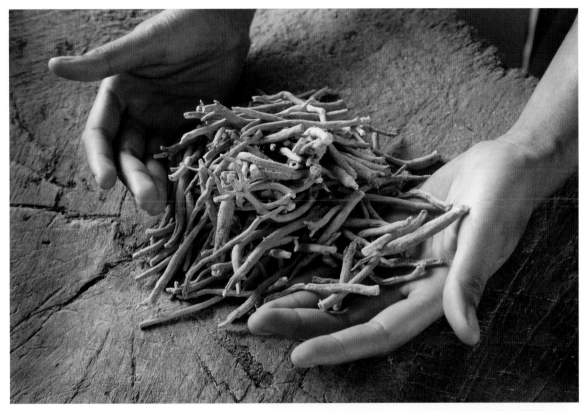

317

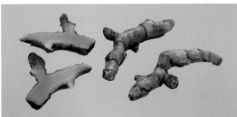

Clockwise from top: Withania somnifera: Also known as the Indian winter cherry, *ashwagandha* root has anti-oxidant properties and is an immune system booster. *Cinnamomum zeylanicum:* The dried leaves and bark of the cinnamon tree are used as a culinary spice, medicinally and as a cosmetic. It is also a brain tonic and aids digestion. *Curcuma domestica:* Turmeric is an all-round Ayurvedic wonder rhizome used by every herbal healer. It detoxifies the liver, balances cholesterol levels and fights allergies.

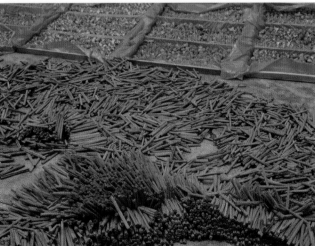

Natural Products

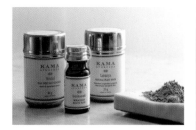

In partnership with the respected AVP in Coimbatore, Kama Ayurveda's range of authentic Ayurvedic products uses original, time-tested, prescriptions for skincare, hair care, body care and Ayurvedic soaps. www.kamaayurveda.com

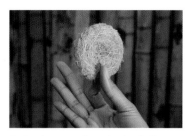

Soukya has a small production facility on site, as well as a herbal store that houses every Ayurvedic herb, root and leaf imaginable. This small loofah, one of their products, is not too harsh on the skin. www.soukya.com

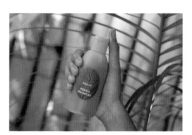

Comprising a small range of skin and hair care products that includes shampoos, scrubs, oils and soaps, Soukya products use organically grown ingredients only. This scented herbal shampoo is very gentle. www.soukya.com

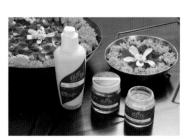

Developed by Ayurvedic doctor Dr Ajit, this Australian brand of skincare products includes a line of shampoos, face packs, cleansers, moisturisers, toners, gels and creams to help clients "feel healthier, look better and age less". www.ayurda.com.au

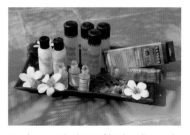

Sansha uses the best of both Indian and overseas ingredients in its range of hand, face and body products. Incorporating Ayurvedic herbals as well as such items as Dead Sea minerals, they are 100 percent natural. www.sanshaayurveda.com

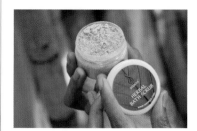

Soukya's products are manufactured to ancient recipes. This home-made bath scrub is made entirely from exfoliating herbs and roots. Packaging is simple with the organic theme running into labels as well as contents. www.soukya.com

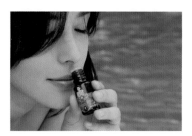

Made to ancient Malay recipes, the Spa Village in Kuala Lumpur, produces a small range of massage oils for use in their highly authentic spa treatments. Utilising local flowers and fruits, they are truly scent-sual. www.spavillage.com

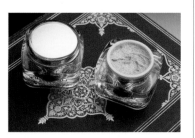

The Diamond collection from the high priestess of herbal healing Shahnaz Husain, uses diamond *bhasma* and plant extracts for sparkling effect (see opposite). It is a modern take on ancient Indian gemstone therapy. www.shahnaz-husain.com

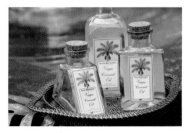

Virgin coconut oil from the Farm at San Benito is cold-processed from fresh mature coconuts. The oil extraction method uses no heat, so the oil is clear, aromatic and 100 percent natural. It is for internal and external use. www.thefarm.com.ph

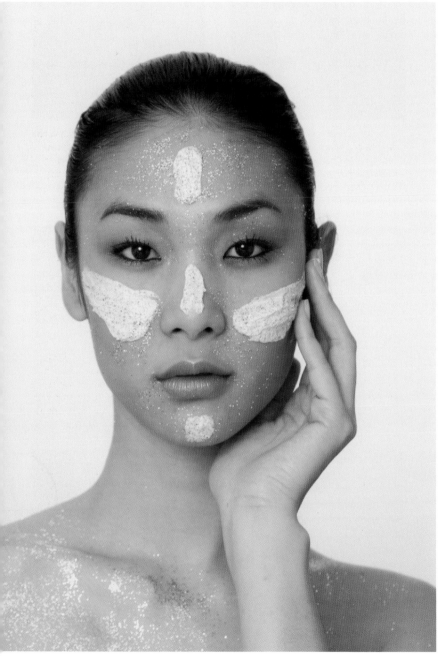

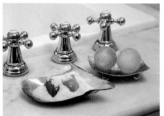

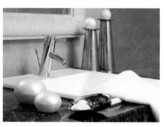

Top: Bath Salts for Inner Peace by UK firm Ila are made from Himalayan salt crystals that are rich in minerals and trace elements easily absorbed by the body. Scented with Damascene rose otto, sandalwood and jasmine essential oils, they strengthen the body's bio-energetic field — and give an indulgent bath treat to boot. www.ila-spa.com

Above: In India and China, crushed pearls have been used to exfoliate, whiten and protect skin from sun's rays for centuries. It's not surprising therefore that Shahnaz Husain has developed two pearly products: a frothy rehydrating and whitening cream and a mask to rejuvenate facial skin at a deep cellular level. www.shahnaz-husain.com

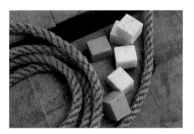

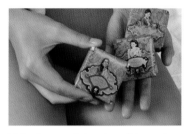

The Oriental Spa range from Lucien Ortscheit is manufactured in Asia. This soap, made from rice oil in a natural manner, comes in its own hand-crafted leaf pouch. It is available in a variety of fragrances. www.orientalspa.de

These little cube soaps with lavender, calendula and rose scents are also part of the Oriental Spa range. Sold in threes and attached by a sweet string, they make wonderful natural presents. www.orientalspa.de

Malaysian spa aficionados will instantly recognise the sweet packaging of these soaps from the Spa Village group of spas. Available in coconut, pomelo and clove, they are handmade to a traditional recipe. www.spavillage.com

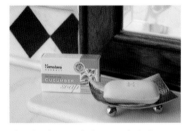

The Himalaya Herbals range includes health care, oral care, hair care, skincare and baby care formulations in the form of soaps, washes, cleansers, shampoos and more. www.himalayanhealthcare.com

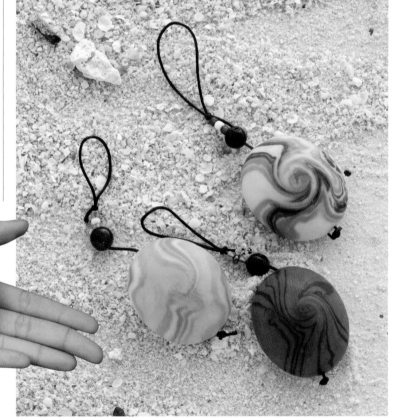

Right:
These little
"rock soaps" are
made from coconut, rice and sesame oil and come in a number of fruity flavours. www.orientalspa.de

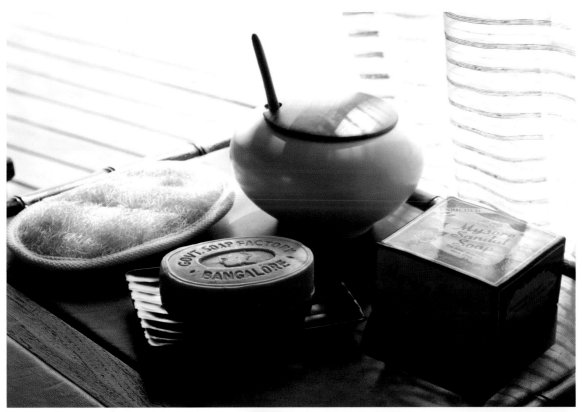

Opposite, inset: A natural organic soap from Soukya.

Above: The Government Sandal Oil Factory in Mysore has been in operation since 1917 and today uses the same processes to produce first-class sandalwood oil as it did when it opened. One thousand kilograms of wood produces only 30 litres of oil, showing how pure the boiling, cooling and distillation procedures are. This beautifully scented soap, only available at government stores, is one of their best-selling products.

Right and far right: Tapping into ancient herbal lore from across Asia, Lucien Ortscheit presents a selection of facial and body pouches specially hand-crafted for home use. Designed to relieve sore and strained muscles as well as tired skin, the pouches release herbal properties after they have been warmed and applied to the skin. Scented with Asian herbs and spices, they are wonderfully revitalising. Soaps are from the same company. www.orientalspa.de

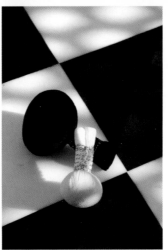

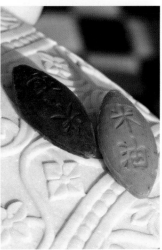

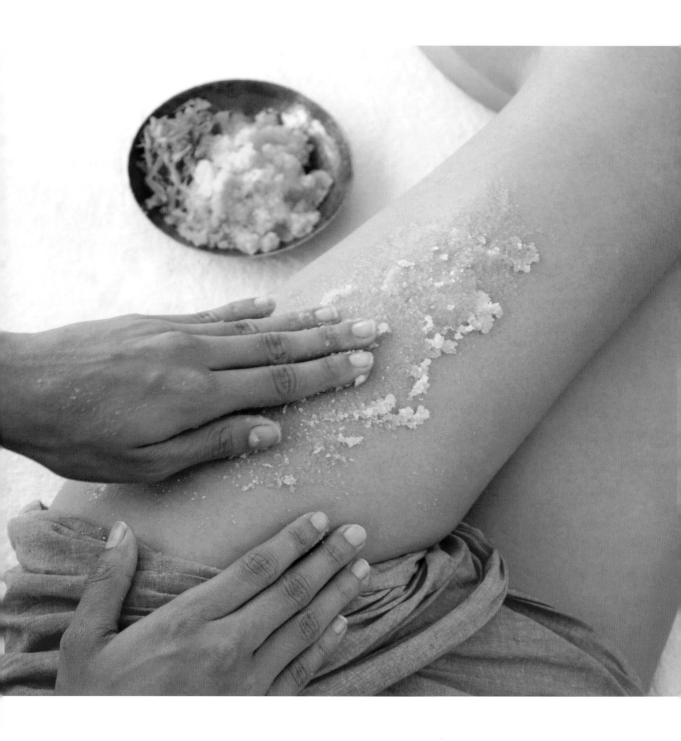

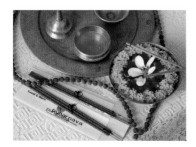

Hand-rolled in the Himalayas, Punarnava incense sticks are free from synthetic substances. They utilise aromatic roots and barks, herbs, spices, flowers and resins to release a distinct, therapeutic aroma. They come in three fragrances: Stability, Energy and Serenity. www.punarnava.com

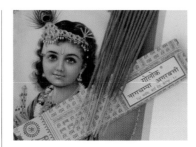

The sandalwood forests around Mysore have long supplied the city with the raw product to make incense sticks, sandalwood oil and carvings. These *agarabathi* (incense sticks) made by Karnataka-based Goloka, and widely available in India, are the result of a 150-hour distillation process.

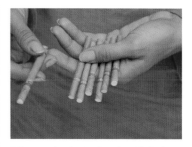

Tobacco, nicotine and tar free Nirdosh Ayurvedic cigarettes were developed by a Mr N M Bhavsar who used the *Charaka Samita* as his guide. They contain liquorice, turmeric, a type of ginger, *tendu* leaves, cinnamon, Bishop's weed and a tree gum. www.nirdosh.co.nz

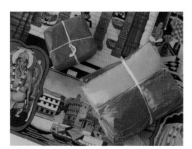

Small bags of red, vermilion and maroon powders in India's numerous bazaars are a common sight. They are used to mark the *tilak* or sacred mark on the forehead — a mark of auspiciousness. Generally made from red vermilion powder (*sindoor*), sandal powder or *kumkum* (red turmeric), they are also used on the hair parting.

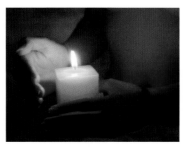

Six Senses spas, whose aim is to balance and invirorate all five senses and one more, carry a wide range of candles and oil burners in their gallery on line and in their stores. A spa at home wouldn't be a spa without one. www.sixsenses.com

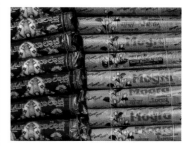

Mogra is a type of jasmine with a highly fragrant, gentle, yet sweet scent. Coming from the *Jasminum sambac* species, it has been used in Indian beauty products since time immemorial. These aromatic *agarabathi* are available in Indian bazaars.

Left: This Ila Body Scrub for Energising and Detoxifying is made from pure Himalayan salt crystals and scented with geranium, rose and wild juniper berry oils. The salts eliminate toxins while the addition of *argan* oil with a natural SPF provides antioxidants and anti-aging properties. www.ila-spa.com

Six Senses spa products are made only from natural ingredients, in harmony with the environment. Their incense cones make for a unique present. www.sixsenses.com

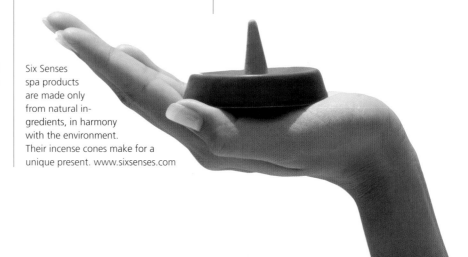

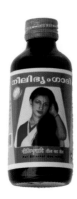

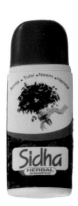

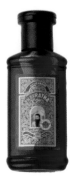

324

One hundred percent natural hair oils are extremely common in India. Often containing extracts of *Eclipta alba* or *bhringaraj* (literally "king of tresses"), such oils nourish the hair, balance the mind, improve surface blood circulation and allegedly improve memory.

Drawing its name from the Siddha form of medicine, this shampoo was launched by Surya Laboratories in 1988. Made from *amla*, *tulsi*, neem and henna, it nourishes the scalp and conditions the hair. Don't be put off by the dark viscous appearance.

Made from extracts from natural herbs, Himani Navratna oil is used as a hair oil to keep the head cool and relieve headaches. It may also be used as a muscle toner or massage oil, and is useful for minor burns and cuts. It's a great tension reliever.

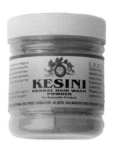

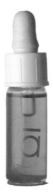

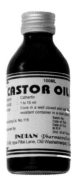

Traditionally, Indians washed their hair with powder, as it doesn't strip the hair of natural oils. This hair wash, made from Ayurvedic herbs including vetiver, *tulsi* and acacia, is gentle and cleansing. It is made by the AVP. www.avpayurveda.com

Ila describes its ethos as "beyond organic" and certainly these Face Oils for Glowing Radiance are extremely pure. Made from *argan* (Moroccan almond), rosehip seed and Damascene rose otto oils, they plump out the face. www.ila-spa.com

Castor oil from Indian Pharmaceuticals is a staple in the medicine cabinet of many Indian homes. Used in a pack or topically, it helps with skin problems, burns and cuts as well as such ailments as abdominal complaints. www.pharmaceutical-india.com

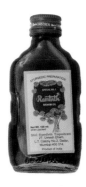

Introduced in 1944, Sri Ramtirth Brahmi Oil is composed from 22 Ayurvedic herbs blended with coconut oil. It promotes hair growth, provides relief from dandruff and helps with joint pains if rubbed into the skin. www.ramtirth.trade-india.com

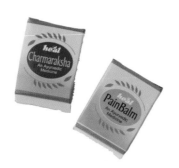

The Heal brand from Ayurvedic giants Arya Vaidya Pharmacy includes skin-care products, soaps and pain balms (pictured here). Made to old Ayurvedic formulations, a small amount of balm applied to the skin acts as quick acting headache and body ache relievers. www.avpayurveda.com

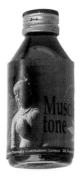

This oil is an over the counter product that is useful for toning muscles. If taken in conjunction with a steam as dictated by Ayurvedic practice, it improves skin and muscle tone, as well as removing toxins from the body. www.avpayurveda.com

325

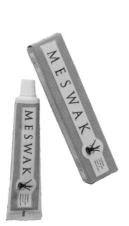

In the traditional Muslim world, the *siwak* or *miswak* was a toothbrush made from a twig. Meswak toothpaste with extracts of the *Salvadora persica* or toothbrush tree, is said to have 70 different health benefits for the entire body. www.balsara.com

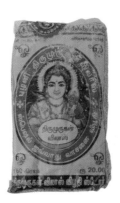

Jute bags of henna powder are plentiful in Indian bazaars: Usually containing 100 percent pure crushed *mehndi* leaves, they are perfect for dyeing hair naturally. Depending on your natural hair colour, results range from auburn to orange or glints of red.

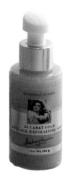

Gold is believed to have powerful anti-aging properties, as it helps to reverse oxidation damage. Here it takes gold leaf form in a range of skincare products from Shahnaz Husain. This exfoliating scrub is an alchemist's dream. www.shahnaz-husain.com

Ayurvedic Preparations and Production

Ayurveda, Siddha, Unani and Tibetan traditional medicine all use materials from the earth in their prescriptions. In most cases, the ingredients are not simply plucked and used, but undergo certain preparatory procedures before they are considered ready for use. Ayurvedic doctors stress the link between freshness and efficacy in the case of herbs and plants, whilst materials from the ground (metals, minerals and so forth) have to undergo complicated, time-consuming purification processes.

In Ayurveda, some preparations are used internally, others are reserved for external use and some can be used for both. For the most part, oils (*thailam*), powders (*choornam*), raw herbal pastes (*kalkam*) and processed herbal pastes (*leham*) are widely used as topical applications. Internal prescriptions include fermented preparations such as *asavam* and *arishtam* (both decoctions, the former made without heat, the latter with heat), medicated ghees or *gritham*, *bhasmas* (incinerated powders) and *gulikam* (pills). None are easy to make.

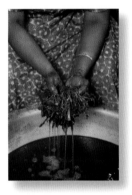

Depending on the size and scale of the Ayurvedic establishment, medicines and oils are either sourced from reputable manufacturing companies or pharmacies, or made on site. It is usually the smaller concerns that grow or locally source their own ingredients, and make their own medicines. In recent years, Kerala has seen a resurgence of the small Ayurvedic homestay, where doctors (usually from a long lineage of Ayurvedic ancestry) offer rooms for four to six long-staying patients: they diagnose, supervise and administer treatments themselves in a highly personal and caring environment, and make their own medications, often to recipes handed down through the generations.

Dr P Sathyanarayanan, a third-generation Ayurvedic doctor but also a qualified doctor from the Ayurvedic College in Coimbatore, runs such an establishment with his wife. "We have centuries of tradition behind us," he explains, "but also modern facilities and a home-away-from-home environment. All our medicines are made on site in our production facility, and we individually custom-make prescriptions for all our patients." Exploring the production facility is an eye-opener: each oil or powder or pill has to go through numerous processes before it is ready for use. The procedures are time-consuming, made-by-hand and labour-intensive, but this "return to basics" in Dr Sathyanarayanan's opinion is the true route for authentic Ayurveda.

Many agree with him. Punarnava, a Coimbatore-based Ayurvedic consultancy that helps link patients with suitable Ayurvedic doctors and homestays, embraces the concept of "living in the present but drawing on traditions from the past to look to the future." Their doctors believe that "real" Ayurveda is a potent combination of ancient knowledge, logical, ethical and spiritual practice, a caring environment, correctly administered procedures and authentically prepared medicines. If all the above are practised, they believe that Ayurveda and Ayurvedic medicines have a bright future.

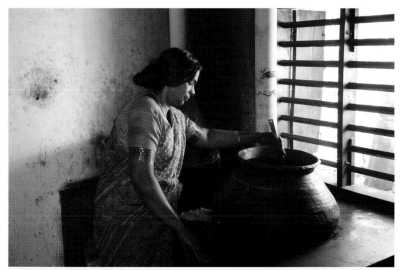

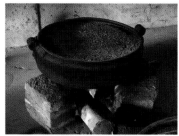

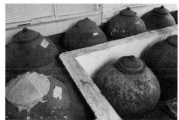

327

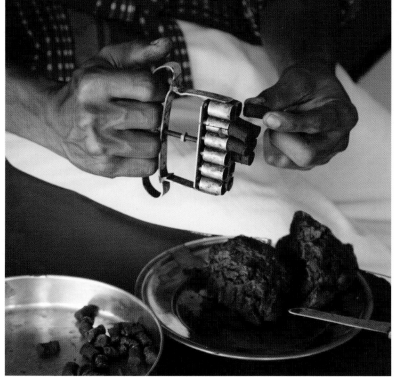

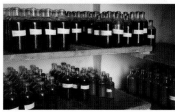

The production facility at Aditya, a small Ayurvedic homestay near Palakkad, is abuzz with activity.

Opposite: Sida cordifolia roots are cut, washed, then crushed, before being boiled and reduced (sometimes many times). The resulting *bala* decoction may be added to milk for a *kshira bala* or is used in oil for *vata* imbalances.

This page, clockwise from top: Stirring roots in a large cauldron. Reducing the mix. Some fermented preparations need to be stored in ceramic pots underneath earth for at least a month before they are ready for use. The storage cupboard at Aditya is constantly replenished. Ancient machinery grinds and reduces ingredients into a thick black paste like consistency. This is then used to make pills or *gulikam*.

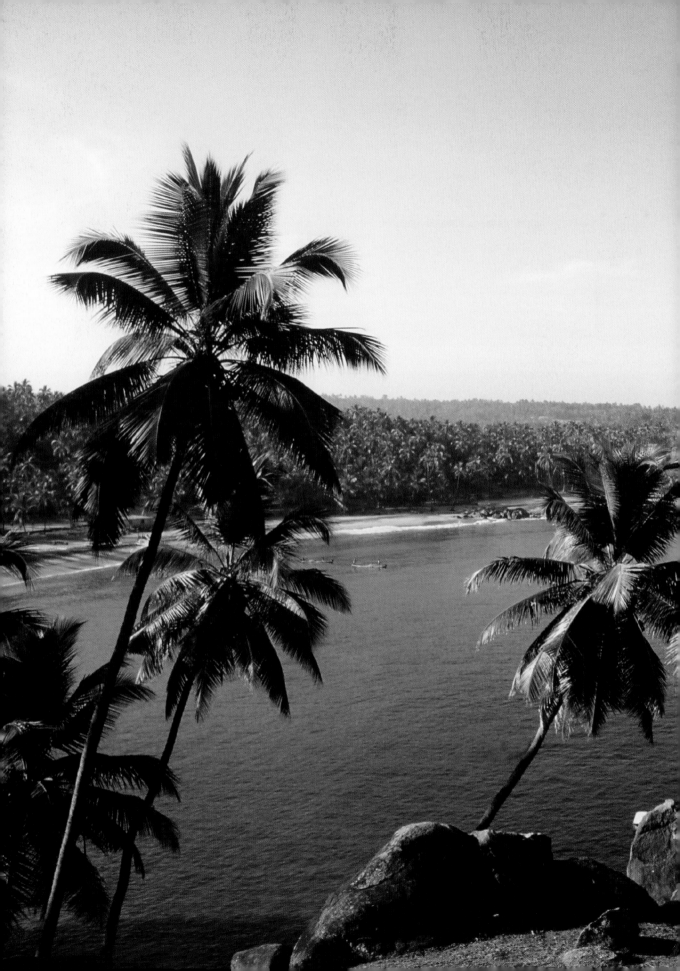

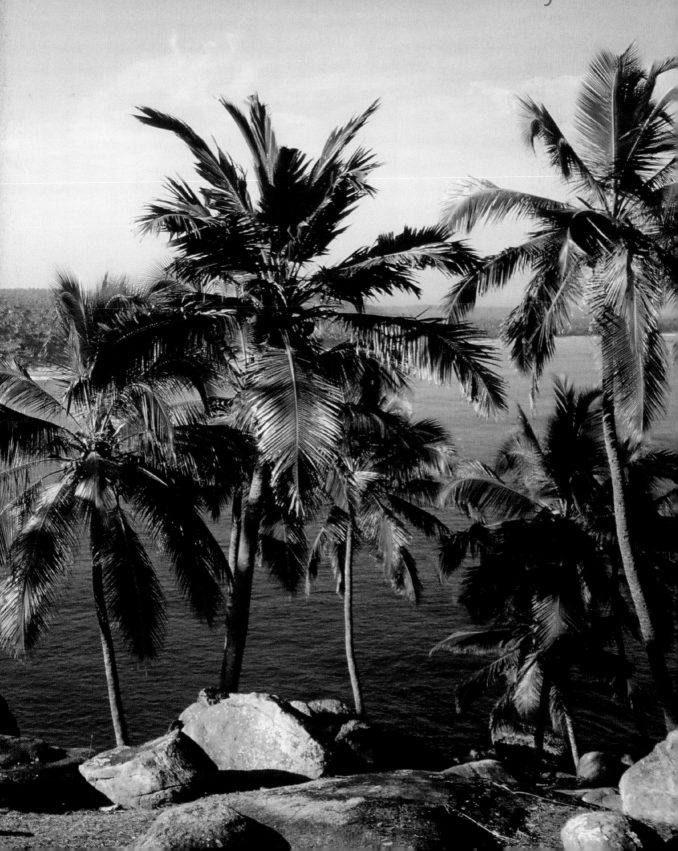

Selected Destinations

Hotels and Resorts with Spas:

Neemrana "non hotel" Hotels
No.13 Nizamuddin East Market,
New Delhi 110 013, India.
Tel: +91 11 24356145, 41825001
Fax: +91 11 24351112
http://www.neemranahotels.com

Neemrana Fort Palace,
Village Neemrana, District Alwar,
Rajasthan 301705, India.
Tel: +91 1494 246006/7/8
Fax: +91 1494 246005

Pataudi Palace,
Village Pataudi, District Gurgaon,
Haryana, India.
Tel: +91 124 2672244
Fax: +91 124 2672976

Park Hotels (corporate office)
Apeejay Surrendra Group
Pragati Bhavan, Jai Singh Road,
New Delhi 110 001, India.
Tel: +91 11 233 61193/94
Fax: +91 11 237 47123
http://www.theparkhotels.com

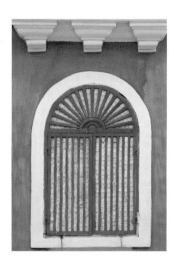

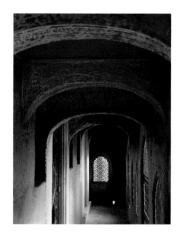

The Park New Delhi
15 Parliament Street,
New Delhi 110 001, India.
Tel: +91 11 2374 3000
Fax:+ 91 11 2374 4000

The Park Bangalore
14/7 Mahatma Gandhi Road,
Bangalore 560 042, India.
Tel: +91 80 2559 4666
Fax: +91 80 2559 4029

The Park Chennai
601 Anna Salai,
Chennai 600 006, India.
Tel: +91 44 4214 4000
Fax: +91 44 4214 4100

Ananda – In The Himalayas (corp office)
IHHR hospitality Pvt. Ltd.,
C-26, Qutab Institutional Area,
New Delhi 110 016, India.
Tel: +91 11 2656 8888
Fax: +91 11 2656 9999
http://www.anandaspa.com

The Oberoi Group (corporate office)
7, Sham Nath Marg,
Delhi 110 054, India.
Tel: +91 11 2389 0505
Fax: +91 11 2389 0568
http://www.oberoihotels.com

Udaivilas
Udaipur 313 001,
Rajasthan, India.
Tel: +91 294 243 3300
Fax: +91 294 243 3200

Rajvilas
Jaipur 303 012,
Rajasthan, India.
Tel: +91 141 268 0101
Fax: +91 141 268 0202

Shangri-La Hotels and Resorts
21/F, CITIC Tower,
1 Tim Mei Avenue,
Central, Hong Kong.
Tel: +852 25993591
Fax: +852 25993615
http://www.shangri-la.com

Aman Resorts (corporate office)
1 Orchard Spring Lane,
#05-01 Tourism Court,
Singapore 247729.
Tel: +65 6887 3337
Fax: +65 6887 3338
http://www.amanresorts.com

Amanbagh
Ajabgarh, Rajasthan, India.
Tel: +91 1465 223333
Fax: +91 1465 223335

Aman-i-Khas
Ranthambhore, Rajasthan, India.
Tel: +91 7462 252052
Fax: +91 7462 252178

Amangalla
Galle, Sri Lanka.
Tel: +94 91 2233388
Fax: +94 91 2233355

Park Hyatt Resort & Spa
Arossim Beach, Cansaulim,
South Goa 403 712, India.
Tel: +91 832 2721234
Fax: +91 832 2721235
http//:www. goa.park.hyatt.com

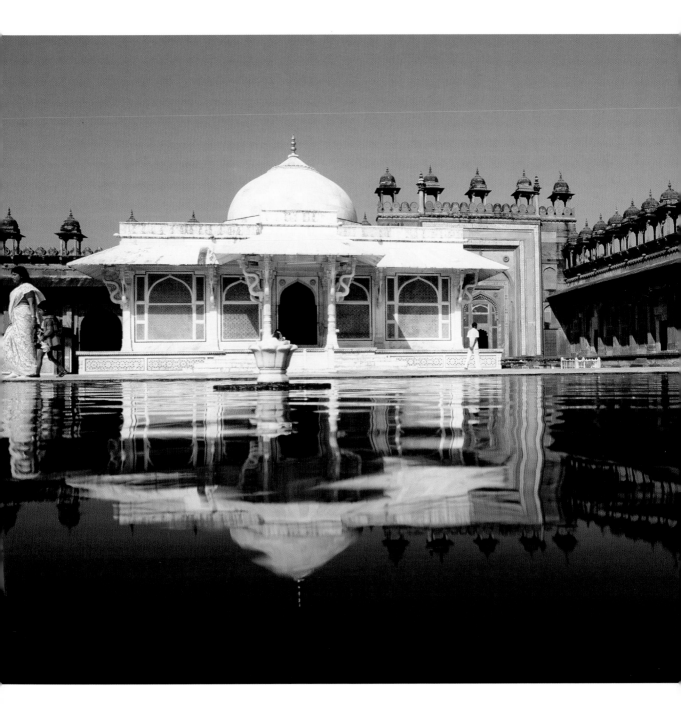

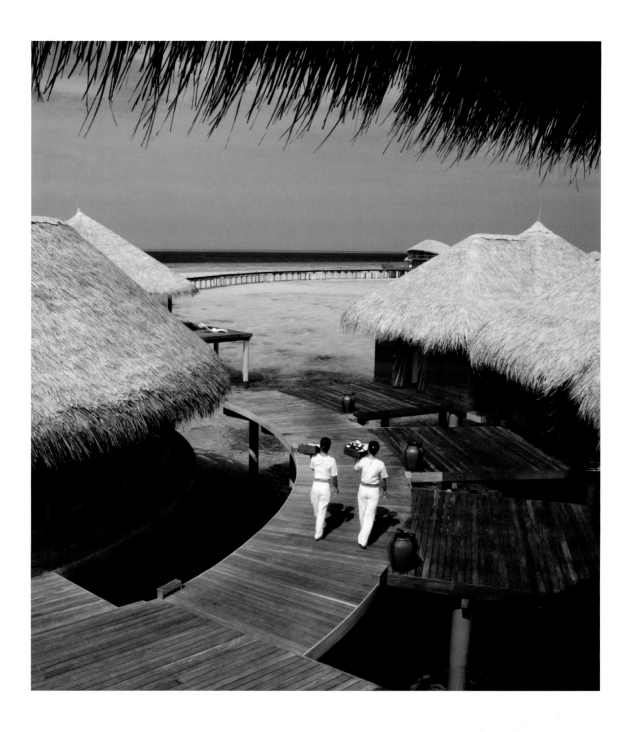

JW Marriott Mumbai
Juhu Tara Road,
Juhu Beach,
Mumbai 400 049, India.
Tel: +91 22 66933000
Fax: +91 22 66933100
http//:www.marriott.com

The Leela Kempinski
Sahar Mumbai 400 059,
India.
Tel: +91 22 6691 1234
Fax: +91 22 6691 1455
www.theleela.com

Taj Hotels, Resorts and Palaces
(corporate office)
Oxford House,
N F Road, Apollo Bunder,
Mumbai 400 001, India.
Tel: +91 22 6665 1272
Fax: +91 22 2281 8849
http://www.tajhotels.com

Taj Lake Palace
Post Box No 5, Lake Pichola,
Udaipur 313 001, India.
Tel: +91 294 242 8800
Fax: +91 294 252 8700

Umaid Bhawan Palace
Jodhpur 342 006, India.
Tel: +91 291 251 0101
Fax: +91291 251 0100

CGH Earth Hotels (corporate office)
Willingdon Island, Cochin,
Kerala 682 003, India.
Tel: +91 484 266 8221, 266 6821
Fax: +91 484 266 8001
http//:www.cghearth.com

Shalimar Spice Garden Resort,
Murikkady PO,
Idukki 685 535,
Kerala, India.
Tel: +91 4869 222132
Fax: +91 4869 223022
http://www.shalimarkerala.com

Kumarakom Lake Resort
KV 4 Panampilly Nagar,
Kochi 36, Kerala, India.
Telefax: +91 484 2323555/2316251
www.klresort.com

Raheem Residency
Beach Road, Alappuzha 688 012,
Kerala, India.
Tel/Fax: +91 477 2239767/2230767
http://www.raheemresidency.com

Mandarin Oriental Hotel Group
(corporate office)
281 Gloucester Road, Causeway Bay,
Hong Kong.
Tel: +852 2895 9288
Fax: +852 2837 3500
http://www.mandarinoriental.com

Mandarin Oriental Dhara Dhevi
51/4 Chiang Mai – Sankampaeng Rd,
Moo 1 T. Tasala A. Muang
Chiang Mai 50000, Thailand.
Tel: +66 53 888 983
Fax: +66 53 262 568

The Oriental, Bangkok
48 Oriental Avenue,
Bangkok 10500, Thailand.
Tel: +66 2 659 9000
Fax: +66 2 659 9284

Pangkor Laut Resort,
Lumut 32200,
Perak, Malaysia.
Tel: +60 5 699 1100
Fax: +60 5 699 1200
http://www.pangkorlautresort.com

Four Seasons Maldives
at Landaa Giraavar
Baa Atoll, Republic of Maldives.
Tel: +960 66 00 888
Fax: +960 66 00 800
http://www.fourseasons.com

Coco Palm Bodu Hithi
North Malé Atoll,
Republic of Maldives.
Tel: +960 664 1122
Fax: +960 664 1133
http://www.cocopalm.com.mv

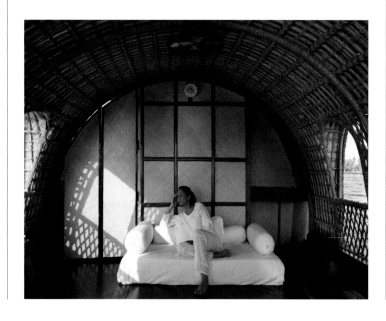

The Villas
Jalan Kunti 118X,
Seminyak,
Bali, Indonesia.
Tel: +62 361 730 840
Fax: +62 361 733 751
http://www.thevillas.net

Uma Paro
Bhutan.
Tel: + 975 8 271597
Fax: + 975 8 271513
http://www.uma.como.bz

Yoga & Meditation Schools & Retreats:

Shreyas Retreat,
Santoshima Farm,
Gollahalli Gate,
Nelamangala,
Bangalore 562123, India.
Tel: +91 80 27737102/103/183
Fax: +91 80 27737016
http://www.shreyasretreat.com

Mysore Mandala Yogashala
581 Dewans Rd,
Mysore 570 004, India.
Tel: +91 821425 6277
http://mandala.ashtanga.org

Ashtanga Yoga Research Institute
#235 8th Cross, 3rd Stage,
Gokulam,
Mysore 570 002, India.
Tel: +91 821 2516 756
http://www.ayri.org

Vipassana Research Institute
Various addresses throughout India
and internationally.
http://www.dhamma.org

Bihar School of Yogashram
Ganga Darshan,
Munger,
Bihar 811 201, India.
Tel: + 91 6344 222430
Fax: + 91 6344 220169

Swaswara Resort
Donibail, Gokarn,
South Kanara District, Karnataka, India.
www.swaswara.com

Salon, Spa and Product Companies:

Shahnaz Husain Group of Companies
M-84A Greater Kailash Part-1,
New Delhi 110048, India.
Tel: +91 11 29245079, 29233578
Fax: +91 11 29233903
http://www.shahnaz-husain.com

Sansha Spas
B-4/290, Safdarjung Enclave,
New Delhi 110 029, India.
Tel: +91 11 26193874/76
Fax : +91 11 2619387
http://www.sanshaayurveda.com

Ayurvedic Hospitals, Homestays and Treatment Centres:

Indus Valley Ayurvedic Center,
Lalithadripura, Mysore Post Box No-3,
Ittigegud, Mysore 570 010,
Karnataka, India.
Tel: +91 821 2473437/2473263
Fax: +91 821 2473590
http//:www.ayurindus.com

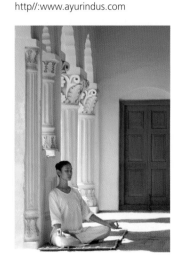

Poomully Aramthampuran's
Ayurveda Mana,
Peringode PO,
Via Kootanadu, Palakkad District,
Kerala, India.
Tel: +91 466 2370660
http://www.ayurvedamana.com

SNA Ayurveda Nursing Home,
East Fort, Thrissur 680 005,
Kerala, India.

Kalari Kovilakom,
Kollengode, Palakkad,
Kerala 678 506, India.
Tel: +91 4923 263737
Fax: +91 4923 263929
http://www.kalarikovilakom.com

The Arya Vaidya Chikitsalayam,
Arya Vaidya Pharmacy (Coimbatore) Ltd,
326 Perumal Koil Street,
Ramanathapuram, Coimbatore 641046,
Tamil Nadu, India.
Tel: +91 422 2313188
Fax: +91 422 2314953
http://www.avpayurveda.com

Keraleeya Ayurveda Samajam
Cheruthuruthy, Shoranur,
Palakkad 679 123,
Kerala, India.
Tel: +91 466 222 2403
Fax: +91 466 222 3383
http//:www.samajam.org

Kerala Ayurveda Ltd,
Athani Post, Ernakulam 683 585,
Kerala, India.
Tel: +91 484 2476301
Fax: +91 484 2474376
http//:www.keralaayurveda.biz

Thulasi Ayurveda Chikitsalayam
Alanallur (PO),
Palakkad District,
Kerala 678 601, India.
Tel: +91 924 263369
Email: ramananddr@ sancharnet.in

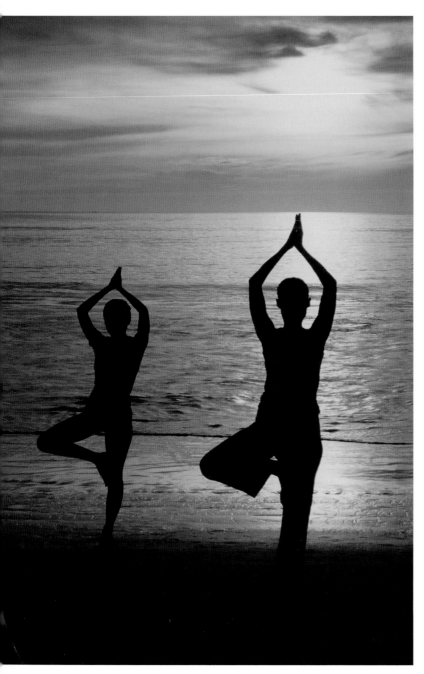

Swaasthya Ayurveda Village
Vijayanagar 1st Stage,
Mysore 570 017, India.
Tel: +91 821 5557557
http://www.swaasthya.com

Ayurvedic consultants:

Punarnava Ayurveda Pte Ltd
A-21, Parsn Galaxy, Parsn Complex,
Nanjundapuram Road,
Coimbatore 641 036,
Tamil Nadu, India.
Tel: +91 422 2311521
Fax: +91 422 4308081
http://www.punarnava-ayurveda.com

Holistic Health Centres:

SOUKYA International Holistic
Health Centre,
Soukya Road, Samethanahalli,
Whitefield,
Bangalore 560 067, India.
Tel: +91 80 7945001/2, 25318405/6
Fax: +91 80 7945010
www.soukya.com

Dance and Martial Arts Schools:

Nrityagram – The Dance Village
Hessaraghatta,
Bangalore 560 088, India.
Tel: +91 80 28466313/4
Fax: +91 80 28466312
http://www.nrityagram.org

Kerala Kalamandalam
Cheruthuruthy,
Thrissur 679 531, Kerala, India.
Tel: +91 4884 226 2418
Fax: +91 4884 226 2019
http://www.kalamandalam.com

CVN Kalari Sangham,
East Fort,
Thiruvananthapuram 695 023,
Kerala, India.
Tel: +91 471 247 4182

335

Acknowledgments

The author and photographer would like to thank the following (in no particular order) for all their invaluable help during the production of this book.

Priti Paul, Priya Paul, Megha Dinesh, Riya Banik and Rupa Thomas at Park Hotels.
Naresh Chandnan, Pushpa Nair, Peter Kerr, Colin Hall, Mark Sands, Dr Sreenarayanan, Damodaran K, Mirjam Rahr and Dinesh Dhanai at Ananda – in the Himalayas.
Sri P R Krishna Kumar at the Arya Vaidya Pharmacy (Coimbatore) Ltd.
Jose Dominique at CGH Earth and Cherry P Cherian, the Ayurvedic team, Tomy Joseph, Siby Abraham, Chef Johnson and Rajasekaran at Kalari Kovilakom.
Shahnaz Husain, Sidhartha Sengupta and Usha Zadoo of Shahnaz Husain Group of Companies.
John Paul, Asa Abraham and Dr Baijuraj at Kumarakom Lake Resort.
Drs Suma and Bhaskaran Vaidyar and Dr Sathyanaravanan at Aditya Ayurveda.
Dr E D Viayananadan and Dr E K Ramanandan at Thulasi Ayurveda Chikitsalayam.
Dr Ramkumar and Dr Indakul at Punarnava.
Mr S Sasunath and Narayanan Namburdiri at Ayurveda Mana.
Talavane Krishna and Prameela Ravindra at Indus Valley Ayurvedic Centre.
Lee Sutton and Noelle Rocque at J W Marriott.
Anjali Nihalchand at Amanresorts and Sally Baughan, Vijay Lakshmi and Sham Lakshmi at Amanbagh.

Dr and Mrs Isaac Mathai, Dr K Shaji, Dr P Ajitha, Dr Shuba, Dr S Usha Devi, Mary Faife, Neela Harish, Ambika, Rekha Manju and Yamuna at Soukya Integrated Health Centre.
Aman Nath, Francis Wacziarg, Thierry Gressier and Mr Ramesh at Neemrana Fort Palace.
Ketaki Narain, Henry Gray, Dr Yogesh, Vettri, Sue Reitz and Dr Renja Raphel of Oberoi Group. Pawan Malik, Nidhi Soodh and N Balaji at Shreyas Retreat.
Tisna Prapansiri of Mandarin Oriental Dhara Devi.
Ian Brewis and Arlene Finch from Shangri-La Group.
Sangeeta Sharma of Sansha Spas.
Lovina Gidwani Jha at Franck Provost.
Chik Lai Ping and Jeff Mong of Pangkor Laut Resort.

Special thanks, also, to Aman Nath for lending us his wonderful collection of prints and pictures to photograph and Soyun Lee who assisted Luca Tettoni in the photography. Also, Namita Gokhale, Pandit Manoj Joshi, Aman Sharif, Sarah Hardy, Kevin McGrath and Loo Tian Yuen, as well as our models Shamita and Mashoom Singha, Yana Odnopozov, Antonica Lovelyne, Candice Pinto, Dipti Gujral, Emy Stames, Atchara Laoruangroch, Tui Sang, Melati, Cindy Burbridge and Byron Bishop – we couldn't have done it without you.

Yoga clothes courtesy of Lucy Pollock and Gili Ravid. For details, see websites: lucy p' clothes that pose @ www.lucyp.co.uk and Anjaly @ www.anjaly.com